Clinical Advances in the Diagnosis and Treatment of Biliary Tract Diseases

Clinical Advances in the Diagnosis and Treatment of Biliary Tract Diseases

Editor

Saburo Matsubara

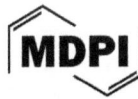

Basel • Beijing • Wuhan • Barcelona • Belgrade • Novi Sad • Cluj • Manchester

Editor
Saburo Matsubara
Department of
Gastroenterology and
Hepatology, Saitama Medical
Center
Saitama Medical University
Saitama, Japan

Editorial Office
MDPI
St. Alban-Anlage 66
4052 Basel, Switzerland

This is a reprint of articles from the Special Issue published online in the open access journal *Journal of Clinical Medicine* (ISSN 2077-0383) (available at: https://www.mdpi.com/journal/jcm/special_issues/Biliary_Tract_Diseases).

For citation purposes, cite each article independently as indicated on the article page online and as indicated below:

Lastname, A.A.; Lastname, B.B. Article Title. *Journal Name* **Year**, *Volume Number*, Page Range.

ISBN 978-3-0365-9318-0 (Hbk)
ISBN 978-3-0365-9319-7 (PDF)
doi.org/10.3390/books978-3-0365-9319-7

© 2023 by the authors. Articles in this book are Open Access and distributed under the Creative Commons Attribution (CC BY) license. The book as a whole is distributed by MDPI under the terms and conditions of the Creative Commons Attribution-NonCommercial-NoDerivs (CC BY-NC-ND) license.

Contents

Yoichi Miyata, Ryota Kogure, Akiko Nakazawa, Rihito Nagata, Tetsuya Mitsui, Riki Ninomiya, et al.
The Efficacy of S-1 as Adjuvant Chemotherapy for Resected Biliary Tract Carcinoma: A Propensity Score-Matching Analysis
Reprinted from: *J. Clin. Med.* **2021**, *10*, 925, doi:10.3390/jcm10050925 1

Yuki Tanisaka, Masafumi Mizuide, Akashi Fujita, Tomoya Ogawa, Masahiro Suzuki, Hiromune Katsuda, et al.
Recent Advances of Interventional Endoscopic Retrograde Cholangiopancreatography and Endoscopic Ultrasound for Patients with Surgically Altered Anatomy
Reprinted from: *J. Clin. Med.* **2021**, *10*, 1624, doi:10.3390/jcm10081624 11

Takashi Sasaki, Tsuyoshi Takeda, Takeshi Okamoto, Masato Ozaka and Naoki Sasahira
Chemotherapy for Biliary Tract Cancer in 2021
Reprinted from: *J. Clin. Med.* **2021**, *10*, 3108, doi:10.3390/jcm10143108 25

Taisuke Obata, Koichiro Tsutsumi, Hironari Kato, Toru Ueki, Kazuya Miyamoto, Tatsuhiro Yamazaki, et al.
Balloon Enteroscopy-Assisted Endoscopic Retrograde Cholangiopancreatography for the Treatment of Common Bile Duct Stones in Patients with Roux-en-Y Gastrectomy: Outcomes and Factors Affecting Complete Stone Extraction
Reprinted from: *J. Clin. Med.* **2021**, *10*, 3314, doi:10.3390/jcm10153314 39

Tsuyoshi Takeda, Takashi Sasaki, Takeshi Okamoto and Naoki Sasahira
Endoscopic Double Stenting for the Management of Combined Malignant Biliary and Duodenal Obstruction
Reprinted from: *J. Clin. Med.* **2021**, *10*, 3372, doi:10.3390/jcm10153372 53

Akihiro Sekine, Kazunari Nakahara, Junya Sato, Yosuke Michikawa, Keigo Suetani, Ryo Morita, et al.
Clinical Outcomes of Early Endoscopic Transpapillary Biliary Drainage for Acute Cholangitis Associated with Disseminated Intravascular Coagulation
Reprinted from: *J. Clin. Med.* **2021**, *10*, 3606, doi:10.3390/jcm10163606 63

Naosuke Kuraoka, Satoru Hashimoto, Shigeru Matsui and Shuji Terai
Outcomes of Endoscopic Ultrasound-Guided Biliary Drainage in a General Hospital for Patients with Endoscopic Retrograde Cholangiopancreatography-Difficult Transpapillary Biliary Drainage
Reprinted from: *J. Clin. Med.* **2021**, *10*, 4105, doi:10.3390/jcm10184105 75

Muneo Ikemura, Ko Tomishima, Mako Ushio, Sho Takahashi, Wataru Yamagata, Yusuke Takasaki, et al.
Impact of the Coronavirus Disease-2019 Pandemic on Pancreaticobiliary Disease Detection and Treatment
Reprinted from: *J. Clin. Med.* **2021**, *10*, 4177, doi:10.3390/jcm10184177 83

Pablo Pérez-Moreno, Ismael Riquelme, Priscilla Brebi and Juan Carlos Roa
Role of lncRNAs in the Development of an Aggressive Phenotype in Gallbladder Cancer
Reprinted from: *J. Clin. Med.* **2021**, *10*, 4206, doi:10.3390/jcm10184206 91

Masanari Sekine, Fumiaki Watanabe, Takehiro Ishii, Takaya Miura, Yudai Koito, Hitomi Kashima, et al.
Investigation of the Indications for Endoscopic Papillectomy and Transduodenal Ampullectomy for Ampullary Tumors
Reprinted from: *J. Clin. Med.* **2021**, *10*, 4463, doi:10.3390/jcm10194463 . . . . **109**

Tadahisa Inoue, Michihiro Yoshida, Yuta Suzuki, Rena Kitano, Fumihiro Okumura and Itaru Naitoh
Long-Term Outcomes of Endoscopic Gallbladder Drainage for Cholecystitis in Poor Surgical Candidates: An Updated Comprehensive Review
Reprinted from: *J. Clin. Med.* **2021**, *10*, 4842, doi:10.3390/jcm10214842 . . . . **119**

Saburo Matsubara, Keito Nakagawa, Kentaro Suda, Takeshi Otsuka, Masashi Oka and Sumiko Nagoshi
Practical Tips for Safe and Successful Endoscopic Ultrasound-Guided Hepaticogastrostomy: A State-of-the-Art Technical Review
Reprinted from: *J. Clin. Med.* **2022**, *11*, 1591, doi:10.3390/jcm11061591 . . . . **131**

Sakue Masuda, Kazuya Koizumi, Makomo Makazu, Haruki Uojima, Jun Kubota, Karen Kimura, et al.
Antibiotic Administration within Two Days after Successful Endoscopic Retrograde Cholangiopancreatography Is Sufficient for Mild and Moderate Acute Cholangitis
Reprinted from: *J. Clin. Med.* **2022**, *11*, 2697, doi:10.3390/jcm11102697 . . . . **153**

Ikuhiro Kobori, Yusuke Hashimoto, Taro Shibuki, Kei Okumura, Masanari Sekine, Aki Miyagaki, et al.
Safe Performance of Track Dilation and Bile Aspiration with ERCP Catheter in EUS-Guided Hepaticogastrostomy with Plastic Stents: A Retrospective Multicenter Study
Reprinted from: *J. Clin. Med.* **2022**, *11*, 4986, doi:10.3390/jcm11174986 . . . . **165**

Saburo Matsubara, Keito Nakagawa, Kentaro Suda, Takeshi Otsuka, Masashi Oka and Sumiko Nagoshi
The Feasibility of Whole-Liver Drainage with a Novel 8 mm Fully Covered Self-Expandable Metal Stent Possessing an Ultra-Slim Introducer for Malignant Hilar Biliary Obstructions
Reprinted from: *J. Clin. Med.* **2022**, *11*, 6110, doi:10.3390/jcm11206110 . . . . **177**

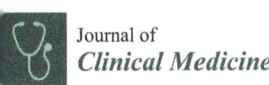

Journal of
Clinical Medicine

Article

The Efficacy of S-1 as Adjuvant Chemotherapy for Resected Biliary Tract Carcinoma: A Propensity Score-Matching Analysis

Yoichi Miyata [1,2,*], Ryota Kogure [3], Akiko Nakazawa [2], Rihito Nagata [4], Tetsuya Mitsui [3], Riki Ninomiya [3], Masahiko Komagome [3], Akira Maki [3], Nobuaki Kawarabayashi [5] and Yoshifumi Beck [3]

1. Department of Surgery, Asahi General Hospital, 1326 I, Asahi-shi, Chiba 289-2511, Japan
2. Department of Surgery, National Defence Medical College, 3-2 Namiki, Tokorozawa-shi, Saitama 359-8513, Japan; nakazawaa-sur@h.u-tokyo.ac.jp
3. Department of Hepatobiliary Pancreatic Surgery, Saitama Medical Centre, Kamoda 1981, Kawagoe-shi, Saitama 350-5500, Japan; ballershigh23and1@yahoo.co.jp (R.K.); tmitchiex@gmail.com (T.M.); rickynino9222@gmail.com (R.N.); komagome@saitama-med.ac.jp (M.K.); akiramaki.md@gmail.com (A.M.); ybeck@saitama-med.ac.jp (Y.B.)
4. Hepato-Biliary-Pancreatic Surgery Division, Department of Surgery, Graduate School of Medicine, The University of Tokyo, Bunkyo-ku, Tokyo 13-8655, Japan; NAGATAR-SUR@h.u-tokyo.ac.jp
5. Department of Surgery, Gyoda General Hospital, Mochida 376, Gyoda-shi, Saitama 361-0056, Japan; kawarabayashi@gyoda-hp.or.jp
* Correspondence: miyata-ham@umin.ac.jp

Abstract: Even though S-1 is a widely used chemotherapeutic agent, there is no evidence for its use in an adjuvant setting for biliary tract carcinoma (BTC). Patients who underwent surgical treatment for BTC between August 2007 and December 2018 were selected. Propensity score matching was performed between patients who received S-1 as adjuvant chemotherapy (S-1 group) and those who underwent surgical treatment alone (observation group). Of 170 eligible patients, 38 patients were selected in each group after propensity score matching. Among those in the matched cohort, both the median recurrence-free survival (RFS) and overall survival (OS) in the S-1 group were significantly longer than those in the observation group (RFS, 61.2 vs. 13.1 months, $p = 0.033$; OS, not available vs. 28.2 months, $p = 0.003$). A multivariate analysis of the OS revealed that perineural invasion and adjuvant S-1 chemotherapy were independent prognostic factors. According to a subgroup analysis of the OS, the S-1 group showed significantly better prognoses than the observation group among patients with perineural invasion ($p < 0.001$). S-1 adjuvant chemotherapy might improve the prognosis of BTC, especially in patients with perineural invasion.

Keywords: adjuvant chemotherapy; biliary tract carcinoma; propensity score matching; retrospective; S-1

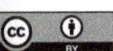

1. Introduction

Biliary tract carcinoma (BTC) is a relatively rare cancer worldwide [1]. According to the World Health Organization classification, BTC includes perihilar and distal extrahepatic bile duct carcinoma and gallbladder carcinoma [2]. The surgical procedure for BTC depends on the location of the lesion. For example, major hepatectomy with extra bile duct resection is performed for perihilar carcinoma, and pancreaticoduodenectomy is the most common approach for distal cholangiocarcinoma. Even though radical resection is required to completely remove the tumour, the recurrence rate is reported to be high, around 50% [3], and the overall survival (OS) rate remains poor.

The benefit of adjuvant chemotherapy after the surgical treatment of several advanced cancers, such as gastric cancer [4–6], colon cancer [7,8], and pancreatic cancer [9], is well established. Various adjuvant chemotherapy regimens are reported to improve the prognosis of patients with such cancers. However, in the case of BTC, the few large randomized trials on adjuvant chemotherapy conducted to date have produced unpromising results [10,11] and the efficacy of adjuvant chemotherapy for BTC remains unknown.

S-1 is an oral anti-cancer drug consisting of tegafur, 5-chloro-2,4-dihydroxypridine, and potassium oxonate [12,13]. The benefit of S-1 as an adjuvant chemotherapy has been reported for gastric cancer [4] and pancreatic cancer [9]. For BTC, several studies have shown that the efficacy of S-1 adjuvant chemotherapy varies [14,15], and its effectiveness remains debatable.

The aim of the present study was to retrospectively investigate the efficacy of S-1 administration as adjuvant chemotherapy after the surgical treatment of BTC. Because the patients with advanced carcinoma received adjuvant chemotherapy, we performed propensity score matching to reduce the inherent bias.

2. Materials and Methods

2.1. Patient Selection

Charts from two institutions were reviewed to select the patients who had undergone surgical treatment for BTC at Saitama Medical Centre and Gyoda General Hospital between August 2007 and December 2018. All the selected patients were pathologically diagnosed with BTC, including gallbladder carcinoma, perihilar cholangiocarcinoma, and distal cholangiocarcinoma. Patients who had received chemotherapies other than S-1 before and/or after their surgical treatment, had undergone R2 resection, or had not been able to receive S-1 adjuvant chemotherapy because they had died from postoperative complications within 90 days after surgery were excluded.

All the clinical, laboratory, radiologic, and pathological data were collected from electronic medical records. The study was conducted according to the guidelines of the Declaration of Helsinki and approved by the Institutional Review Board of Saitama Medical Centre, Saitama Medical University (No. 2002), and Gyoda General Hospital (No. 2019-1).

2.2. Treatment Strategy and Follow Up

The surgical treatment strategy was planned in accordance with the clinical status, such as pancreaticoduodenectomy for distal cholangiocarcinoma or major hepatectomy with extra bile duct resection for perihilar cholangiocarcinoma and gallbladder carcinoma. All the patients underwent adequate regional lymph node dissection, including the removal of hilar and pericholedochal nodes in the hepatoduodenal ligament, posterior and anterior pancreaticoduodenal nodes, and nodes along the common hepatic artery [16]. Intraoperative pathological examination of the proximal and/or distal biliary tract margins was performed to confirm carcinoma-free margins using frozen tissue sections. If the biliary tract margin was positive for carcinoma, then additional biliary tract resection was performed until the margin was free (or to the maximum extent possible) from carcinoma.

Patients in each institution were followed up after their surgical treatment every 3 to 6 months, which consisted of basic blood examinations, including the carbohydrate antigen 19-9 (CA19-9) level, and imaging examinations were usually performed with contrast-enhanced computed tomography. Additional imaging examinations were performed if recurrence was suspected. The end of the follow-up period was set as March 2019 or the date of death.

2.3. Administration Criteria of Adjuvant S-1 Chemotherapy

We considered the administration of S-1 (TS-1; Taiho, Tokyo, Japan) as adjuvant chemotherapy for patients to whom any of the following pathological findings applied: positive for lymphatic invasion and/or venous invasion and/or perineural invasion; positive for lymph node metastases, microscopic residual tumor, T status of T3 or T4. The patients also satisfied all of following criteria: Eastern Cooperative Oncology Group performance status (PS) of less than 2, adequate bone marrow function (leukocyte count $\geq$ 3000 cells per cubic millimeter, hemoglobin concentration $\geq$ 8.0 g/dL, and platelet count $\geq$ 100,000 cells per cubic millimeter), adequate liver function (total bilirubin concentration $\leq$ 2.0 mg/dL, asparate aminotransferase concentration $\leq$ 100 IU/L, and alanine aminotransferase concentration $\leq$ 100 IU/L), adequate renal function (serum creatinine concentration $\leq$ 1.5 mg/dL).

These patients received oral S-1 twice daily at a dose matched to their body surface area (BSA) as follows: BSA < 1.25 m^2, 80 mg/day; 1.25 m^2 ≤ BSA < 1.50 m^2, 100 mg/day; and 1.50 m^2 ≤ BSA, 120 mg/day [13]. S-1 was administered for 28 days, followed by 14 days of rest in each 42-day cycle. Adjuvant S-1 chemotherapy was performed as long as possible unless the patients' condition were intolerable such as PS was higher than 2, or liver and/or renal disfunction. The patients who experienced recurrence were given adequate treatment, including the best supportive care.

2.4. Statistical Analysis

All the pathological diagnoses were recorded in accordance with the 8th edition of the Union for International Cancer Control TMN classification [16]. OS was defined as the interval from the date of surgical treatment to the date of death from any cause or the end of the follow-up period. Recurrence-free survival (RFS) was defined as the interval from the date of surgical treatment to the date of confirmed recurrence. The interval from the surgical treatment to the date of death or end of the follow-up period for patients without recurrence was also defined as RFS.

Continuous data were expressed as the median with range. Quantitative and categorized variables were compared using Wilcoxon's rank-sum test and the chi-squared test, respectively. RFS and OS were estimated using the Kaplan–Meier method, and differences in survival curves were compared using the log-rank test. The multivariate analysis of OS was performed using a Cox proportional-hazards model to the factors statistically significant on univariate analysis, and the results were expressed as the hazard ratio (HR) and 95% confidence interval (95% CI).

Potential co-variables included in the propensity score matching were age, CA19-9 level, tumour (perihilar and distal extrahepatic bile duct carcinoma and gallbladder carcinoma), tumour differentiation, lymphatic invasion, venous invasion, perineural invasion, T status, N status, R status, and postoperative complications in accordance with the Clavien–Dindo classification [17]. Propensity scores were estimated using a logistic regression model, and the C-statistic for evaluating the goodness of fit was calculated. A one-to-one nearest-neighbour matching algorithm was applied with a calliper of 0.2.

p values ≤ 0.050 were considered statistically significant. All the statistical analyses were performed using JMP software (version 9.0.0; SAS Institute, Cary, NC, USA).

3. Results

3.1. Patient Characteristics in the Entire Cohort

During the study periods, 252 patients underwent surgical treatment for BTC. One patient who received chemotherapy before surgery, 23 who received adjuvant chemotherapies other than S-1, 24 treated with R2 resection, and 19 who died within 90 days after surgery without receiving S-1 adjuvant chemotherapy were excluded. Three patients who did not meet the administration criteria received adjuvant S-1 chemotherapy and 12 patients who met the administration criteria received surgical treatment alone were also excluded. Finally, 170 patients were designated as the entire cohort (Figure 1).

The median age of the entire cohort was 74 (range, 42 to 90) years, and 106 (62%) were male. There were 116 (68%) cases of cholangiocarcinoma (49 (29%) hilar cholangiocarcinoma and 67 [39%] distal cholangiocarcinoma) and 54 (32%) cases of gallbladder carcinoma. Hepatectomy was required in 51 (30%) patients (35 (21%) major hepatectomy and 16 (9%) hepatopancreaticoduodenectomy) and 70 patients underwent pancreaticoduodenectomy. Lymphatic invasion, venous invasion, perineural invasion, and lymph node metastases were observed in 87 (51%), 102 (60%), 113 (66%), and 71 (42%) patients, respectively. R0 resection was achieved in 122 (72%) patients. S-1 adjuvant chemotherapy was administered in 77 (45%) patients, and the median duration of S-1 administration was 10.6 (range, 1.9 to 59.3) months. The profiles and tumour characteristics of the patients who received S-1 adjuvant chemotherapy (S-1 group) and surgical treatment alone (observation group) are shown in Table 1. The median age of the S-1 group was significantly lower than that of the observation group ($p < 0.001$). Lymphatic invasion, venous invasion, and perineural invasion were observed significantly more often in the S-1 group than in the observation group ($p = 0.001, 0.001$, and 0.005, respectively). The proportion of patients with a T status of "T3 and T4" and N1 disease was also higher in the S-1 group ($p < 0.001$ for each). The R0 resection rate was comparable between two groups ($p = 0.255$).

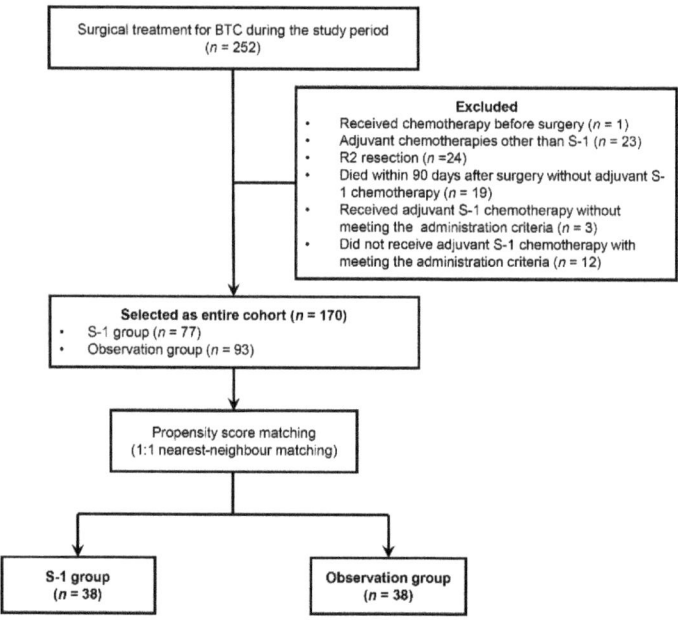

Figure 1. Flow chart of the patients included the study.

Table 1. Profiles and tumour characteristics of the patients in each group of the entire cohort.

	S-1 Group $n = 77$	Observation Group $n = 93$	p Value
Age [y]	70 (44–87)	75 (42–90)	<0.001 *
Gender, male	48 (62)	58 (62)	0.997
Diagnosis			
Hilar cholangiocarcinoma	20 (26)	29 (31)	
Distal cholangiocarcinoma	39 (51)	28 (30)	0.018 *
Gallbladder carcinoma	18 (23)	36 (39)	
Serum CA19-9 [U/mL]	91 (1–33,564)	53 (1–2524)	0.133
Hepatectomy	23 (30)	28 (30)	0.973
Clavien-Dindo classification, III–V	35 (45)	31 (33)	0.107
Pathological findings			
Tumor differentiation, well	25 (32)	37 (40)	0.230
Lymphatic invasion	50 (65)	37 (40)	0.001 *
Venous invasion	57 (74)	45 (48)	0.001 *
Perineural invasion	61 (79)	52 (56)	0.005 *
T status, T3 and T4	46 (60)	29 (31)	<0.001 *
N status, N1	48 (62)	23 (25)	<0.001 *
R status, R0	53 (69)	69 (74)	0.255

* Statistical significance ($p < 0.050$). Values in parentheses are the percentages for categorical data or range for continuous data. CA19-9, carbohydrate antigen 19-9.

The median RFS and OS of the entire cohort were 34.0 and 86.7 months, respectively. The median length of the follow-up interval was 50.6 months. Kaplan–Meier curves of the RFS and OS are shown in Figure S1.

3.2. Patient Characteristics and Survival in the Matched Cohort

After propensity score matching, 76 patients (38 in both the S-1 and observation groups) were selected. The C-statistic for the goodness of fit was 0.818. Table 2 shows the profiles and tumour characteristics of the patients in each group in the matched cohort. Hilar cholangiocarcinoma, distal cholangiocarcinoma, and gallbladder carcinoma were present in 11 (29%), 18 (47%), and 9 (24%) patients in the S-1 group, respectively, and in 10 (26%), 17 (45%), and 11 (29%) patients in the observation group, respectively ($p = 0.871$).

Table 2. Profiles and tumour characteristics of the patients in each group of the matched cohort.

	S-1 Group $n = 38$	Observation Group $n = 38$	p Value
Age [y]	72 (52–82)	74 (42–85)	0.640
Gender, male	25 (66)	22 (58)	0.479
Diagnosis			
Hilar cholangiocarcinoma	11 (29)	10 (26)	
Distal cholangiocarcinoma	18 (47)	17 (45)	0.871
Gallbladder carcinoma	9 (24)	11 (29)	
Serum CA19-9 [U/mL]	64 (1–1807)	68 (1–2524)	0.593
Hepatectomy	11 (29)	13 (34)	0.622
Clavien-Dindo classification, III–V	16 (42)	17 (45)	0.817
Pathological findings			
Tumor differentiation, well	14 (37)	14 (37)	1.000
Lymphatic invasion	25 (66)	23 (61)	0.634
Venous invasion	25 (66)	26 (68)	0.807
Perineural invasion	29 (76)	27 (71)	0.602
T status, T3 and T4	20 (53)	21 (55)	0.818
N status, N1	17 (45)	16 (42)	0.817
R status, R0	29 (76)	28 (74)	0.791

Values in parentheses are the percentages for categorical data or range for continuous data. CA19-9, carbohydrate antigen 19-9.

The median interval from surgical treatment to the initiation of adjuvant S-1 chemotherapy was 63 (range, 21 to 146) days, and the median duration of S-1 administration was 11.1 (range, 1.9 to 59.3) months.

The both median RFS and OS was significantly longer in the S-1 group than observation group (RFS, 61.2 vs. 13.1 months, $p = 0.033$; OS, not available vs. 28.2 months, $p = 0.003$) (Figure 2).

3.3. Univariate and Multivariate Analysis of OS in the Matched Cohort

The univariate and multivariate analysis of OS in the matched cohort is shown in Table 3. According to the univariate analysis, adjuvant S-1 chemotherapy as well as venous invasion and perineural invasion were significant predictors. The multivariate analysis revealed the presence of perineural invasion (Hazard ratio [HR] = 6.038, 95% CI, 1.709–29.153, $p = 0.004$) without adjuvant S-1 chemotherapy (HR = 4.370, 95% CI, 1.989–10.298, $p < 0.001$) was an independent poor prognostic factor.

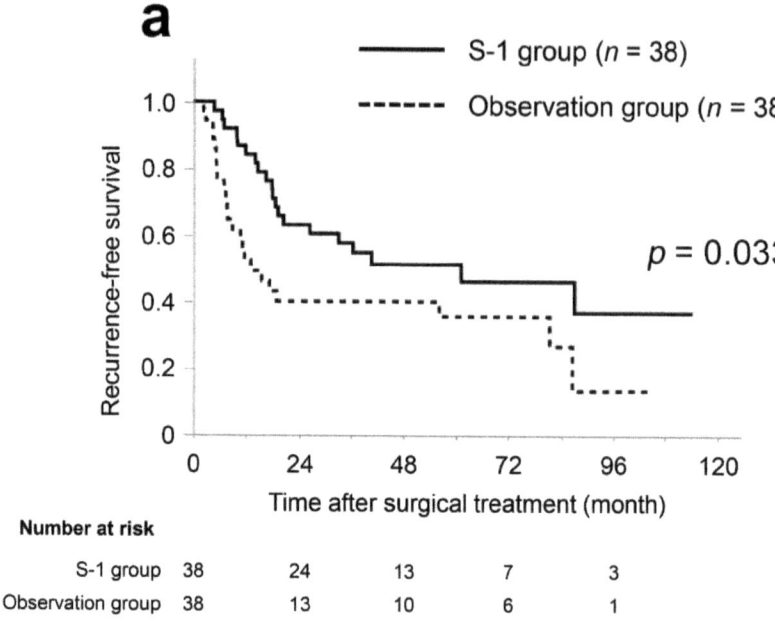
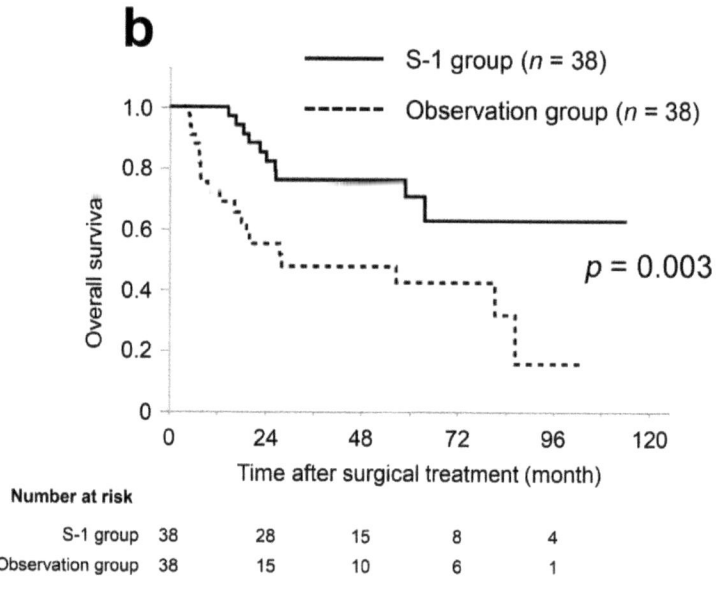

Figure 2. Kaplan–Meier curves of recurrence-free survival (**a**) and overall survival (**b**) in the matched cohort. The survival duration in the S-1 group was significantly longer than that in the observation group both in recurrence-free survival and overall survival ($p = 0.033$ and $p = 0.003$, respectively).

Table 3. Univariate and multivariate analysis of overall survival in the matched cohort.

Variable		n	Median (Months)	Univariate p Value [†]	Multivariate HR	95% CI	p Value [‡]
Age [y]	<65	16	86.7	0.274			
	≥65	60	63.8				
Preoperative CA19-9 [U/mL]	<37	23	86.7	0.317			
	≥37	53	58.9				
Clavien-Dindo classification	I–II	43	86.7	0.666			
	III–V	33	63.8				
Differentiation	well	28	86.7	0.134			
	not well	48	58.9				
Lymphatic invasion	no	28	86.7	0.341			
	yes	51	81.5				
Venous invasion	no	25	86.7	0.024 *	1.342	0.510–4.102	0.568
	yes	51	56.7				
Perineural invasion	no	20	86.7	0.007 *	6.038	1.709–29.153	0.004 *
	yes	56	56.7				
T status	T0–T2	35	86.7	0.053			
	T3 and T4	41	58.9				
N status	N0	43	86.7	0.110			
	N1	33	81.5				
R status	R0	57	81.5	0.569			
	R1	19	28.2				
Adjuvant S-1	yes	42	NA	0.003 *	4.370	1.989–10.298	<0.001 *
	no	42	28.2				

* Statistical significance ($p < 0.050$). [†] log rank test. [‡] Cox proportional-hazards model. NA, not available; HR, hazard ratio; 95% CI, 95% confidence interval.

3.4. Subgroup Analysis of the Prognostic Impact of S-1 Adjuvant Chemotherapy

To evaluate the prognostic impact of adjuvant S-1 chemotherapy for patients with poor prognostic factors of perineural invasion, we compared the OS of the patients with perineural invasion between the S-1 group and the observation group. The profiles and tumour characteristics of the patients with perineural invasion are shown in Table S1. The median OS of the patients with perineural invasion in S-1 group was significantly better than that of the observation group (not available vs. 18.1 months, $p < 0.001$) (Figure 3).

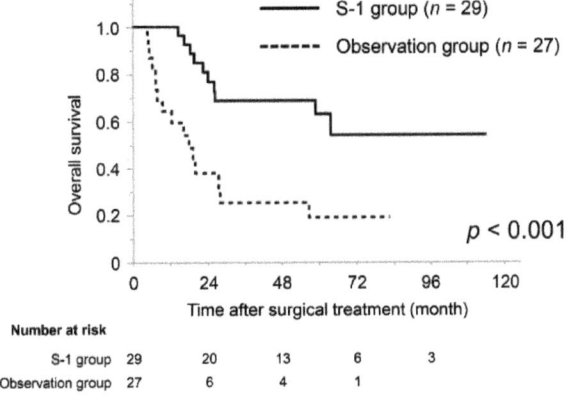

Figure 3. Kaplan–Meier curves for the overall survival of matched cohort patients with perineural invasion. The overall survival of the S-1 group was significantly better than that of the observation group ($p < 0.001$).

4. Discussion

This study investigated the postoperative outcomes of BTC resection with the administration of S-1 as adjuvant chemotherapy. Given that patients considered to be at a high risk of recurrence would likely receive adjuvant chemotherapy, we performed a propensity score-matching analysis to reduce patient selection bias. In our matching cohort, both the RFS and OS of the patients in the S-1 group were significantly longer than those in the observation group. Furthermore, adjuvant S-1 chemotherapy might contribute to the improved prognosis of patients with perineural invasion.

Several studies have reported on adjuvant chemotherapy for BTC [10,11,15,18–26]. The multicentre randomized phase III trial PRODIGE 12-ACCORD 18 conducted by a French group failed to show the efficacy of gemcitabine and oxaliplatin (GEMOX) in treating BTC patients in an adjuvant setting [10]. Additionally, the randomized phase III trial BCAT from Japan also failed to show a significant efficacy of adjuvant gemcitabine chemotherapy [11]. The results of the present study differ from those reported by these two large randomized studies. One explanation may be related to the different adjuvant chemotherapeutic agents used, whereby S-1 appears to achieve a better outcome when compared with gemcitabine in an adjuvant setting [14].

The efficacy of S-1 as adjuvant chemotherapy is well established for gastric cancer [4] and pancreatic cancer [9]. Regarding BTC, some studies showed that adjuvant S-1 improved the prognosis [14,15]. Given that S-1 contains the 5-fluorouracil (5-FU) prodrug tegafur [13], previous studies using 5-FU as adjuvant chemotherapy for BTC [21,23] have also suggested the potential efficacy of S-1. Recently, a multicentre randomized phase III trial of adjuvant chemotherapy for BTC (BILCAP) reported the efficacy of capecitabine, one of the prodrugs of 5-FU, with an OS of 53 months in the adjuvant group versus 36 months in the observation group ($p = 0.028$) [24]. It was reported that the allelic variants of CYP2A6, which is the metabolic enzyme of 5FU, were different between Caucasian and East Asian populations, but the pharmacokinetics of S-1 were not significantly different [27]. All of these previous studies support our current positive data for the use of S-1 in an adjuvant setting.

There are various reports on the prognostic factors after resection for BTC [28–30]. Perineural invasion [31,32] was reported to be one of the poor prognostic factors. In our series, the patients with perineural invasion showed a poor prognosis and thus might benefit from adjuvant chemotherapy with S-1. Further studies are required to investigate the extent of benefit from adjuvant chemotherapy for BTC.

The present study has several limitations. The first was its retrospective nature. Although we analysed our data using propensity score matching, some selection bias may have remained. Second, our series contained a heterogeneous group of BTC patients and a small sample size. A future study with a homogeneous group of BTC patients and a larger sample size is required to confirm our results. Finally, the administration protocol of adjuvant S-1 was not unified, particularly the duration of administration. Further controlled prospective research is necessary, and the final results of the JCOG 1202 study [33], a randomized phase III trial of adjuvant S-1 therapy versus observation alone in resected BTC patients, are awaited.

In conclusion, we reported the efficacy of S-1 as adjuvant chemotherapy after the resection of BTC using a propensity score matching analysis, and our results suggest that this approach might improve patients' prognoses, especially in patients with perineural invasion.

Supplementary Materials: The following are available online at https://www.mdpi.com/2077-0383/10//925/s1: Figure S1: Kaplan–Meier curves of recurrence-free survival and overall survival in the entire cohort, Table S1: Profiles and tumour characteristics of the patients with perineural invasion in each group of the matched cohort.

Author Contributions: Conceptualization, Y.M.; methodology, Y.M.; formal analysis, Y.M.; investigation, Y.M.; resources, R.K., A.N., R.N. (Rihito Nagata), T.M., Y.M., R.N. (Riki Ninomiya), M.K., A.M., N.K., and Y.B.; data curation, Y.M.; writing—original draft preparation, Y.M.; writing—review and editing, Y.B.; supervision, Y.B.; project administration, Y.M. and Y.B. All authors have read and agreed to the published version of the manuscript.

Funding: This research received no external funding.

Institutional Review Board Statement: The study was conducted according to the guidelines of the Declaration of Helsinki, and approved by the Institutional Review Board of Saitama Medical Centre, Saitama Medical University (approval no.: 2002; approval date: 1 November 2018) and Gyoda General Hospital (approval no.: 2019-1; approval date: 12 November 2019).

Informed Consent Statement: Informed consent was obtained from all the subjects involved in the study.

Data Availability Statement: The data presented in this study are available in the article.

Acknowledgments: We thank Hugh McGonigle and Melissa Crawford.

Conflicts of Interest: The authors declare no conflict of interest.

References

1. Bray, F.; Ferlay, J.; Soerjomataram, I.; Siegel, R.L.; Torre, L.A.; Jemal, A. Global cancer statistics 2018: GLOBOCAN estimates of incidence and mortality worldwide for 36 cancers in 185 countries. *CA Cancer J. Clin.* **2018**, *68*, 394–424. [CrossRef]
2. Bosman, F.T.; Carneiro, F.; Hruban, R.H.; Theise, N.D. *WHO Classification of Tumours of the Digestive System*, 4th ed.; IARC: Lyon, France, 2010.
3. Miyazaki, Y.; Kokudo, T.; Amikura, K.; Kageyama, Y.; Takahashi, A.; Ohkohchi, N.; Sakamoto, H. Survival of surgery for recurrent biliary tract cancer: A single-center experience and systematic review of literature. *Jpn. J. Clin. Oncol.* **2017**, *47*, 206–212. [CrossRef]
4. Sakuramoto, S.; Sasako, M.; Yamaguchi, T.; Kinoshita, T.; Fujii, M.; Nashimoto, A.; Furukawa, H.; Nakajima, T.; Ohashi, Y.; Imamura, H.; et al. Adjuvant chemotherapy for gastric cancer with S-1, an oral fluoropyrimidine. *N. Engl. J. Med.* **2007**, *357*, 1810–1820. [CrossRef]
5. Bang, Y.J.; Kim, Y.W.; Yang, H.K.; Chung, H.C.; Park, Y.K.; Lee, K.H.; Lee, K.W.; Kim, Y.H.; Noh, S.I.; Cho, J.Y.; et al. Adjuvant capecitabine and oxaliplatin for gastric cancer after D2 gastrectomy (CLASSIC): A phase 3 open-label, randomised controlled trial. *Lancet* **2012**, *379*, 315–321. [CrossRef]
6. Japanese Gastric Cancer Association. Japanese gastric cancer treatment guidelines 2014 (ver. 4). *Gastric Cancer* **2017**, *20*, 1–19. [CrossRef]
7. NIH Consensus Conference. Adjuvant therapy for patients with colon and rectal cancer. *JAMA* **1990**, *264*, 1444–1450. [CrossRef]
8. Hashiguchi, Y.; Muro, K.; Saito, Y.; Ito, Y.; Ajioka, Y.; Hamaguchi, T.; Hasegawa, K.; Hotta, K.; Ishida, H.; Ishiguro, M.; et al. Japanese Society for Cancer of the Colon and Rectum (JSCCR) guidelines 2019 for the treatment of colorectal cancer. *Int. J. Clin. Oncol.* **2020**, *25*, 1–42. [CrossRef]
9. Uesaka, K.; Boku, N.; Fukutomi, A.; Okamura, Y.; Konishi, M.; Matsumoto, I.; Kaneoka, Y.; Shimizu, Y.; Nakamori, S.; Sakamoto, H.; et al. Adjuvant chemotherapy of S-1 versus gemcitabine for resected pancreatic cancer: A phase 3, open-label, randomised, non-inferiority trial (JASPAC 01). *Lancet* **2016**, *388*, 248–257. [CrossRef]
10. Edeline, J.; Benabdelghani, M.; Bertaut, A.; Watelet, J.; Hammel, P.; Joly, J.P.; Boudjema, K.; Fartoux, L.; Bouhier-Leporrier, K.; Jouve, J.L.; et al. Gemcitabine and Oxaliplatin Chemotherapy or Surveillance in Resected Biliary Tract Cancer (PRODIGE 12-ACCORD 18-UNICANCER GI): A Randomized Phase III Study. *J. Clin. Oncol.* **2019**, *37*, 658–667. [CrossRef] [PubMed]
11. Ebata, T.; Hirano, S.; Konishi, M.; Uesaka, K.; Tsuchiya, Y.; Ohtsuka, M.; Kaneoka, Y.; Yamamoto, M.; Ambo, Y.; Shimizu, Y.; et al. Randomized clinical trial of adjuvant gemcitabine chemotherapy versus observation in resected bile duct cancer. *Br. J. Surg.* **2018**, *105*, 192–202. [CrossRef]
12. Shirasaka, T.; Shimamato, Y.; Ohshimo, H.; Yamaguchi, M.; Kato, T.; Yonekura, K.; Fukushima, M. Development of a novel form of an oral 5-fluorouracil derivative (S-1) directed to the potentiation of the tumor selective cytotoxicity of 5-fluorouracil by two biochemical modulators. *Anticancer Drugs* **1996**, *7*, 548–557. [CrossRef]
13. Shirasaka, T. Development history and concept of an oral anticancer agent S-1 (TS-1): Its clinical usefulness and future vistas. *Jpn. J. Clin. Oncol.* **2009**, *39*, 2–15. [CrossRef] [PubMed]
14. Kobayashi, S.; Terashima, T.; Shiba, S.; Yoshida, Y.; Yamada, I.; Iwadou, S.; Horiguchi, S.; Takahashi, H.; Suzuki, E.; Moriguchi, M.; et al. Multicenter retrospective analysis of systemic chemotherapy for unresectable combined hepatocellular and cholangiocarcinoma. *Cancer Sci.* **2018**, *109*, 2549–2557. [CrossRef]
15. Okabayashi, T.; Shima, Y.; Iwata, J.; Morita, S.; Sumiyoshi, T.; Sui, K.; Shimada, Y.; Iiyama, T. Characterization of Prognostic Factors and the Efficacy of Adjuvant S-1 Chemotherapy in Patients with Post-surgery Extrahepatic Bile Duct Cancer. *Anticancer Res.* **2017**, *37*, 7049–7056. [CrossRef]
16. Brierley, J.D.; Gospodarowicz, M.K.; Wittekind, C. *International Union Against Cancer (UICC): TNM Classification of Malignant Tumors*; Wiley: New York, NY, USA, 2017.
17. Dindo, D.; Demartines, N.; Clavien, P.A. Classification of surgical complications: A new proposal with evaluation in a cohort of 6336 patients and results of a survey. *Ann. Surg.* **2004**, *240*, 205–213. [CrossRef]

18. Bergeat, D.; Turrini, O.; Courtin-Tanguy, L.; Truant, S.; Darnis, B.; Delpero, J.R.; Mabrut, J.Y.; Regenet, N.; Sulpice, L. Impact of adjuvant chemotherapy after pancreaticoduodenectomy for distal cholangiocarcinoma: A propensity score analysis from a French multicentric cohort. *Langenbecks Arch. Surg.* **2018**, *403*, 701–709. [CrossRef]
19. Murakami, Y.; Uemura, K.; Sudo, T.; Hayashidani, Y.; Hashimoto, Y.; Nakamura, H.; Nakashima, A.; Sueda, T. Adjuvant gemcitabine plus S-1 chemotherapy improves survival after aggressive surgical resection for advanced biliary carcinoma. *Ann. Surg.* **2009**, *250*, 950–956. [CrossRef] [PubMed]
20. Murakami, Y.; Uemura, K.; Sudo, T.; Hayashidani, Y.; Hashimoto, Y.; Nakamura, H.; Nakashima, A.; Sueda, T. Gemcitabine-based adjuvant chemotherapy improves survival after aggressive surgery for hilar cholangiocarcinoma. *J. Gastrointest. Surg.* **2009**, *13*, 1470–1479. [CrossRef]
21. Kim, Y.S.; Jeong, C.Y.; Song, H.N.; Kim, T.H.; Kim, H.J.; Lee, Y.J.; Hong, S.C. The efficacy of fluoropyrimidine-based adjuvant chemotherapy on biliary tract cancer after R0 resection. *Chin. J. Cancer* **2017**, *36*, 9. [CrossRef]
22. Yin, L.; Xu, Q.; Li, J.; Wei, Q.; Ying, J. The efficiency and regimen choice of adjuvant chemotherapy in biliary tract cancer: A STROBE-compliant retrospective cohort study. *Medicine* **2018**, *97*, e13570. [CrossRef] [PubMed]
23. Neoptolemos, J.P.; Moore, M.J.; Cox, T.F.; Valle, J.W.; Palmer, D.H.; McDonald, A.C.; Carter, R.; Tebbutt, N.C.; Dervenis, C.; Smith, D.; et al. Effect of adjuvant chemotherapy with fluorouracil plus folinic acid or gemcitabine vs observation on survival in patients with resected periampullary adenocarcinoma: The ESPAC-3 periampullary cancer randomized trial. *JAMA* **2012**, *308*, 147–156. [CrossRef] [PubMed]
24. Primrose, J.N.; Fox, R.P.; Palmer, D.H.; Malik, H.Z.; Prasad, R.; Mirza, D.; Anthony, A.; Corrie, P.; Falk, S.; Finch-Jones, M.; et al. Capecitabine compared with observation in resected biliary tract cancer (BILCAP): A randomised, controlled, multicentre, phase 3 study. *Lancet Oncol.* **2019**, *20*, 663–673. [CrossRef]
25. Nassour, I.; Mokdad, A.A.; Porembka, M.R.; Choti, M.A.; Polanco, P.M.; Mansour, J.C.; Minter, R.M.; Wang, S.C.; Yopp, A.C. Adjuvant Therapy Is Associated with Improved Survival in Resected Perihilar Cholangiocarcinoma: A Propensity Matched Study. *Ann. Surg. Oncol.* **2018**, *25*, 1193–1201. [CrossRef] [PubMed]
26. Kemp Bohan, P.M.; Kirby, D.T.; Chick, R.C.; Bader, J.O.; Clifton, G.T.; Vreeland, T.J.; Nelson, D.W. Adjuvant Chemotherapy in Resectable Gallbladder Cancer is Underutilized Despite Benefits in Node-Positive Patients. *Ann. Surg. Oncol.* **2020**. [CrossRef]
27. Chuah, B.; Goh, B.C.; Lee, S.C.; Soong, R.; Lau, F.; Mulay, M.; Dinolfo, M.; Lim, S.E.; Soo, R.; Furuie, T.; et al. Comparison of the pharmacokinetics and pharmacodynamics of S-1 between Caucasian and East Asian patients. *Cancer Sci.* **2011**, *102*, 478–483. [CrossRef]
28. Matsukuma, S.; Tokumitsu, Y.; Shindo, Y.; Matsui, H.; Nagano, H. Essential updates to the surgical treatment of biliary tract cancer. *Ann. Gastroenterol. Surg.* **2019**, *3*, 378–389. [CrossRef]
29. Beetz, O.; Klein, M.; Schrem, H.; Gwiasda, J.; Vondran, F.W.R.; Oldhafer, F.; Cammann, S.; Klempnauer, J.; Oldhafer, K.J.; Kleine, M. Relevant prognostic factors influencing outcome of patients after surgical resection of distal cholangiocarcinoma. *BMC Surg.* **2018**, *18*, 56. [CrossRef] [PubMed]
30. Petrova, E.; Ruckert, F.; Zach, S.; Shen, Y.; Weitz, J.; Grutzmann, R.; Wittel, U.A.; Makowiec, F.; Hopt, U.T.; Bronsert, P.; et al. Survival outcome and prognostic factors after pancreatoduodenectomy for distal bile duct carcinoma: A retrospective multicenter study. *Langenbecks Arch. Surg.* **2017**, *402*, 831–840. [CrossRef]
31. Bhuiya, M.R.; Nimura, Y.; Kamiya, J.; Kondo, S.; Fukata, S.; Hayakawa, N.; Shionoya, S. Clinicopathologic studies on perineural invasion of bile duct carcinoma. *Ann. Surg.* **1992**, *215*, 344–349. [CrossRef] [PubMed]
32. Yamaguchi, R.; Nagino, M.; Oda, K.; Kamiya, J.; Uesaka, K.; Nimura, Y. Perineural invasion has a negative impact on survival of patients with gallbladder carcinoma. *Br. J. Surg.* **2002**, *89*, 1130–1136. [CrossRef]
33. Nakachi, K.; Konishi, M.; Ikeda, M.; Mizusawa, J.; Eba, J.; Okusaka, T.; Ishii, H.; Fukuda, H.; Furuse, J. A randomized Phase III trial of adjuvant S-1 therapy vs. observation alone in resected biliary tract cancer: Japan Clinical Oncology Group Study (JCOG1202, ASCOT). *Jpn. J. Clin. Oncol.* **2018**, *48*, 392–395. [CrossRef] [PubMed]

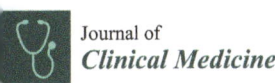

Review

Recent Advances of Interventional Endoscopic Retrograde Cholangiopancreatography and Endoscopic Ultrasound for Patients with Surgically Altered Anatomy

Yuki Tanisaka *, Masafumi Mizuide, Akashi Fujita, Tomoya Ogawa, Masahiro Suzuki, Hiromune Katsuda, Youichi Saito, Kazuya Miyaguchi, Tomoaki Tashima, Yumi Mashimo and Shomei Ryozawa

Department of Gastroenterology, Saitama Medical University International Medical Center, 1397-1, Yamane, Hidaka, Saitama 350-1298, Japan; mizuide1971@yahoo.co.jp (M.M.); a.fujita0628@gmail.com (A.F.); t.ogawa0210@icloud.com (T.O.); msuzgast@tmd.ac.jp (M.S.); hk0112@saitama-med.ac.jp (H.K.); stm_ys41@yahoo.co.jp (Y.S.); kaz.hr77@gmail.com (K.M.); tomo3029@saitama-med.ac.jp (T.T.); ymashimo@saitama-med.ac.jp (Y.M.); ryozawa@saitama-med.ac.jp (S.R.)
* Correspondence: tanisaka1205@gmail.com; Tel.: +81-42-984-4111

Abstract: Endoscopic retrograde cholangiopancreatography (ERCP) is considered to be the gold standard for diagnosis and interventions in biliopancreatic diseases. However, ERCP in patients with surgically altered anatomy (SAA) appears to be more difficult compared to cases with normal anatomy. Since the production of a balloon enteroscope (BE) for small intestine disorders, BE had also been used for biliopancreatic diseases in patients with SAA. Since the development of BE-assisted ERCP, the outcomes of procedures, such as stone extraction or drainage, have been reported as favorable. Recently, an interventional endoscopic ultrasound (EUS), such as EUS-guided biliary drainage (EUS-BD), has been developed and is available mainly for patients with difficult cases of ERCP. It is a good option for patients with SAA. The effectiveness of interventional EUS for patients with SAA has been reported. Both BE-assisted ERCP and interventional EUS have advantages and disadvantages. The choice of procedure should be individualized to the patient's condition or the expertise of the endoscopists. The aim of this review article is to discuss recent advances in interventional ERCP and EUS for patients with SAA.

Keywords: endoscopic retrograde cholangiopancreatography; altered anatomy; ERCP; balloon enteroscope; single balloon enteroscopy; double balloon enteroscopy; endoscopic ultrasound; EUS; interventional EUS; EUS-BD

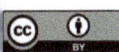

1. Introduction

There is a large variety of biliary tract diseases, such as bile duct stones and benign/malignant biliary strictures. They lead to hepatobiliary dysfunction, cholangitis, and eventually liver failure requiring appropriate therapy. Since its introduction in 1968, endoscopic retrograde cholangiopancreatography (ERCP) is thought to be the gold standard for diagnosis and interventions in biliopancreatic diseases. It has been reported that ERCP-related procedures have achieved success in approximately 95% of cases [1,2]. However, it is technically challenging to perform ERCP in patients with surgically altered anatomy (SAA), such as Roux-en-Y gastrectomy, hepaticojejunostomy with Roux-en-Y, pancreaticoduodenectomy, or Billroth II gastrectomy. First of all, the afferent limb, increased intestinal curvature, or postoperative adhesions hinder accessibility of the target site, such as the papilla or the hepatico/pancreatojejunal anastomosis. Next, selective biliary cannulation and subsequent procedures, such as stone extraction or drainage, are more difficult in patients with SAA than cases with normal anatomy. Outcomes using a conventional duodenoscope have not been satisfactory [3,4]. Hence, alternative treatments, such as percutaneous transhepatic biliary drainage (PTBD), have been widely applied to patients with SAA [5,6]. One study from a tertiary referral endoscopy center reported that the afferent loop intubation and cannulation success rates using side-viewing duodenoscope in patients with Billroth II gastrectomy were 86.7% (618/713 patients) and 93.8% (580/613 patients). The main reason for intubation failure was a long and angulated afferent loop [7]. Another systematic review and meta-analysis reported that the afferent loop intubation and cannulation success rates using a forward-viewing endoscope in patients with Billroth II gastrectomy were 91.1% and 92.3%. The subgroup analysis of the forward-viewing endoscope showed that the success rates of afferent loop intubation using the forward-viewing endoscope with cap-fitting (92.5%) was higher than the forward-viewing endoscope without cap-fitting (88.6%). The success rates of cannulation using the forward-viewing endoscope with cap-fitting (93.7%) was higher than the forward-viewing endoscope without cap-fitting (89.2%) [8]. These studies showed the usefulness of a conventional side or forward-viewing scope in patients with Billroth II gastrectomy. However, these scopes cannot achieve the afferent loop intubation in 10% of patients due to a long and angulated afferent loop.

Since the introduction of the balloon enteroscope (BE) for small bowel disorders [9], balloon-assisted ERCP, such as single-balloon enteroscopy (SBE)-assisted ERCP, or double-balloon enteroscopy (DBE)-assisted ERCP, have been developed for patients with SAA. Despite the evident effectiveness of BE-assisted ERCP, it is still more challenging to perform than ERCP in patients with normal anatomy in terms of scope insertion, biliary cannulation, and subsequent diagnostic and interventional procedures, such as forceps biopsy, stone extraction, and stent placement. Recently, interventional endoscopic ultrasound (EUS), such as EUS-guided biliary drainage (EUS-BD) or EUS-guided antegrade intervention, have been available for difficult cases of ERCP, making it a good option for patients with SAA. In this review, we discuss recent advances in interventional ERCP and EUS for patients with SAA.

2. Balloon Enteroscope

Table 1 shows the specifications of the SBE and DBE presently available. The BEs are advanced by holding and shortening the intestine with an inflated balloon. The difference of SBE and DBE is the number of balloons (Figure 1). A balloon is attached to the tip of the over-tube for SBE. DBE equips two balloons. One is attached to the tip of the endoscope while another is attached to the tip of the over-tube. Moreover, the working channel port in SBE appears in an 8 o'clock direction on the endoscopic screen. In contrast, it shows in a 5.30 o'clock direction for DBE.

Table 1. Specifications of single-balloon enteroscopy (SBE) and double-balloon enteroscopy (DBE).

Company	Olympus	Olympus	Fujifilm	Fujifilm
	SIF-Q260	SIF-H290S	EN-580T	EI-580BT
Angle of view	140°	140°	140°	140°
Outer diameter (mm)	9.2	9.2	9.4	9.4
Working length (mm)	2000	1520	2000	1550
Working channel diameter (mm)	2.8	3.2	3.2	3.2
Passive bending	No	Yes	No	No
High-force transmission	No	Yes	No	No
The adaptive bending	No	No	No	Yes
Advanced force transmission	No	No	No	Yes

SBE, single-balloon enteroscopy. DBE, double-balloon enteroscopy.

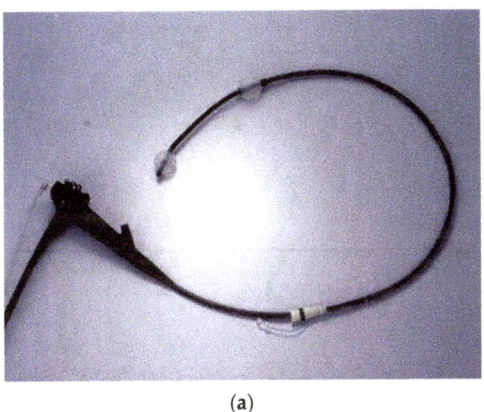 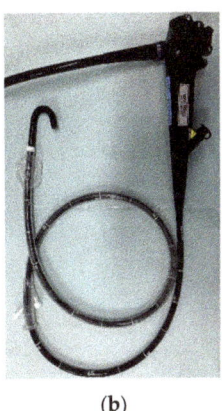

(a) (b)

Figure 1. Balloon enteroscope: (a) double-balloon enteroscopy and (b) single-balloon enteroscopy.

Use of conventional SBE and DBE is limited by their long working length of 200 cm. Therefore, only a few ERCP accessories are available. Recently, a short-type SBE (short SBE) and DBE (short DBE) with a working length of 152 cm (short SBE) and 155 cm (short DBE), and with a working channel diameter of 3.2 mm is available to increase accessories that can be used for BE-assisted ERCP. Moreover, the short SBE permits the function of passive bending and high-force transmission [10], and the short DBE permits the function of adaptive bending and advanced force transmission [11]. When using SBE, if the scope is at the intestinal tract wall when passing through a sharp flexure, then the passive bending section allows the scope to smoothly bend along the bend of the wall, making it possible to move forward. High-force transmission capabilities make it possible to perform torque operations efficiently and to provide better scope control. Therefore, it is also useful for bile duct cannulation and subsequent treatment procedures. In short, DBE, adaptive bending, and advanced force transmission provide a similar role to passive bending and high-force transmission. These features have contributed to overcoming the difficulties of scope insertion to the target site or biliary cannulation.

In general, ERCP-related procedures using BE are performed under conscious sedation, such as intravenous midazolam and pethidine. During scope insertion, patients are positioned in the prone position. However, for difficult cases, the position may be changed or abdominal pressure may be used. In case the BE forms a loop during insertion, the small intestine is fixed using the inflated balloon and shortened by withdrawing the BE. It is useful and safe for scope insertion to use carbon dioxide. In some difficult cases, such as long afferent limbs seen in Roux-en-Y reconstruction cases, it is difficult to proceed to the target site using short BE. Hence, a change to a conventional-type enteroscope (working length of 200 cm) is required [12]. A transparent hood is useful not only for scope insertion but also for subsequent procedures, such as biliary cannulation [13]. Since postoperative adhesions tend to occur in patients with SAA, endoscopists could feel adhesions during scope insertion or shortening. It must be taken into consideration that there is an increased risk of perforation during scope insertion in patients with SAA than in anatomically normal cases. After achievement of scope insertion to the target site, biliary cannulation is performed using a catheter with a guidewire for cholangiography and deep cannulation. After biliary cannulation, endoscopic diagnosis/interventions, such as stone extraction, stent placement, and biopsy/cytology for diagnosis are performed.

Although endoscopic sphincterotomy (EST) is one of the common procedures in ERCP, it can be particularly troublesome in patients with SAA (Billroth II gastrectomy or Roux-en-Y gastrectomy). It is considered to be difficult because the correct direction of the incision is sometimes uncertain due to the upside-down position in these patients. If the incision is made in the wrong direction, perforation could occur. One study from a tertiary referral endoscopy center evaluated 40 cases of the endoscopic papillary large balloon (over 10-mm) dilation (EPLBD) without EST for stone extraction in patients with Billroth II gastrectomy. Stones were successfully removed in all cases. Acute complications from EPLBD included mild pancreatitis in two patients (5.0%) [14]. This result showed the usefulness and safety of EPLBD without EST. If an endoscopist feels difficult to perform EST in patients with Billroth II gastrectomy or Roux-en-Y gastrectomy, EPLBD without EST may be recommended.

3. Single Balloon-Assisted ERCP

Table 2 shows outcomes of SBE-assisted ERCP procedures in patients with SAA [12,13,15–22]. The latest systematic review and meta-analysis reported that the pooled data reaching the target site, biliary cannulation, and procedural success rates were 86.6%, 90%, and 75.8%. Adverse events occurred in 6.6% of the procedures [23]. Fatal pancreatitis and intestinal perforation requiring surgical operation were included in the report. Although these were acceptable adverse event rates, we must be mindful that fatal adverse events can occur. It was also reported that bilateral stenting (partial stent-in-stent placement method) using self-expandable metallic stents for patients with hilar bile duct cancer was possible by use of short SBE [24].

Table 2. Outcomes of single balloon enteroscopy (SBE)-assisted endosopic retrograde cholangiopancreatography (ERCP) procedure in patients with surgically altered anatomy (SAA).

Authors	Year	Reaching the Target Site Success, % (n)	Biliary Cannulation Success, % (n)	Procedural Success, % (n)
Wang et al. [15]	2010	81.3 (13/16)	92.3 (12/13)	75.0 (12/16)
Shah et al. [16]	2013	68.9 (31/45)	87.1 (27/31)	60.0 (27/45)
Lenze et al. [17]	2014	73.1 (19/26)	78.9 (15/19)	57.7 (15/26)
Trindade et al. [13]	2015	87.5 (49/56)	89.8 (44/49)	71.4 (40/56)
Kawamura et al. [18]	2015	88.9 (24/27)	83.3 (20/24)	70.4 (19/27)
Yamauchi et al. [19]	2015	90.5 (76/84)	89.5 (68/76)	77.4 (65/84)
Ishii et al. [20]	2016	91.9 (113/123)	94.1 (95/101)	88.1 (96/109)
Yane et al. [21]	2017	92.6 (188/203)	N/A	81.8 (166/203)
Tanisaka et al. [12]	2019	94.8 (181/191)	92.3 (167/181)	85.9 (164/191)
Sawas et al. [22]	2020	86.0 (37/43)	83.8 (31/37)	69.8 (30/43)

SBE, single-balloon enteroscopy. ERCP, endoscopic retrograde cholangiopancreatography. SAA, surgically altered anatomy. N/A, not available.

Selective biliary cannulation seems to be more difficult in patients with SAA than patients with normal anatomy. The reason is the following: the papilla appears inverted, the view of the papilla tends to be tangential, SBE is forward-viewing, and the elevator system is not equipped. There are several tips for biliary cannulation using SBE. As previously mentioned, the use of a transparent hood is effective for biliary cannulation [13]. Moreover, it was reported that suction of the papilla into the transparent cap facilitated biliary cannulation [25]. The retroflex position contributes to gaining a better view of the papilla in patients with Roux-en-Y gastrectomy. [20,26]. To achieve the retroflex position, the endoscope is advanced while using the upper angle at the inferior duodenal angle. The scope provides a J-turn form (Figure 2). Moreover, cannulation techniques, such as the double-guidewire method, insertion along the pancreatic duct (PD) stent [27], and use of the unique cannula equipped double-lumen [28] are useful.

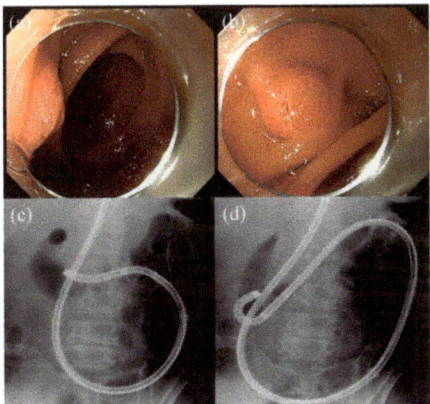

Figure 2. Retroflex position: (**a,c**). The papilla is positioned tangential, so it is difficult for biliary cannulation. (**b,d**) The endoscope is advanced while using the up angle at the inferior duodenal angle. As a result, it provides a better view of the papilla.

Some studies have reported factors affecting procedural results. One study reported that pancreatic indications, first ERCP attempt, and no transparent hood affected procedural failure [21]. Another study reported that malignant biliary obstruction, first ERCP attempt, and Roux-en-Y reconstruction affected procedural failure [12]. Figure 3 demonstrates endoscopic stone extraction using short SBE for patients with SAA.

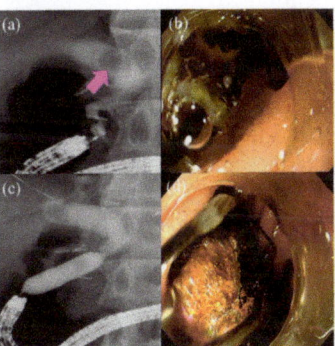

Figure 3. Endoscopic stone extraction using short single-balloon enteroscopy (short SBE) for patients with surgically altered anatomy (SAA): (**a**) Cholangiography showing a 15-mm biliary stone (pink arrow) in the distal bile duct. (**b,c**) Endoscopic papillary large balloon dilation was performed for stone extraction. The balloon was inflated up to 13-mm. (**d**) Stone extraction was completed without crushing.

4. Double Balloon-Assisted ERCP

Table 3 shows the outcomes of DBE-assisted ERCP procedures in patients with SAA [29–38]. The latest systematic review and meta-analysis reported that the pooled data reaching the target site, biliary cannulation, and procedural success rates were 90%, 94%, and 93%. Adverse events occurred in 4% [39]. One case of intestinal perforation requiring surgery was included in the report. A single-center large cohort study reported that Billroth II gastrectomy (B-II) and the native papilla were notable risk factors for complications [40]. In that report, especially cases of B-II with an extremely short afferent loop between the gastro-jejunal anastomosis and Treitz ligament, had a risk of perforation because B-II with an extremely short afferent loop tend to receive a strong force while proceeding a scope into the afferent loop. This kind of perforation could also occur in SBE.

Table 3. Outcomes of double balloon endoscopy (DBE)-assisted ERCP procedure in patients with surgically altered anatomy (SAA).

Authors	Year	Reaching the Target Site Success, % (n)	Biliary Cannulation Success, % (n)	Procedural Success, % (n)
Aabakken et al. [29]	2007	94.4 (17/18)	88.2 (15/17)	83.3 (15/18)
Emmett et al. [30]	2007	85.0 (17/20)	94.1 (16/17)	80.0 (16/20)
Shimatani et al. [31]	2009	97.1 (100/103)	98.0 (98/100)	95.1 (98/103)
Cho et al. [32]	2011	86.2 (25/29)	96.0 (24/25)	82.8 (24/29)
Tsutsumi et al. [33]	2015	98.6 (71/72)	100 (71/71)	98.6 (71/72)
Cheng et al. [34]	2015	94.8 (73/77)	94.5 (69/73)	87.0 (67/77)
Shimatani et al. [35]	2016	97.7 (304/311)	96.4 (293/304)	92.3 (287/311)
Liu et al. [36]	2017	75.6 (65/86)	92.3 (60/65)	69.8 (60/86)
Kashani et al. [37]	2018	93.8 (121/129)	N/A	88.4 (114/129)
Uchida et al. [38]	2020	94.3 (759/805)	N/A	90.7 (730/805)

DBE, double-balloon enteroscopy. ERCP, endoscopic retrograde cholangiopancreatography. SAA, surgically altered anatomy. N/A, not available.

There are several technical tips for DBE. As previously mentioned, the retroflex position is also useful for biliary cannulation using DBE. Since the working channel port shows up in a 5:30 o'clock direction on the endoscopic screen, positioning and fixing the papilla in a 6 o'clock direction is effective to perform endoscopic sphincterotomy safely [41]. This position provides the oral protrusion and the hooding fold, which are landmarks of the direction of bile duct in performing endoscopic sphincterotomy. Furthermore, it enables confirmation whether common bile duct stones are present or not between the balloon and common bile duct during endoscopic papillary large balloon dilation [42].

Factors affecting procedural results using DBE have also been reported. One study noted that patients with surgery during childhood, biliary atresia, and second operation post-transplant were factors affecting procedure results in patients with Roux-en-Y reconstruction [36]. Another study reported that Roux-en-Y reconstruction and the first-time procedure affected the outcomes and adverse events [38]. In the report, a physician in training did not significantly affect the outcomes.

5. Other Device-Assisted ERCP

There are several reports of ERCP using other devices. Motorized spiral enteroscopy (PSF-1, Olympus Medical Systems, Tokyo, Japan) with a working length of 168 cm, and with a working channel diameter of 3.2 mm is available from 2015. The drive motor located in the endoscope handle is activated by foot pedals and controls the direction and speed of rotation of a coupler located in the middle of the endoscope's insertion tube. The single-use spiral assembly is composed of corrugated tubing with an atraumatic plastic spiral bonded to its exterior. It relies on rotation of the spiral component to "pleat" or "un-pleat" the bowel either on or off the insertion tube as the spiral thread rotates in a clockwise or counterclockwise direction, respectively [43–45]. It has been evaluated in prospective clinical trials and shown to be safe and effective for deep enteroscopy [45]. Moreover, in view of ERCP, it allows the uses of standard ERCP-accessories in the same way as short SBE and DBE. Actually, there is one report published regarding motorized spiral enteroscopy-assisted ERCP in a patient with SAA, showing successful and rapid enteroscopic access, cannulation, and balloon dilation therapy [46]. Although further studies are needed, it could be the upcoming ERCP technology in pa-tients with SAA.

Moreover, laparoscopy-assisted ERCP (LA-ERCP) is accomplished by placing a trocar in the remnant stomach under laparoscopic guidance followed by insertion of the conventional duodenoscope through the trocar to reach the papilla. ERCP is then carried out in a standard method. The advantage of LA-ERCP is that the duodenoscope, which is used for ERCP when normal anatomy is available. It was reported that LA-ERCP achieved high success rates [47,48]. A multicenter study reported that the procedural success, and adverse events rates were 98%, and 18% (laparoscopy related, 10%, ERCP related, 7%, both, 1%) [49]. Although there is a high success rate, the overall adverse event rate was high due to the added laparoscopy-related events.

6. Interventional EUS

Despite the high effectiveness reported for BE-assisted ERCP in patients with SAA, it has several challenges for successful completion of procedures. Alternative treatment modalities are needed for some cases. Percutaneous transhepatic biliary drainage (PTBD) has been traditionally performed in these patients despite PTBD being associated with a higher adverse event rate than ERCP [50]. PTBD is conventionally performed using the following three-step approach: (1) external drainage with confirmation of clinical improvement, (2) stent deployment with maintenance of the external drainage tube, and (3) external drainage tube removal after the confirmation of proper drainage through the stent. Although PTBD is one of the alternatives, it may be impractical for urgent cases due to the requirement of serial dilation and track maturation [51]. Moreover, external drainage tube trouble could be caused. However, PTBD is possible to perform stone extraction effectively and safely, so we can choose PTBD as the alternatives for cases of difficult stone extraction using BE.

Recently, interventional EUS has been in the spotlight as an alternative therapy for patients with difficult ERCP, such as scope insertion and biliary cannulation. Interventional EUS may be a first-line treatment in some cases, such as malignant cases with cancer invasion of the small intestines or papilla [12].

There are several drainage methods for interventional EUS [52]. The first method is the EUS-guided hepaticogastrostomy (EUS-HGS). Generally, the left intrahepatic bile duct (B 2 or 3) is punctured to make the drainage route. After cholangiography and guidewire insertion, the fistula is dilated using a dilation device followed by the placement of a biliary stent [53]. If the stomach has been resected, such as in Roux-en-Y gastrectomy cases, a puncture is performed from the jejunal limb. The second method is EUS-guided antegrade stenting (EUS-AG). After puncture of the left intrahepatic bile duct, a guidewire is directed to the papilla or hepaticojejunal anastomosis, and the biliary stent is placed via an antegrade route [54]. Moreover, the EUS-guided rendezvous technique (EUS-RV) is also a useful alternative procedure [55]. In cases of difficult biliary cannulation using a BE, after the left intrahepatic bile duct (B2 or B3) is punctured, the guidewire is directed beyond the papilla or hepaticojejunal anastomosis. As a result, the guidewire is positioned into the duodenum or jejunum. Afterward, a scope exchange from the echoendoscope to BE is carried out. The guidewire is grasped using a forceps device and pulled into the working channel. Finally, biliary cannulation through the papilla or anastomotic site is successful.

Table 4 shows outcomes of EUS-guided biliary drainage (EUS-BD) [56–64]. The latest systematic review and meta-analysis reported that the pooled technical success rates and clinical success rates were 91.5% and 87%, respectively. Adverse events occurred in 17.9%. The main adverse events were bile leakage (4.1%), stent migration (3.9%), and infections (3.8%) [65]. Although there were high success rates using interventional EUS, adverse events were higher than BE-assisted ERCP. Therefore, EUS-BD should be performed carefully and endoscopists should take into consideration that severe adverse events could develop. Figure 4 provides the successful EUS-HGS in a patient with SAA. Although SBE-assisted ERCP was initially performed, it failed due to cancer invasion of the small intestine.

Table 4. Outcomes of endoscopic ultrasound (EUS)-guided biliary drainage.

Authors	Year	Technical Success, % (n)	Clinical Success, % (n)	Adverse Events, % (n)
Shah et al. [56]	2011	70.5 (62/88)	70.5 (62/88)	6.8 (6/88)
Khashab et al. [57]	2013	94.3 (33/35)	91.4 (32/35)	11.4 (4/35)
Park et al. [58]	2013	91.1 (41/45)	86.7 (39/45)	8.9 (4/45)
Kawakubo et al. [59]	2014	95.3 (61/64)	N/A	18.8 (12/64)
Gupta et al. [60]	2014	88.5 (207/234)	N/A	34.6 (81/234)
Dhir et al. [61]	2015	93.3 (97/104)	89.4 (93/104)	8.7 (9/104)
Kahaleh et al. [62]	2016	91.4 (32/35)	88.6 (31/35)	25.7 (9/35)
Tsuchiya et al. [63]	2018	100 (19/19)	94.7 (18/19)	36.8 (7/19)
Minaga et al. [64]	2019	85.2 (46/54)	85.2 (46/54)	18.5 (10/54)

EUS, endoscopic ultrasound. N/A, not available.

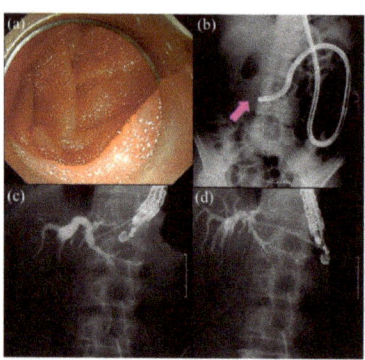

Figure 4. Endoscopic ultrasound-guided hepaticogastrostomy for patients with surgically altered anatomy (SAA) showing a failed case of single-balloon enteroscopy-assisted (SBE) endoscopic retrograde cholangiopancreatography (ERCP). (**a**) It was impossible to reach the papilla due to cancer invasion of the duodenum. (**b**) Fluoroscopic image showing duodenal obstruction due to cancer invasion (pink arrow). (**c**) Endoscopic ultrasound-guided hepaticogastrostomy is performed. First, B 3 is punctured using a 19-gauge needle. After puncture, we performed cholangiography to confirm the position of the guidewire. (**d**) Finally, a biliary stent was placed.

7. Comparison between BE-Assisted ERCP and Interventional EUS

Some papers have conducted a comparison between BE-assisted ERCP and EUS-BD in patients with SAA. A multicenter retrospective study reported that clinical success was 88% in the EUS-BD group. It was 59.1% in the BE-assisted ERCP group (odds ratio [OR] 2.83, $p = 0.03$). The EUS-BD group completed the procedure in a shorter amount of time than the BE-assisted ERCP group (55 min vs. 95 min, $p < 0.0001$). However, adverse events occurred more often in the EUS-BD group (20% vs. 4%, $p = 0.01$) [66]. An international multicenter study compared EUS-BD and BE-assisted ERCP in patients with Roux-en-Y gastric bypass and showed that the technical success rate of EUS-BD was superior to BE-assisted ERCP (100% vs. 60%). Adverse events occurred comparably [67]. These comparison studies had lower success rates than studies in Tables 2 and 3. These comparison studies' population were almost all R-Y reconstruction. Studies in Tables 2 and 3 included Billroth II gastrectomy and pancreaticoduodenectomy, which are considered to be easier than R-Y. Therefore, these success rates for BE would be lower than Tables 2 and 3.

Although interventional EUS provided a higher success rate and shorter procedure time, adverse events tended to be high. A fatal complication, such as aberrant stent displacement into the abdominal cavity, has been reported [68]. Dedicated devices used by EUS-BD are warranted for safety. Hence, the choice between BE-assisted ERCP and interventional EUS depends on the postoperative reconstruction, patient's condition, or the expertise of the endoscopist.

8. Conclusions

We discussed recent advances in interventional ERCP and EUS for patients with SAA. Both BE-assisted ERCP and interventional EUS have advantages and disadvantages. The choice of procedure should be individualized to the patient's condition or the expertise of the endoscopist. We propose the following interventional strategy for patients with SAA (Figure 5). First, if tumor invasion to the small intestine can be adequately predicted prior to the procedure by cross-sectional imaging, such as computed tomography, the most appropriate technique for the case, such as PTBD or EUS-BD, can be selected as alternative interventions. During the procedure, if the target site (papilla or hepaticojejunal anastomosis) cannot be reached using a BE, laparoscopy-assisted ERCP, PTBD, or EUS-BD will be required to complete the treatment procedure. In case of failed biliary cannulation or an intended procedure, reattempting BE-assisted ERCP, PTBD, or EUS-BD should be selected according to the previous treatment.

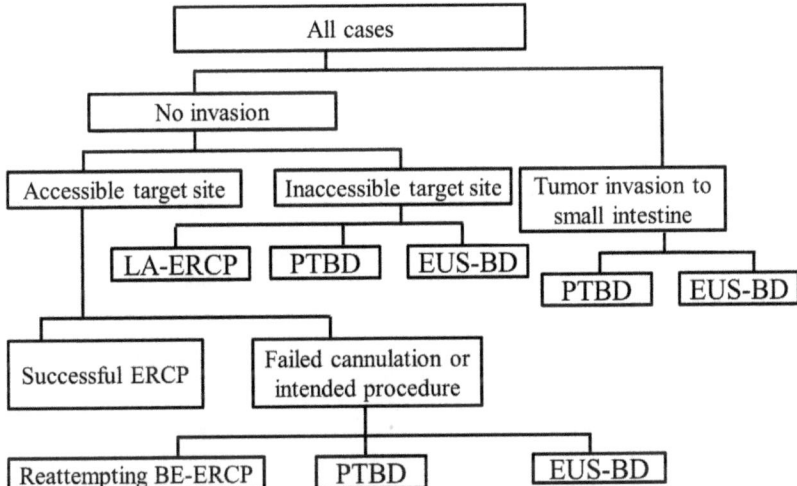

Figure 5. Flowchart of our proposed interventional strategy for patients with surgically altered anatomy (SAA). ERCP, endoscopic retrograde cholangiopancreatography. EUS-BD, endoscopic ultrasound-guided biliary drainage. PTBD, percutaneous transhepatic biliary drainage. LA-ERCP, laparoscopy-assisted ERCP. BE-ERCP, balloon enteroscope-assisted ERCP.

Further improvement of both BE-assisted ERCP and interventional EUS are needed to perform effective and safe procedures for patients with SAA.

Author Contributions: The paper was authored by Y.T., who designed and drafted the article. M.M., A.F., T.O., M.S., H.K., Y.S., K.M., T.T., Y.M., and S.R. provided a critical revision of the article for important intellectual content. Y.T. finally approved the article for submission. The final version of the manuscript was approved by all authors. All authors have read and agreed to the published version of the manuscript.

Funding: This research received no external funding.

Institutional Review Board Statement: Not applicable.

Informed Consent Statement: Not applicable.

Data Availability Statement: Data sharing not applicable.

Conflicts of Interest: The authors declare no conflict of interest.

References

1. Freeman, M.L.; Guda, N.M. ERCP cannulation: A review of reported techniques. *Gastrointest. Endosc.* **2005**, *61*, 112–125. [CrossRef]
2. Suissa, A.; Yassin, K.; Lavy, A.; Lachter, J.; Chermech, I.; Karban, A.; Tamir, A.; Eliakim, R. Outcome and early complications of ERCP: A prospective single center study. *Hepatogastroenterology* **2005**, *52*, 352–355. [PubMed]
3. Elton, E.; Hanson, B.L.; Qaseem, T.; Howell, D.A. Diagnostic and therapeutic ERCP using an enteroscope and a pediatric colonoscope in long-limb surgical bypass patients. *Gastrointest. Endosc.* **1998**, *47*, 62–67. [CrossRef]
4. Wright, B.E.; Cass, O.W.; Freeman, M.L. ERCP in patients with long-limb Roux-en-Y gastrojejunostomy and intact papilla. *Gastrointest. Endosc.* **2002**, *56*, 225–232. [CrossRef]
5. Teplick, S.K.; Flick, P.; Brandon, J.C. Transhepatic cholangiography in patients with suspected biliary disease and nondilated intrahepatic bile ducts. *Gastrointest. Radiol.* **1991**, *16*, 193–197. [CrossRef]
6. Ko, G.Y.; Sung, K.B.; Yoon, H.K.; Kim, K.R.; Gwon, D.I.; Lee, S.G. Percutaneous transhepatic treatment of hepaticojejunal anastomotic biliary strictures after living donor liver transplantation. *Liver Transpl.* **2008**, *14*, 1323–1332. [CrossRef] [PubMed]
7. Bove, V.; Tringali, A.; Familiari, P.; Gigante, G.; Boškoski, I.; Perri, V.; Mutignani, M.; Costamagna, G. ERCP in patients with prior Billroth II gastrectomy: Report of 30 years' experience. *Endoscopy* **2015**, *47*, 611–616. [CrossRef]
8. Park, T.Y.; Bang, C.S.; Choi, S.H.; Yang, Y.J.; Shin, S.P.; Suk, K.T.; Baik, G.H.; Kim, D.J.; Yoon, J.H. Forward-viewing endoscope for ERCP in patients with Billroth II gastrectomy: A systematic review and meta-analysis. *Surg. Endosc.* **2018**, *32*, 4598–4613. [CrossRef]
9. Yamamoto, H.; Sekine, Y.; Sato, Y.; Higashizawa, T.; Miyata, T.; Iino, S.; Ido, K.; Sugano, K. Total enteroscopy with a nonsurgical steerable double-balloon method. *Gastrointest. Endosc.* **2001**, *53*, 216–220. [CrossRef]
10. Tanisaka, Y.; Ryozawa, S.; Mizuide, M.; Kobayashi, M.; Fujita, A.; Minami, K.; Kobatake, T.; Omiya, K.; Iwano, H.; Araki, R. Usefulness of the "newly designed" short-type single-balloon enteroscope for ERCP in patients with Roux-en-Y gastrectomy: A pilot study. *Endosc. Int. Open* **2018**, *6*, E1417–E1422. [CrossRef]
11. Shimatani, M.; Tokuhara, M.; Kato, K.; Miyamoto, S.; Masuda, M.; Sakao, M.; Fukata, N.; Miyoshi, H.; Ikeura, T.; Takaoka, M.; et al. Utility of newly developed short-type double-balloon endoscopy for endoscopic retrograde cholangiography in postoperative patients. *J. Gastroenterol. Hepatol.* **2017**, *32*, 1348–1354. [CrossRef]
12. Tanisaka, Y.; Ryozawa, S.; Mizuide, M.; Harada, M.; Fujita, A.; Ogawa, T.; Nonaka, K.; Tashima, T.; Araki, R. Analysis of the factors involved in procedural failure: Endoscopic retrograde cholangiopancreatography using a short-type single-balloon enteroscope for patients with surgically altered gastrointestinal anatomy. *Dig. Endosc.* **2019**, *31*, 682–689. [CrossRef]
13. Trindade, A.J.; Mella, J.M.; Slattery, E.; Cohen, J.; Dickstein, J.; Garud, S.S.; Chuttani, R.; Pleskow, D.K.; Sawhney, M.S.; Berzin, T.M. Use of a cap in single-balloon enteroscopy-assisted endoscopic retrograde cholangiography. *Endoscopy* **2015**, *47*, 453–456. [CrossRef]
14. Jang, H.W.; Lee, K.J.; Jung, M.J.; Jung, J.W.; Park, J.Y.; Park, S.W.; Song, S.Y.; Chung, J.B.; Bang, S. Endoscopic papillary large balloon dilatation alone is safe and effective for the treatment of difficult choledocholithiasis in cases of Billroth II gastrectomy: A single center experience. *Dig. Dis. Sci.* **2013**, *58*, 1737–1743. [CrossRef]
15. Wang, A.Y.; Sauer, B.G.; Behm, B.W.; Ramanath, M.; Cox, D.G.; Ellen, K.L.; Shami, V.M.; Kahaleh, M. Single-balloon enteroscopy effectively enables diagnostic and therapeutic retrograde cholangiography in patients with surgically altered anatomy. *Gastrointest. Endosc.* **2010**, *71*, 641–649. [CrossRef]
16. Shah, R.J.; Smolkin, M.; Yen, R.; Ross, A.; Kozarek, R.A.; Howell, D.A.; Bakis, G.; Jonnalagadda, S.S.; Al-Lehibi, A.A.; Hardy, A.; et al. A multicenter, U.S. experience of single-balloon, double-balloon, and rotational overtube-assisted enteroscopy ERCP in patients with surgically altered pancreaticobiliary anatomy (with video). *Gastrointest. Endosc.* **2013**, *77*, 593–600. [CrossRef] [PubMed]
17. Lenze, F.; Meister, T.; Matern, P.; Heinzow, H.S.; Domschke, W.; Ullerich, H. Single-balloon enteroscopy-assisted endoscopic retrograde cholangiopancreaticography in patients with surgically altered anatomy: Higher failure rate in malignant biliary obstruction—A prospective single center cohort analysis. *Scand. J. Gastroenterol.* **2014**, *49*, 766–771. [CrossRef] [PubMed]
18. Kawamura, T.; Uno, K.; Suzuki, A.; Mandai, K.; Nakase, K.; Tanaka, K.; Yasuda, K. Clinical usefulness of a short-type, prototype single-balloon enteroscope for endoscopic retrograde cholangiopancreatography in patients with altered gastrointestinal anatomy: Preliminary experiences. *Dig. Endosc.* **2015**, *27*, 82–86. [CrossRef] [PubMed]
19. Yamauchi, H.; Kida, M.; Okuwaki, K.; Miyazawa, S.; Iwai, T.; Tokunaga, S.; Takezawa, M.; Imaizumi, H.; Koizumi, W. Passive-bending, short-type single-balloon enteroscope for endoscopic retrograde cholangiopancreatography in Roux-en-Y anastomosis patients. *World J. Gastroenterol.* **2015**, *21*, 1546–1553. [CrossRef] [PubMed]
20. Ishii, K.; Itoi, T.; Tonozuka, R.; Itokawa, F.; Sofuni, A.; Tsuchiya, T.; Tsuji, S.; Ikeuchi, N.; Kamada, K.; Umeda, J.; et al. Balloon enteroscopy-assisted ERCP in patients with Roux-en-Y gastrectomy and intact papillae (with videos). *Gastrointest. Endosc.* **2016**, *83*, 377–386. [CrossRef]
21. Yane, K.; Katanuma, A.; Maguchi, H.; Takahashi, K.; Kin, T.; Ikarashi, S.; Sano, I.; Yamazaki, H.; Kitagawa, K.; Yokoyama, K.; et al. Short-type single-balloon enteroscope-assisted ERCP in postsurgical altered anatomy: Potential factors affecting procedural failure. *Endoscopy* **2017**, *49*, 69–74. [CrossRef] [PubMed]

2. Sawas, T.; Storm, A.C.; Bazerbachi, F.; Fleming, C.J.; Vargas, E.J.; Chandrasekhara, V.; Andrews, J.C.; Levy, M.J.; Martin, J.A.; Petersen, B.T.; et al. An innovative technique using a percutaneously placed guidewire allows for higher success rate for ERCP compared to balloon enteroscopy assistance in Roux-en-Y gastric bypass anatomy. *Surg. Endosc.* **2020**, *34*, 806–813. [CrossRef]
3. Tanisaka, Y.; Ryozawa, S.; Mizuide, M.; Araki, R.; Fujita, A.; Ogawa, T.; Tashima, T.; Noguchi, T.; Suzuki, M.; Katsuda, H. Status of single-balloon enteroscopy-assisted endoscopic retrograde cholangiopancreatography in patients with surgically altered anatomy: Systematic review and meta-analysis on biliary interventions. *Dig. Endosc.* **2020**. [CrossRef] [PubMed]
4. Tanisaka, Y.; Ryozawa, S.; Mizuide, M.; Fujita, A.; Ogawa, T.; Tashima, T.; Noguchi, T.; Suzuki, M.; Katsuda, H.; Araki, R. Usefulness of self-expandable metal stents for malignant biliary obstruction using a short-type single-balloon enteroscope in patients with surgically altered anatomy. *J. Hepatobiliary Pancreat. Sci.* **2021**, *28*, 272–279. [CrossRef] [PubMed]
5. Zimmer, V. Mission (nearly) impossible: ERCP using an oblique cap with suction cannulation in a diffusely strictured duodenal stump after Billroth II with Braun enteroenterostomy. *Endoscopy* **2020**, *52*, E63–E65. [CrossRef]
6. Tanisaka, Y.; Ryozawa, S.; Mizuide, M.; Fujita, A.; Ogawa, T.; Harada, M.; Noguchi, T.; Suzuki, M.; Araki, R. Biliary Cannulation in Patients with Roux-en-Y Gastrectomy: An Analysis of the Factors Associated with Successful Cannulation. *Intern. Med.* **2020**, *59*, 1687–1693. [CrossRef]
7. Tanisaka, Y.; Ryozawa, S.; Mizuide, M.; Fujita, A.; Harada, M.; Ogawa, T. Novel technique using pancreatic duct stent facilitates difficult biliary cannulation in patients with Roux-en-Y anatomy (with video). *JGH Open* **2019**, *4*, 296–298. [CrossRef]
8. Takenaka, M.; Minaga, K.; Kamata, K.; Yamao, K.; Yoshikawa, T.; Ishikawa, R.; Okamoto, A.; Yamazaki, T.; Nakai, A.; Omoto, S.; et al. Efficacy of a modified double-guidewire technique using an uneven double lumen cannula (uneven method) in patients with surgically altered gastrointestinal anatomy (with video). *Surg. Endosc.* **2020**, *34*, 1432–1441. [CrossRef]
9. Aabakken, L.; Bretthauer, M.; Line, P.D. Double-balloon enteroscopy for endoscopic retrograde cholangiography in patients with a Roux-en-Y anastomosis. *Endoscopy* **2007**, *39*, 1068–1071. [CrossRef]
10. Emmett, D.S.; Mallat, D.B. Double-balloon ERCP in patients who have undergone Roux-en-Y surgery: A case series. *Gastrointest. Endosc.* **2007**, *66*, 1038–1041. [CrossRef]
11. Shimatani, M.; Matsushita, M.; Takaoka, M.; Koyabu, M.; Ikeura, T.; Kato, K.; Fukui, T.; Uchida, K.; Okazaki, K. Effective "short" double-balloon enteroscope for diagnostic and therapeutic ERCP in patients with altered gastrointestinal anatomy: A large case series. *Endoscopy* **2009**, *41*, 849–854. [CrossRef]
12. Cho, S.; Kamalaporn, P.; Kandel, G.; Kortan, P.; Marcon, N.; May, G. 'Short' double-balloon enteroscope endoscopic retrograde cholangiopancreatography in patients with a surgically altered upper gastrointestinal tract. *Can. J. Gastroenterol.* **2011**, *25*, 615–619. [CrossRef]
13. Tsutsumi, K.; Kato, H.; Muro, S.; Yamamoto, N.; Noma, Y.; Horiguchi, S.; Harada, R.; Okada, H.; Yamamoto, K. ERCP using a short double-balloon enteroscope in patients with prior pancreatoduodenectomy: Higher maneuverability supplied by the efferent-limb route. *Surg. Endosc.* **2015**, *29*, 1944–1951. [CrossRef] [PubMed]
14. Cheng, C.L.; Liu, N.J.; Tang, J.H.; Yu, M.C.; Tsui, Y.N.; Hsu, F.Y.; Lee, C.S.; Lin, C.H. Double-balloon enteroscopy for ERCP in patients with Billroth II anatomy: Results of a large series of papillary large-balloon dilation for biliary stone removal. *Endosc. Int. Open* **2015**, *3*, E216–E222. [CrossRef]
15. Shimatani, M.; Hatanaka, H.; Kogure, H.; Tsutsumi, K.; Kawashima, H.; Hanada, K.; Matsuda, T.; Fujita, T.; Takaoka, M.; Yano, T.; et al. Diagnostic and Therapeutic Endoscopic Retrograde Cholangiography Using a Short-Type Double-Balloon Endoscope in Patients With Altered Gastrointestinal Anatomy: A Multicenter Prospective Study in Japan. *Am. J. Gastroenterol.* **2016**, *111*, 1750–1758. [CrossRef]
16. Liu, K.; Joshi, V.; Saxena, P.; Kaffes, A.J. Predictors of success for double balloon-assisted endoscopic retrograde cholangiopancreatography in patients with Roux-en-Y anastomosis. *Dig. Endosc.* **2017**, *29*, 190–197. [CrossRef] [PubMed]
17. Kashani, A.; Abboud, G.; Lo, S.K.; Jamil, L.H. Double balloon enteroscopy-assisted endoscopic retrograde cholangiopancreatography in Roux-en-Y gastric bypass anatomy: Expert vs. novice experience. *Endosc. Int. Open* **2018**, *6*, E885–E891. [CrossRef] [PubMed]
18. Uchida, D.; Tsutsumi, K.; Kato, H.; Matsumi, A.; Saragai, Y.; Tomoda, T.; Matsumoto, K.; Horiguchi, S.; Okada, H. Potential Factors Affecting Results of Short-Type Double-Balloon Endoscope-Assisted Endoscopic Retrograde Cholangiopancreatography. *Dig. Dis. Sci.* **2020**, *65*, 1460–1470. [CrossRef] [PubMed]
19. Anvari, S.; Lee, Y.; Patro, N.; Soon, M.S.; Doumouras, A.G.; Hong, D. Double-balloon enteroscopy for diagnostic and therapeutic ERCP in patients with surgically altered gastrointestinal anatomy: A systematic review and meta-analysis. *Surg. Endosc.* **2021**, *35*, 18–36. [CrossRef]
20. Tokuhara, M.; Shimatani, M.; Mitsuyama, T.; Masuda, M.; Ito, T.; Miyamoto, S.; Fukata, N.; Miyoshi, H.; Ikeura, T.; Takaoka, M.; et al. Evaluation of complications after endoscopic retrograde cholangiopancreatography using a short type double balloon endoscope in patients with altered gastrointestinal anatomy: A single-center retrospective study of 1,576 procedures. *J. Gastroenterol. Hepatol.* **2020**, *35*, 1387–1396. [CrossRef]
21. Shimatani, M.; Takaoka, M.; Okazaki, K. Tips for double balloon enteroscopy in patients with Roux-en-Y reconstruction and modified child surgery. *J. Hepatobiliary Pancreat. Sci.* **2014**, *21*, E22–E28. [CrossRef] [PubMed]
22. Shimatani, M.; Takaoka, M.; Mitsuyama, T.; Miyoshi, H.; Ikeura, T.; Okazaki, K. Complication of endoscopic papillary large-balloon dilation using double-balloon endoscopy for biliary stones in a postoperative patient. *Endoscopy* **2014**, *46* (Suppl. 1), E390. [CrossRef]

43. Beyna, T.; Schneider, M.; Pullmann, D.; Gerges, C.; Kandler, J.; Neuhaus, H. Motorized spiral colonoscopy: A first single-center feasibility trial. *Endoscopy* **2018**, *50*, 518–523. [CrossRef] [PubMed]
44. Neuhaus, H.; Beyna, T.; Schneider, M.; Devière, J. Novel motorized spiral enteroscopy: First clinical case. *VideoGIE* **2016**, *1*, 32–33. [CrossRef] [PubMed]
45. Beyna, T.; Arvanitakis, M.; Schneider, M.; Gerges, C.; Böing, D.; Devière, J.; Neuhaus, H. Motorised spiral enteroscopy: First prospective clinical feasibility study. *Gut* **2021**, *70*, 261–267.
46. Beyna, T.; Schneider, M.; Höllerich, J.; Neuhaus, H. Motorized spiral enteroscopy-assisted ERCP after Roux-en-Y reconstructive surgery and bilioenteric anastomosis: First clinical case. *VideoGIE* **2020**, *5*, 311–313. [CrossRef] [PubMed]
47. Lopes, T.L.; Clements, R.H.; Wilcox, C.M. Laparoscopy-assisted ERCP: Experience of a high-volume bariatric surgery center (with video). *Gastrointest. Endosc.* **2009**, *70*, 1254–1259. [CrossRef] [PubMed]
48. Saleem, A.; Levy, M.J.; Petersen, B.T.; Que, F.G.; Baron, T.H. Laparoscopic assisted ERCP in Roux-en-Y gastric bypass (RYGB) surgery patients. *J. Gastrointest. Surg.* **2012**, *16*, 203–208. [CrossRef]
49. Abbas, A.M.; Strong, A.T.; Diehl, D.L.; Brauer, B.C.; Lee, I.H.; Burbridge, R.; Zivny, J.; Higa, J.T.; Falcão, M.; El Hajj, I.I.; et al. Multicenter evaluation of the clinical utility of laparoscopy-assisted ERCP in patients with Roux-en-Y gastric bypass. *Gastrointest. Endosc.* **2018**, *87*, 1031–1039. [CrossRef]
50. Inamdar, S.; Slattery, E.; Bhalla, R.; Sejpal, D.V.; Trindade, A.J. Comparison of adverse events for endoscopic vs percutaneous biliary drainage in the treatment of malignant biliary tract obstruction in an inpatient national cohort. *JAMA Oncol.* **2016**, *2*, 112–117. [CrossRef]
51. Choi, E.K.; Chiorean, M.V.; Coté, G.A.; El Hajj, I.I.; Ballard, D.; Fogel, E.L.; Watkins, J.L.; McHenry, L.; Sherman, S.; Lehman, G.A. ERCP via gastrostomy vs. double balloon enteroscopy in patients with prior bariatric Roux-en-Y gastric bypass surgery. *Surg. Endosc.* **2013**, *27*, 2894–2899. [CrossRef]
52. Katanuma, A.; Hayashi, T.; Kin, T.; Toyonaga, H.; Honta, S.; Chikugo, K.; Ueki, H.; Ishii, T.; Takahashi, K. Interventional endoscopic ultrasonography in patients with surgically altered anatomy: Techniques and literature review. *Dig. Endosc.* **2020**, *32*, 263–274. [CrossRef]
53. Nakai, Y.; Sato, T.; Hakuta, R.; Ishigaki, K.; Saito, K.; Saito, T.; Takahara, N.; Hamada, T.; Mizuno, S.; Kogure, H.; et al. Long-term outcomes of a long, partially covered metal stent for EUS-guided hepaticogastrostomy in patients with malignant biliary obstruction (with video). *Gastrointest. Endosc.* **2020**, *92*, 623–631. [CrossRef]
54. Iwashita, T.; Yasuda, I.; Doi, S.; Uemura, S.; Mabuchi, M.; Okuno, M.; Mukai, T.; Itoi, T.; Moriwaki, H. Endoscopic ultrasound-guided antegrade treatments for biliary disorders in patients with surgically altered anatomy. *Dig. Dis. Sci.* **2013**, *58*, 2417–2422. [CrossRef]
55. Matsubara, S.; Nakagawa, K.; Suda, K.; Otsuka, T.; Isayama, H.; Nakai, Y.; Oka, M.; Nagoshi, S. A Proposed Algorithm for Endoscopic Ultrasound-Guided Rendezvous Technique in Failed Biliary Cannulation. *J. Clin. Med.* **2020**, *9*, 3879. [CrossRef]
56. Shah, J.N.; Marson, F.; Weilert, F.; Bhat, Y.M.; Nguyen-Tang, T.; Shaw, R.E.; Binmoeller, K.F. Single-operator, single-session EUS-guided anterograde cholangiopancreatography in failed ERCP or inaccessible papilla. *Gastrointest. Endosc.* **2012**, *75*, 56–64. [CrossRef] [PubMed]
57. Khashab, M.A.; Valeshabad, A.K.; Modayil, R.; Widmer, J.; Saxena, P.; Idrees, M.; Iqbal, S.; Kalloo, A.N.; Stavropoulos, S.N. EUS-guided biliary drainage by using a standardized approach for malignant biliary obstruction: Rendezvous versus direct transluminal techniques (with videos). *Gastrointest. Endosc.* **2013**, *78*, 734–741. [CrossRef] [PubMed]
58. Park, D.H.; Jeong, S.U.; Lee, B.U.; Lee, S.S.; Seo, D.W.; Lee, S.K.; Kim, M.H. Prospective evaluation of a treatment algorithm with enhanced guidewire manipulation protocol for EUS-guided biliary drainage after failed ERCP (with video). *Gastrointest. Endosc.* **2013**, *78*, 91–101. [CrossRef] [PubMed]
59. Kawakubo, K.; Isayama, H.; Kato, H.; Itoi, T.; Kawakami, H.; Hanada, K.; Ishiwatari, H.; Yasuda, I.; Kawamoto, H.; Itokawa, F.; et al. Multicenter retrospective study of endoscopic ultrasound-guided biliary drainage for malignant biliary obstruction in Japan. *J. Hepatobiliary Pancreat. Sci.* **2014**, *21*, 328–334. [CrossRef] [PubMed]
60. Gupta, K.; Perez-Miranda, M.; Kahaleh, M.; Artifon, E.L.; Itoi, T.; Freeman, M.L.; de-Serna, C.; Sauer, B.; Giovannini, M.; InEBD Study Group. Endoscopic ultrasound-assisted bile duct access and drainage: Multicenter, long-term analysis of approach, outcomes, and complications of a technique in evolution. *J. Clin. Gastroenterol.* **2014**, *48*, 80–87. [CrossRef] [PubMed]
61. Dhir, V.; Itoi, T.; Khashab, M.A.; Park, D.H.; Yuen Bun Teoh, A.; Attam, R.; Messallam, A.; Varadarajulu, S.; Maydeo, A. Multicenter comparative evaluation of endoscopic placement of expandable metal stents for malignant distal common bile duct obstruction by ERCP or EUS-guided approach. *Gastrointest. Endosc.* **2015**, *81*, 913–923. [CrossRef] [PubMed]
62. Kahaleh, M.; Perez-Miranda, M.; Artifon, E.L.; Sharaiha, R.Z.; Kedia, P.; Peñas, I.; De la Serna, C.; Kumta, N.A.; Marson, F.; Gaidhane, M.; et al. International collaborative study on EUS-guided gallbladder drainage: Are we ready for prime time? *Dig. Liver. Dis.* **2016**, *48*, 1054–1057. [CrossRef] [PubMed]
63. Tsuchiya, T.; Teoh, A.Y.B.; Itoi, T.; Yamao, K.; Hara, K.; Nakai, Y.; Isayama, H.; Kitano, M. Long-term outcomes of EUS-guided choledochoduodenostomy using a lumen-apposing metal stent for malignant distal biliary obstruction: A prospective multicenter study. *Gastrointest. Endosc.* **2018**, *87*, 1138–1146. [CrossRef] [PubMed]
64. Minaga, K.; Ogura, T.; Shiomi, H.; Imai, H.; Hoki, N.; Takenaka, M.; Nishikiori, H.; Yamashita, Y.; Hisa, T.; Kato, H.; et al. Comparison of the efficacy and safety of endoscopic ultrasound-guided choledochoduodenostomy and hepaticogastrostomy for malignant distal biliary obstruction: Multicenter, randomized, clinical trial. *Dig. Endosc.* **2019**, *31*, 575–582. [CrossRef] [PubMed]

65. Dhindsa, B.S.; Mashiana, H.S.; Dhaliwal, A.; Mohan, B.P.; Jayaraj, M.; Sayles, H.; Singh, S.; Ohning, G.; Bhat, I.; Adler, D.G. EUS-guided biliary drainage: A systematic review and meta-analysis. *Endosc. Ultrasound* **2020**, *9*, 101–109.
66. Khashab, M.A.; El Zein, M.H.; Sharzehi, K.; Marson, F.P.; Haluszka, O.; Small, A.J.; Nakai, Y.; Park, D.H.; Kunda, R.; Teoh, A.Y.; et al. EUS-guided biliary drainage or enteroscopy-assisted ERCP in patients with surgical anatomy and biliary obstruction: An international comparative study. *Endosc. Int. Open* **2016**, *4*, E1322–E1327. [CrossRef] [PubMed]
67. Bukhari, M.; Kowalski, T.; Nieto, J.; Kunda, R.; Ahuja, N.K.; Irani, S.; Shah, A.; Loren, D.; Brewer, O.; Sanaei, O.; et al. An international, multicenter, comparative trial of EUS-guided gastrogastrostomy-assisted ERCP versus enteroscopy-assisted ERCP in patients with Roux-en-Y gastric bypass anatomy. *Gastrointest. Endosc.* **2018**, *88*, 486–494. [CrossRef]
68. Weilert, F.; Binmoeller, K.F.; Marson, F.; Bhat, Y.; Shah, J.N. Endoscopic ultrasound-guided anterograde treatment of biliary stones following gastric bypass. *Endoscopy* **2011**, *43*, 1105–1108. [CrossRef]

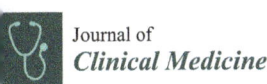

Review

Chemotherapy for Biliary Tract Cancer in 2021

Takashi Sasaki *, Tsuyoshi Takeda, Takeshi Okamoto, Masato Ozaka and Naoki Sasahira

Department of Hepato-Biliary-Pancreatic Medicine, Cancer Institute Hospital of Japanese Foundation for Cancer Research, 3-8-31, Ariake, Koto-ku, Tokyo 135-8550, Japan; tsuyoshi.takeda@jfcr.or.jp (T.T.); takeshi.okamoto@jfcr.or.jp (T.O.); masato.ozaka@jfcr.or.jp (M.O.); naoki.sasahira@jfcr.or.jp (N.S.)
* Correspondence: sasakit-tky@umin.ac.jp; Tel.: +81-3-3520-0111; Fax: +81-3-3520-0141

Abstract: Biliary tract cancer refers to a group of malignancies including cholangiocarcinoma, gallbladder cancer, and ampullary cancer. While surgical resection is considered the only curative treatment, postoperative recurrence can sometimes occur. Adjuvant chemotherapy is used to prolong prognosis in some cases. Many unresectable cases are also treated with chemotherapy. Therefore, systemic chemotherapy is widely introduced for the treatment of biliary tract cancer. Evidence on chemotherapy for biliary tract cancer is recently on the increase. Combination chemotherapy with gemcitabine and cisplatin is currently the standard of care for first-line chemotherapy in advanced cases. Recently, FOLFOX also demonstrated efficacy as a second-line treatment. In addition, efficacies of isocitrate dehydrogenase inhibitors and fibroblast growth factor receptor inhibitors have been shown. In the adjuvant setting, capecitabine monotherapy has become the standard of care in Western countries. In addition to conventional cytotoxic agents, molecular-targeted agents and immunotherapy have been evaluated in multiple clinical trials. Genetic testing is used to check for genetic alterations and molecular-targeted agents and immunotherapy are introduced based on tumor characteristics. In this article, we review the latest evidence of chemotherapy for biliary tract cancer.

Keywords: biliary tract cancer; cholangiocarcinoma; chemotherapy; cytotoxic agents; molecular targeted agents; immunotherapy; precision medicine; genetic testing

1. Introduction

Biliary tract cancer is a heterogeneous group of highly aggressive cancers including intrahepatic/perihilar/distal cholangiocarcinoma, gallbladder cancer, and ampullary cancer [1]. Biliary tract cancer is common in Japan, Southeast Asia, South America, and India [2,3]. Cholangiocarcinoma has been increasing worldwide, while the incidence of gallbladder cancer has been decreasing in recent years [4–6]. In Japan, the incidence and mortality of biliary tract cancer have plateaued over the last decade, with an annual incidence and mortality of approximately 22,000 and 18,000, respectively [7]. This cancer is still the sixth leading cause of cancer-related death. In Japan, more than 45% of new cases are diagnosed over the age of 80.

While surgical resection is considered the only curative treatment, postoperative recurrence can sometimes occur. Data from the biliary tract cancer registry in Japan revealed that five-year survival rates were 39.8% for gallbladder cancer, 24.2% for perihilar cholangiocarcinoma, 39.1% for distal cholangiocarcinoma, and 61.3% for ampullary cancer [8]. Adjuvant chemotherapy is sometimes introduced to achieve long-term survival for resected cases with poor prognostic factors. Many unresectable cases are also treated with chemotherapy. As surgery for biliary tract cancer is a highly invasive procedure, surgery may be avoided in potentially resectable cases due to old age or comorbidities. Therefore, systemic chemotherapy is widely introduced for the treatment of biliary tract cancer. Recently, evidence on chemotherapy for biliary tract cancer is on the increase. In addition to conventional cytotoxic agents, molecular-targeted agents and immunotherapy have widely been introduced in this field. Genetic testing is used to check for genetic alterations and molecular-targeted agents and immunotherapy are introduced based on tumor characteristics. Here, we review the latest evidence on chemotherapy for biliary tract cancer.

2. First-Line Chemotherapy for Advanced Biliary Tract Cancer

Standard chemotherapy for biliary tract cancer was not established until about 2000. Until then, chemotherapy for pancreatic cancer had been used as a reference. The efficacy of chemotherapy was confirmed in a randomized control study conducted before 2000 which compared chemotherapy to best supportive care in advanced pancreatic and biliary tract cancers [9]. Subsequently, a randomized controlled study comparing chemotherapy and best supportive care for unresectable gallbladder cancer was reported from India in 2010, confirming the usefulness of chemotherapy [10]. Between 2000 and 2010, gemcitabine and 5-fluorouracil were considered the key drugs for the treatment of advanced cases. A pooled analysis of clinical trials conducted between 1985 and 2006 identified gemcitabine, fluoropyrimidines, and cisplatin as the key active agents and concluded that gemcitabine combined with platinum compounds represented the provisional standard of chemotherapy for advanced biliary tract cancer [11].

The combination chemotherapy of gemcitabine and platinum compounds demonstrated good efficacy in advanced cases. A randomized phase II study (ABC-01) comparing the doublet of gemcitabine and cisplatin to gemcitabine alone was reported from the United Kingdom [12]. The doublet regimen was associated with improved tumor control and progression-free survival. Based on this result, the study was extended to a phase III study (ABC-02) to verify the prognostic effect of the combination chemotherapy relative to gemcitabine monotherapy [13]. Four hundred ten patients were randomized to receive either gemcitabine and cisplatin combination chemotherapy or gemcitabine alone. The primary endpoint was overall survival. The median overall survival was 11.7 months in the combination group and 8.1 months in the monotherapy group (hazard ratio, 0.64; $p < 0.001$). The median progression-free survivals of the combination and monotherapy groups were 8.0 months and 5.0 months, respectively ($p < 0.001$). The rate of tumor control among patients in the combination group was significantly increased (81.4% vs. 71.8%, $p = 0.049$). Although neutropenia occurred more frequently in the combination group, combination chemotherapy with gemcitabine and cisplatin was considered a feasible regimen for advanced biliary tract cancer. This combination chemotherapy was also evaluated in Japanese patients and similar efficacy was confirmed in a multicenter, randomized phase II study (BT-22) [14]. Treatment was repeated for up to 24 weeks in the ABC-02 study and up to 48 weeks in the BT-22 study. In a meta-analysis of these two studies, the efficacy of gemcitabine and cisplatin combination chemotherapy was confirmed in patients with good performance status (performance status of 0 or 1) and in patients with cholangiocarcinoma or gallbladder cancer [15]. On the other hand, the superiority of this combination chemotherapy was not shown in patients with poor performance status or ampullary cancer. The major grade 3/4 adverse events of gemcitabine and cisplatin combination chemotherapy were neutropenia and anemia. We also need to pay attention to renal dysfunction and hearing loss. Oxaliplatin is another platinum compound known to cause less renal damage and therefore does not require aggressive hydration, unlike cisplatin. Oxaliplatin is sometimes used as a substitute for cisplatin. However, the non-inferiority of gemcitabine and oxaliplatin combination chemotherapy, when compared to gemcitabine and cisplatin combination chemotherapy, has not been proven. One randomized controlled study comparing these two regimens was conducted in India [16]. A total of 243 patients with unresectable gallbladder cancer were randomly assigned to one of these two regimens. The median overall survivals of gemcitabine and oxaliplatin combination chemotherapy and gemcitabine and cisplatin combination chemotherapy were 9.0 months and 8.3 months, respectively (hazard ratio, 0.78; $p = 0.057$). Because the predetermined statistical threshold was not met, the study failed to prove non-inferiority.

Moreover, this study was underpowered to determine the superiority of gemcitabine and oxaliplatin combination chemotherapy.

Several randomized controlled studies have been conducted in pursuit of treatment regimens that are superior to the standard treatment of gemcitabine and platinum compounds. Some involved combination chemotherapies which added a third drug to the doublet, while others involved a novel regimen. Table 1 summarizes previous randomized controlled studies on first-line chemotherapy for advanced biliary tract cancer. No additional benefits of epidermal growth factor receptor and vascular endothelial growth factor receptor inhibitors have been observed to date [17]. On the other hand, good results have been obtained with S-1, which is widely used in Japan [18,19].

Table 1. Randomized controlled studies on first-line chemotherapy for advanced biliary tract cancer.

Authors	Year	Regimen	Phase	Result	N	RR	Median PFS	Median OS
Valle et al. [13]	2010	GemCis / GEM	3	Positive	204 / 206	26.1% / 15.5%	8.0 M / 5.0 M	11.7 M / 8.1 M
Sharma et al. [10]	2010	GEMOX / 5FU + FA / BSC	3	Positive	26 / 28 / 27	30.7% / 14.3% / 0%	8.5 M / 3.5 M / 2.8 M	9.5 M / 4.6 M / 4.5 M
Lee et al. [17]	2012	GEMOX + Erlotinib / GEMOX	3	Negative	135 / 133	29.6% / 15.8%	5.8 M / 4.2 M	9.5 M / 9.5 M
Sharma et al. [16]	2019	GEMOX / GemCis	3	Negative	119 / 124	25.2% / 23.4%	5.0 M / 4.0 M	9.0 M / 8.3 M
Morizane et al. [18]	2019	GEM + S-1 / GemCis	3	Positive	179 / 175	29.8% / 32.4%	6.8 M / 5.8 M	15.1 M / 13.4 M
Sakai et al. [19]	2018	GemCis + S-1 / GemCis	3	Positive	123 / 123	41.5% / 15.0%	7.4 M / 5.5 M	13.5 M / 12.6 M
Kim et al. [20]	2019	Cape + Oxaliplatin / GEMOX	3	Positive	108 / 114	15.7% / 24.6%	5.8 M / 5.3 M	10.6 M / 10.4 M
Phelip et al. [21]	2020	mFOLFIRINOX / GemCis	2/3	Negative	94 / 96	25.0% / 19.4%	6.2 M / 7.4 M	11.7 M / 14.3 M
Kang et al. [22]	2012	S-1 + CDDP / GemCis	rP2	Positive	47 / 49	23.8% / 19.6%	5.4 M / 5.7 M	9.9 M / 10.1 M
Lee et al. [23]	2015	Cape + CDDP / GemCis	rP2	Positive	44 / 49	27.3% / 6.1%	5.2 M / 3.6 M	10.7 M / 8.6 M
Malka et al. [24]	2014	GEMOX + Cmab / GEMOX	rP2	Negative	76 / 74	23.1% / 29.0%	6.0 M / 5.3 M	11.0 M / 12.4 M
Chen et al. [25]	2015	GEMOX + Cmab / GEMOX	rP2	Negative	62 / 60	27.4% / 16.7%	6.7 M / 4.1 M	10.6 M / 9.8 M
Leone et al. [26]	2016	GEMOX + Pmab / GEMOX	rP2	Negative	45 / 44	24.4% / 18.2%	7.7 M / 5.5 M	9.5 M / 9.9 M
Vogel et al. [27]	2018	GemCis + Pmab / GemCis	rP2	Negative	62 / 28	45.2% / 39.3%	6.5 M / 8.3 M	12.8 M / 20.1 M
Valle et al. [28]	2015	GemCis + Cediranib / GemCis	rP2	Negative	62 / 62	44.1% / 18.5%	7.7 M / 7.4 M	14.1 M / 11.9 M
Moehler et al. [29]	2014	GEM + Sorafenib / GEM	rP2	Negative	52 / 50	14.3% / 10.0%	3.0 M / 4.9 M	8.4 M / 11.2 M

Table 1. Cont.

Authors	Year	Regimen	Phase	Result	N	RR	Median PFS	Median OS
Santoro et al. [30]	2015	GEM + Vandetanib	rP2	Negative	58	19.3%	3.8 M	9.5 M
		GEM			56	13.5%	4.9 M	10.2 M
		Vandetanib			59	3.6%	3.5 M	7.6 M
Schnizari et al. [31]	2017	FOLFOX4	rP2	Positive	25	28.0%	5.2 M	13.0 M
		5FU + LV			23	21.7%	2.8 M	7.5 M
Markussen et al. [32]	2020	GEMOX + Cape	rP2	Negative	47	17.0%	5.7 M	8.7 M
		GemCis			49	16.3%	7.3 M	12.0 M
dos Santos et al. [33]	2020	CPT-11 + CDDP	rP2	Positive	24	35%	5.3 M	11.9 M
		GemCis			23	31.8%	7.8 M	9.8 M

N; number, RR; response rate, PFS; progression-free survival, OS; overall survival, M; months, rP2; randomized phase II study, GemCis; gemcitabine + cisplatin, GEM; gemcitabine, GEMOX; gemcitabine + oxaliplatin, 5FU; 5-fluorouracil, FA; folinic acid, BSC; best supportive care, CDDP; cisplatin, Cape; capecitabine, mFOLFIRINOX; modified FOLFIRINOX (5-fluorouracil + leucovorin + irinotecan + oxaliplatin), Cmab; cetuximab, Pmab; panitumumab; FOLFOX; 5-fluorouracil + leucovorin + oxaliplatin, LV; leucovorin, CPT-11; irinotecan.

S-1 is an oral fluoropyrimidine derivative used mainly in Asian countries. The combination of gemcitabine and S-1 was widely evaluated in phase II and randomized phase II studies in Japan [34–37]. Based on these results, a randomized phase III study comparing gemcitabine and S-1 combination chemotherapy with gemcitabine and cisplatin combination chemotherapy was conducted in Japan [18]. This study was conducted to evaluate the non-inferiority of gemcitabine and S-1 combination chemotherapy compared to gemcitabine and cisplatin combination chemotherapy. Patients with advanced biliary tract cancer were randomly assigned either gemcitabine and S-1 combination chemotherapy or gemcitabine and cisplatin combination chemotherapy. The primary endpoint was overall survival. The median overall survivals were 15.1 months and 13.4 months, respectively (hazard ratio 0.945, $p = 0.046$ for non-inferiority). Because the toxicities of gemcitabine and S-1 combination chemotherapy were deemed acceptable, this new doublet also became the standard of care for patients with advanced biliary tract cancer. The major grade 3/4 adverse event of gemcitabine and S-1 combination chemotherapy was neutropenia. We also need to pay attention to diarrhea, oral mucositis, maculopapular rash, and skin hyperpigmentation. S-1 was also evaluated as the triplet with gemcitabine and cisplatin. Based on the good result of a phase II study evaluating the efficacy of gemcitabine + cisplatin + S-1 combination chemotherapy [38], a phase III study was conducted to confirm the superiority of this triplet over gemcitabine and cisplatin combination chemotherapy in Japan [19]. Two hundred forty-six patients with advanced biliary tract cancer were randomized 1:1 to receive either the triplet or the doublet chemotherapy. The primary endpoint was overall survival. The median overall survivals of gemcitabine + cisplatin + S-1 combination chemotherapy and gemcitabine + cisplatin combination chemotherapy were 13.5 months and 12.6 months, respectively (hazard ratio 0.791, $p = 0.046$). This adverse event's profile of the triplet chemotherapy was also acceptable. The major grade 3/4 adverse event of triplet chemotherapy was also neutropenia. This triplet is also needed to pay attention to diarrhea, stomatitis, and rash. Therefore, gemcitabine + cisplatin + S-1 combination chemotherapy is currently considered a standard regimen for advanced cases.

In summary, the global standard first-line chemotherapy for advanced biliary tract cancer is still gemcitabine and cisplatin combination chemotherapy. In Japan, gemcitabine + S-1 combination chemotherapy and gemcitabine + cisplatin + S-1 combination chemotherapy are also considered alternatives of gemcitabine + cisplatin combination chemotherapy in the first-line setting.

3. Second-Line Chemotherapy for Advanced Biliary Tract Cancer

The usefulness of second-line chemotherapy has been reported based on a systematic review and large retrospective studies, but standard treatment has not been established [39–45]. In Japan, S-1 is widely used as monotherapy in the clinical setting [46,47]. To establish the standard treatment of second-line chemotherapy, various treatments such as molecular-targeted agents and immunotherapy are being developed in addition to conventional cytotoxic agents [48]. Recently, several randomized phase II and phase III studies were reported, some of which showed positive results. Table 2 summarizes previous randomized controlled studies of second-line or third-line chemotherapy for advanced biliary tract cancer.

Table 2. Randomized controlled studies on second-line or third-line chemotherapy for advanced biliary tract cancer.

Authors	Year	Regimen	Phase	Result	N	RR	Median PFS	Median OS
Abou-Alfa et al. [49]	2020	Ivosidenib	3	Positive	124	2.4%	2.7 M	10.8 M
		BSC			61	0%	1.4 M	9.7 M
Lamarca et al. [50]	2021	FOLFOX	3	Positive	81	4.9%	4.0 M	6.2 M
		ASC			81	-	-	5.3 M
Jalve et al. [51]	2020	Cape + Varlitinib	2/3	Negative	64	9.4%	2.8 M	7.8 M
		Cape			63	4.8%	2.8 M	7.5 M
Cereda et al. [52]	2016	Cape + MMC	rP2	Negative	29	3.4%	2.3 M	8.1 M
		Cape			28	0%	2.1 M	9.5 M
Zheng et al. [53]	2018	Cape + Irinotecan	rP2	Positive	30	13.3%	3.7 M	10.1 M
		Irinotecan			30	6.7%	2.4 M	7.3 M
Kim et al. [54]	2020	Trametinib	rP2	Negative	24	8.3%	1.4 M	4.3 M
		5FU + LV or Cape			20	10.0%	3.3 M	6.6 M
Demols et al. [55]	2020	Regorafenib	rP2	Positive	33	0%	3.0 M	5.3 M
		BSC			33	0%	1.5 M	5.1 M
Ueno et al. [56]	2021	S-1 + Resminostat	rP2	Negative	50	6.0%	2.9 M	7.8 M
		S-1			51	9.8%	3.0 M	7.5 M
Ramaswamy et al. [57]	2021	Cape + Irinotecan	rP2	Negative	49	6.1%	2.3 M	5.2 M
		Irinotecan			49	0%	3.1 M	6.3 M
Yoo et al. [58]	2021	5FU + LV + nal-IRI	rP2	Positive	88	14.8%	7.1 M	8.6 M
		5FU + LV			86	5.8%	1.4 M	5.5 M

N; number, RR; response rate, PFS; progression-free survival, OS; overall survival, M; months, rP2; randomized phase 2 study, BSC; best supportive care, FOLFOX; 5-fluorouracil + leucovorin + oxaliplatin, ASC; active symptom control, Cape; capecitabine, MMC; mitomycin-C, 5FU; 5-fluorouracil, LV; leucovorin, nal-IRI; nano-liposomal irinotecan.

A phase III study (ABC-06) comparing FOLFOX (5-fluorouracil + leucovorin + oxaliplatin) and active symptom control was conducted in the United Kingdom [50]. Patients with advanced biliary tract cancer treated previously with gemcitabine and cisplatin combination chemotherapy were included. Enrolled patients were randomized to receive either FOLFOX or active symptom control, which was the equivalent of best supportive care. Patients in the active symptom control group could receive FOLFOX after radiographic disease progression was confirmed. The primary endpoint was overall survival. The median overall survivals of FOLFOX and active symptom control groups were 6.2 months and 5.3 months, respectively (hazard ratio 0.69, $p = 0.031$). The benefit of FOLFOX was consistent across subgroups, including those with platinum sensitivity during first-line chemotherapy. The major grade 3/4 adverse events of FOLFOX were neutropenia, fatigue, and catheter-related infection. We also need to pay attention to peripheral neuropathy. This study was the first prospective phase III study that confirmed the benefit of chemotherapy after combination chemotherapy with gemcitabine and cisplatin. Another positive phase III study that showed the efficacy of second-line chemotherapy was the ClarIDHy study. This study was a global phase III study comparing ivosidenib and best supportive care.

Ivosidenib is a first-in-class, oral, targeted, small-molecule inhibitor of mutant isocitrate dehydrogenase (IDH) 1 protein. IDH1 mutations occur in up to 20% of cholangiocarcinomas. Patients with advanced cholangiocarcinoma who had received 1–2 prior therapies were enrolled in this study. Patients were randomly assigned to either the ivosidenib group or the best supportive care group. The primary endpoint was progression-free survival. The median progression-free survivals of the ivosidenib and best supportive care groups were 2.7 months and 1.4 months, respectively (hazard ratio 0.37, $p < 0.001$). The major grade 3/4 adverse events of ivosidenib were reported as ascites. This study was the first prospective phase III study that demonstrated a clinical benefit in targeting a molecularly defined subgroup of cholangiocarcinoma and in evaluating genetic profiles of biliary tract cancer. In 2021, the result of a randomized phase II study (NIFTY) comparing 5-fluorouracil + leucovorin + nano-liposomal irinotecan and 5-fluorouracil + leucovorin was reported [58]. This triplet chemotherapy is now known as the NAPOLI regimen and is widely used for second-line chemotherapy in advanced pancreatic cancer. The additional benefit of nano-liposomal irinotecan was demonstrated in this study. Two other randomized phase II studies also showed positive results with capecitabine and irinotecan combination chemotherapy and with regorafenib monotherapy. However, the number of patients enrolled in these studies was relatively small. Therefore, further evaluation is required to establish more solid evidence on these two regimens.

Biliary tract cancers are a heterogeneous group of cancers with different genetic alteration profiles [59–62]. Potential clinically actionable alterations, defined as oncogenic driver alterations with matched therapeutic agents either under investigation or approved in other tumor types, were identified in 44.5% of patients, showing promise for precision medicine in this field [62]. Common genes implicated in biliary tract cancer tumorigenesis include IDH1, IDH2, fibroblast growth factor receptor (FGFR) 1, FGFR2, FGFR3, and human epidermal growth factor receptor (HER) 2. Encouraging results were seen in patients with identified mutational targets, especially in tumors harboring FGFR2 fusions, HER2, and IDH mutations. The efficacy of an IDH1 inhibitor (ivosidenib) was shown in a phase III study [49]. Several FGFR inhibitors have been evaluated in phase II studies [63–66]. FGFR2 rearrangements were reported in 7.4% and 3.6% of Japanese intrahepatic cholangiocarcinoma and perihilar cholangiocarcinoma patients, respectively [67]. Based on the results of a phase II study (FIGHT-202) [65], pemigatinib was approved in many countries for patients with FGFR2 fusion or rearrangement. The major grade 3/4 adverse events of pemigatinib were hypophosphatemia, arthralgia, stomatitis, hyponatremia, abdominal pain, and fatigue.

The efficacies of pembrolizumab for microsatellite instability (MSI)-high solid tumors [68] and neurotrophic tyrosine receptor kinase (NTRK) inhibitors (entrectinib and larotrectinib) for solid tumors with NTRK fusion have also been reported [69,70]. Only a few biliary tract cancer patients were included in these studies, owing to the rarity of these alterations. MSI-high biliary tract cancer was reported in 2.22% and 1.50% of Japanese cholangiocarcinoma and gallbladder cancer patients, respectively [71]. NTRK fusion positivity was reported in only 0.18% of biliary tract cancers [72]. The efficacy and safety of pembrolizumab were evaluated in KEYNOTE-028 and KEYNOTE-158 [73]. Pembrolizumab provides durable antitumor activity in 6–13% of patients with advanced biliary tract cancer regardless of programmed cell death 1 ligand 1 (PD-L1) expression and has manageable toxicity. Other immune checkpoint inhibitors were also evaluated in phase I or II studies involving both naïve and refractory advanced biliary tract cancer [74–79]. The results of these studies were promising, and further large-scale evaluation is underway. When using these immune checkpoint inhibitors, appropriate management of immune-related adverse events is required.

In summary, FOLFOX is becoming the standard second-line chemotherapy for refractory cases. The presence of IDH mutations, FGFR fusion/rearrangement and NTRK fusion, as well as MSI status, should be confirmed to consider treatment with relevant inhibitors or immune checkpoint inhibitors where applicable. It is also important to consider participation in clinical studies if molecular-targeted agents matched with identified gene alterations are available.

4. Adjuvant Chemotherapy for Resected Biliary Tract Cancer

While surgical resection is regarded as the only treatment with a chance of curing biliary tract cancer, postoperative recurrence can sometimes occur. However, standard adjuvant chemotherapy has not been established to date.

Several phase III studies have been reported on adjuvant chemotherapy for resected biliary tract cancer. The first phase III study evaluated the efficacy of adjuvant chemotherapy of 5-fluorouracil + mitomycin-C versus surgery alone in patients with resected pancreaticobiliary carcinoma [80]. Results indicated that gallbladder carcinoma patients who underwent noncurative resection may derive some benefit from systemic chemotherapy. However, alternative modalities must be developed for patients with carcinomas of the pancreas, bile duct, or ampulla of Vater. Several prospective phase III studies focused on adjuvant chemotherapy for biliary tract cancer were subsequently conducted, as summarized in Table 3.

Table 3. Randomized controlled studies of adjuvant chemotherapy for resected biliary tract cancer.

Authors	Year	Biliary Site	Regimen	Phase	Result	N	Median RFS	Median OS
Neoptolemos et al. [81]	2012	EHCC, AC	5FU + FA GEM Surgery alone	3	Marginal	143 141 144	23.0 M 29.1 M 19.5 M	38.9 M 45.7 M 35.2 M
Ebata et al. [82]	2018	EHCC	GEM Surgery alone	3	Negative	117 108	36.0 M 39.9 M	62.3 M 63.8 M
Edeline et al. [83]	2019	ICC, EHCC, GBC	GEMOX Surgery alone	3	Negative	94 99	30.4 M 18.5 M	75.8 M 50.8 M
Primrose et al. [84]	2019	ICC, EHCC, GBC	Capecitabine Surgery alone	3	Marginal	223 224	24.4 M 17.5 M	51.1 M 36.4 M

N; number, RFS; recurrent-free survival, OS; overall survival, M; months, EHCC; extrahepatic cholangiocarcinoma, AC; ampullary cancer, ICC; intrahepatic cholangiocarcinoma, GBC; gallbladder cancer, 5FU; 5-fluorouracil, FA; folinic acid, GEM; gemcitabine, GEMOX; gemcitabine + oxaliplatin.

ESPAC-3 was a phase III study that evaluated the efficacy of adjuvant chemotherapy using 5-fluorouracil + folinic acid or gemcitabine monotherapy against surgery alone [81]. Patients with extrahepatic cholangiocarcinoma and ampullary cancer were enrolled in this study. This study did not show superiority of adjuvant chemotherapy over surgery alone based on an intention-to-treat analysis. However, sensitivity analysis adjusted for prognostic factors showed improved prognosis in both the adjuvant chemotherapy group and the gemcitabine monotherapy group compared to the surgery alone group. BCAT was a phase III study conducted to evaluate the efficacy of adjuvant chemotherapy using gemcitabine against surgery alone [82]. This Japanese study was limited to extrahepatic cholangiocarcinoma patients. Treatment outcomes of surgery alone were extremely good, and no additional benefits of gemcitabine were observed. PRODIGE 12-ACCORD 18 was a French phase III study that compared adjuvant gemcitabine and oxaliplatin combination chemotherapy with surgery alone [83]. All types of biliary tract cancer other than ampullary cancer were included. The efficacy of adjuvant combination chemotherapy was not demonstrated in this negative study. BILCAP was a British phase III study that compared adjuvant capecitabine and surgery alone [84]. While capecitabine monotherapy failed to show improvement based on an intention-to-treat analysis, significant improvement was demonstrated in a per-protocol analysis. The major grade 3/4 adverse events of capecitabine were hand-foot syndrome, diarrhea and fatigue. Because of this promising result, the American Society of Clinical Oncology guideline recommends adjuvant capecitabine monotherapy for resected biliary tract cancer [85].

In summary, capecitabine monotherapy of six months for adjuvant chemotherapy is considered standard treatment for resected biliary tract cancer in Western counties. Until prospective studies show otherwise, surgery alone remains the standard of care in Japan.

5. Ongoing Clinical Trials for Biliary Tract Cancer

Currently, effective chemotherapy for biliary tract cancer is extremely limited, and the development of new therapies is urgently needed. There are a large number of ongoing prospective studies for biliary tract cancer [86–91]. Based on promising early-phase study results, phase III studies are underway [92–94]. A list of major ongoing randomized controlled studies for biliary tract cancer is provided in Table 4. In addition to conventional treatments using cytotoxic agents, a wide variety of drugs such as molecular-targeted agents and immune checkpoint inhibitors are being investigated. Despite the low frequency of genetic alterations, precision medicine with molecular-targeted agents holds promise for selected patients. Umbrella and basket studies are increasingly being conducted, based on the need to build a mechanism to provide drugs suited to each genetic alteration regardless of tumor origin. The efficacy of immunotherapy combined with conventional treatment is also being investigated. In addition, a new large-scale trial for neoadjuvant chemotherapy is underway. Many new therapies that enhance the effectiveness of current regimens have been validated in late-phase clinical trials such as those listed in Table 4. On the other hand, many new drugs have been validated in other, slightly earlier phase clinical trials. It is hoped that such drugs will advance to late-phase clinical trials sooner. Like other cancers, it is also expected that molecular-targeted drugs and immunotherapy that matched cancer genetic characteristics, such as first-line FGFR inhibitors, can produce much better treatment than current standard treatments.

Table 4. Major ongoing clinical studies for biliary tract cancer.

Regimen	N	Phase	Trial ID
First-line chemotherapy			
NUC-1031 (Acelarin) + CDDP vs. GemCis (NuTide:121)	828	3	NCT04163900
GemCis + Pembrolizumab vs. GemCis (KEYNOTE-966)	788	3	NCT04003636
GemCis + Durvalumab vs. GemCis (TOPAZ-1)	757	3	NCT03875235
Pemigatinib vs. GemCis (FIGHT-302)	432	3	NCT03656536
GEMOX + KN035 vs. GEMOX (KN035-BTC)	390	3	NCT03478488
Infigratinib vs. GemCis (PROOF 301 trial)	384	3	NCT037773302
GemCis + nab-paclitaxel vs. GemCis (SWOG/S1815)	268	3	NCT03768414
Futibatinib vs. GemCis (FOENIX-CCA3)	216	3	NCT04093362
GemCis + Bintrafusp alfa vs. GemCis	512	2/3	NCT04066491
Second-line chemotherapy			
TQB2450 + Anlotinib vs. Cape + Oxaliplatin or Cape + GEM	392	3	NCT04809142
Surufatinib vs. Cape	298	2/3	NCT03873532
Adjuvant chemotherapy			
GemCis vs. Surgery alone or Cape (ACTICCA-1)	781	3	NCT02170090
GEM + Cape vs. Cape (AdBTC-1)	460	3	NCT03779035
S-1 vs. Surgery alone (ASCOT)	350	3	UMIN000011688
Neoadjuvant chemotherapy			
Neoadjuvant & adjuvant GemCis vs. Adjuvant CTx (GAIN)	300	3	NCT03673072
Neoadjuvant GCS vs. Surgery first (NABICAT)	300	3	jRCTs031200388

CDDP; cisplatin, GemCis; gemcitabine + cisplatin, GEMOX; gemcitabine + oxaliplatin, Cape; capecitabine, GEM; gemcitabine, CTx; chemotherapy, GCS; gemcitabine + cisplatin + S-1.

6. Conclusions

Figure 1 shows the proposed treatment algorithm of chemotherapy for advanced biliary tract cancer in 2021. It is necessary to arrange this algorithm according to the medical situation in each country.

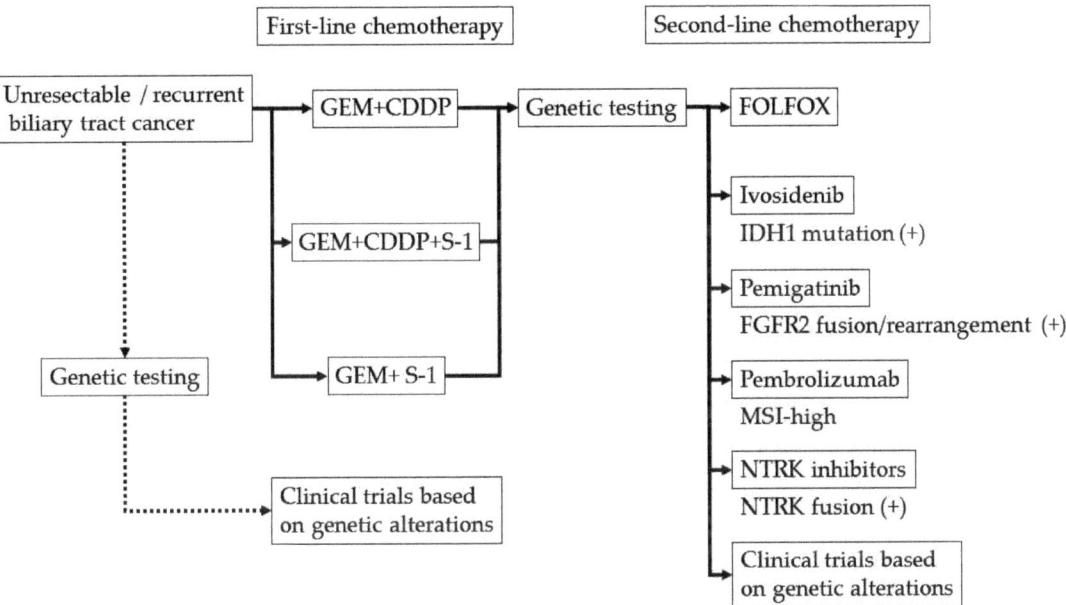

Figure 1. Proposed treatment algorithm of chemotherapy for advanced biliary tract cancer. GEM; gemcitabine, CDDP; cisplatin, FOLFOX; 5-fluorouracil + leucovorin + oxaliplatin, IDH; isocitrate dehydrogenase, FGFR; fibroblast growth factor receptor, MSI; microsatellite instability, NTRK; neurotrophic tyrosine receptor kinase.

Biliary tract cancer is considered a population with various genetic alterations. Genetic alterations are often measured before starting second- or third-line chemotherapy only in patients who are able to get enough tissue samples. If the effectiveness of molecular-targeted drugs and immunotherapy based on the characteristics of cancer is shown at first-line setting, it is thought that the trend of investigating genetic alterations from the time of diagnosis will accelerate in the future. In addition, to overcome the problem that biliary tract cancer is sometimes difficult to get enough tissue samples, there are great expectations for liquid biopsy in this field. Furthermore, there is an urgent need to develop more drugs that match genetic alterations and establish a system to deliver the drugs to the matched patients in clinical practice.

While evidence relating to chemotherapy for biliary tract cancer had been limited, numerous clinical studies have been conducted in the last decade and evidence is steadily accumulating. Many large-scale clinical studies are still underway, some of which may lead to improved treatment outcomes going forward.

Author Contributions: Writing—original draft preparation, T.S.; writing—review and editing, T.T., T.O., supervision, M.O., N.S. All authors have read and agreed to the published version of the manuscript.

Funding: This research received no external funding.

Informed Consent Statement: Not applicable.

Data Availability Statement: Not applicable.

Conflicts of Interest: T.S. has received honoraria from Taiho Pharmaceutical Co., Ltd., Yakult Honsha Co., Ltd., Eisai Co., Ltd. T.T. has received honoraria from Taiho Pharmaceutical Co., Ltd. M.O. has received honoraria from Taiho Pharmaceutical Co., Ltd., Yakult Honsha Co., Ltd., Eisai Co., Ltd., AstraZeneca, ONO Pharmaceutical Co., Ltd., Chugai Pharmaceutical Co., Novartis, MSD. N.S. has received research grants from Taiho Pharmaceutical Co., Ltd., Chugai Pharmaceutical Co., Ltd., and has received honoraria Chugai Pharmaceutical Co., Ltd., Eisai Co., Ltd. The other author declares no conflicts of interest.

References

1. Valle, J.W.; Kelley, R.K.; Nervi, B.; Oh, D.Y.; Zhu, A.X. Biliary tract cancer. *Lancet* **2021**, *397*, 428–444. [CrossRef]
2. Siegel, R.L.; Miller, K.D.; Fuchs, H.E.; Jemal, A. Cancer Statistics, 2021. *CA. Cancer J. Clin.* **2021**, *71*, 7–33. [CrossRef] [PubMed]
3. Sung, H.; Ferlay, J.; Siegel, R.L.; Laversanne, M.; Soerjomataram, I.; Jemal, A.; Bray, F. Global Cancer Statistics 2020: GLOBOCAN Estimates of Incidence and Mortality Worldwide for 36 Cancers in 185 Countries. *CA. Cancer J. Clin.* **2021**, *71*, 209–249. [CrossRef]
4. Florio, A.A.; Ferlay, J.; Znaor, A.; Ruggieri, D.; Alvarez, C.S.; Laversanne, M.; Bray, F.; McGlynn, K.A.; Petrick, J.L. Global trends in intrahepatic and extrahepatic cholangiocarcinoma incidence from 1993 to 2012. *Cancer* **2020**, *126*, 2666–2678. [CrossRef] [PubMed]
5. Gad, M.M.; Saad, A.M.; Faisaluddin, M.; Gaman, M.A.; Ruhban, I.A.; Jazieh, K.A.; Al-Husseini, M.J.; Simons-Linares, C.R. Epidemiology of Cholangiocarcinoma; United States Incidence and Mortality Trends. *Clin. Res. Hepatol. Gastroenterol.* **2020**, *44*, 885–893. [CrossRef] [PubMed]
6. Rawla, P.; Sunkara, T.; Thandra, K.C.; Barsouk, A. Epidemiology of gallbladder cancer. *Clin. Exp. Hepatol.* **2019**, *5*, 93–102. [CrossRef] [PubMed]
7. Cancer Registry and Statistics. Cancer Information Service, National Cancer Center, Japan (Vital Statistics of Japan). Available online: https://ganjoho.jp/reg_stat/statistics/dl/index.html (accessed on 1 June 2021).
8. Ishihara, S.; Horiguchi, A.; Miyakawa, S.; Endo, I.; Miyazaki, M.; Takada, T. Biliary tract cancer registry in Japan from 2008 to 2013. *J. Hepatobiliary Pancreat. Sci.* **2016**, *23*, 149–157. [CrossRef] [PubMed]
9. Glimelius, B.; Hoffman, K.; Sjödén, P.O.; Jacobsson, G.; Sellström, H.; Enander, L.K.; Linné, T.; Svensson, C. Chemotherapy improves survival and quality of life in advanced pancreatic and biliary cancer. *Ann. Oncol.* **1996**, *7*, 593–600. [CrossRef]
10. Sharma, A.; Dwary, A.D.; Mohanti, B.K.; Deo, S.V.; Pal, S.; Sreenivas, V.; Raina, V.; Shukla, N.K.; Thulkar, S.; Garg, P.; et al. Best supportive care compared with chemotherapy for unresectable gall bladder cancer: A randomized controlled study. *J. Clin. Oncol.* **2010**, *28*, 4581–4586. [CrossRef]
11. Eckel, F.; Schmid, R.M. Chemotherapy in advanced biliary tract carcinoma: A pooled analysis of clinical trials. *Br. J. Cancer* **2007**, *96*, 896–902. [CrossRef]
12. Valle, J.W.; Wasan, H.; Johnson, P.; Jones, E.; Dixon, L.; Swindell, R.; Baka, S.; Maraveyas, A.; Corrie, P.; Falk, S.; et al. Gemcitabine alone or in combination with cisplatin in patients with advanced or metastatic cholangiocarcinomas or other biliary tract tumours: A mulitcentre randomized phase II study—The UK ABC-01 Study. *Br. J. Cancer* **2009**, *101*, 621–627. [CrossRef]
13. Valle, J.; Wasan, H.; Palmer, D.H.; Cunningham, D.; Anthoney, A.; Maraveyas, A.; Madhusudan, S.; Iveson, T.; Hughes, S.; Pereira, S.P.; et al. Cisplatin plus gemcitabine versus gemcitabine for biliary tract cancer. *N. Engl. J. Med.* **2010**, *362*, 1273–1281. [CrossRef] [PubMed]
14. Okusaka, T.; Nakachi, K.; Fukutomi, A.; Mizuno, N.; Ohkawa, S.; Funakoshi, M.; Nagino, M.; Kondo, S.; Nagaoka, S.; Funai, J.; et al. Gemcitabine alone or in combination with cisplatin in patients with biliary tract cancer: A comparative multicentre study in Japan. *Br. J. Cancer* **2010**, *103*, 469–474. [CrossRef]
15. Valle, J.W.; Furuse, J.; Jitlal, M.; Beare, S.; Mizuno, N.; Wasan, H.; Bridgewater, J.; Okusaka, T. Cisplatin and gemcitabine for advanced biliary tract cancer: A meta-analysis of two randomized trials. *Ann. Oncol.* **2014**, *25*, 391–398. [CrossRef] [PubMed]
16. Sharma, A.; Kalyan Mohanti, B.; Pal Chaudhary, S.; Sreenivas, V.; Kumar Sahoo, R.; Kumar Shukla, N.; Thulkar, S.; Pal, S.; Deo, S.V.; Pathy, S.; et al. Modified gemcitabine and oxaliplatin or gemcitabine + cisplatin in uresectable gallbladder cancer: Results of a phase III randomized controlled trial. *Eur. J. Cancer* **2019**, *123*, 162–170. [CrossRef]
17. Lee, J.; Park, S.H.; Chang, H.M.; Kim, J.S.; Choi, H.J.; Lee, M.A.; Jang, J.S.; Jeung, H.C.; Kang, J.H.; Lee, H.W.; et al. Gemcitabine and oxaliplatin with or without erlotinib in advanced biliary-tract cancer: A multicentre, open-label, randomized, phase 3 study. *Lancet Oncol.* **2012**, *13*, 181–188. [CrossRef]
18. Morizane, C.; Okusaka, T.; Mizusawa, J.; Katayama, H.; Ueno, M.; Ikeda, M.; Ozaka, M.; Okano, N.; Sugimori, K.; Fukutomi, A.; et al. Combination gemcitabine plus S-1 versus gemcitabine plus cisplatin for advanced/recurrent biliary tract cancer: The FUGA-BT (JCOG1113) randomized phase III clinical trial. *Ann. Oncol.* **2019**, *30*, 1950–1958. [CrossRef] [PubMed]
19. Sakai, D.; Kanai, M.; Kobayashi, S.; Eguchi, H.; Baba, H.; Seo, S.; Taketomi, A.; Takayama, T.; Yamaue, H.; Ishioka, C.; et al. Randomized phase III study of gemcitabine, cisplatin plus S-1 (GCS) versus gemcitabine, cisplatin (GC) for advanced biliary tract cancer (KHBO1401-MITSUBA). *Ann. Oncol.* **2018**, *29* (Suppl. 8), viii205–viii270. [CrossRef]
20. Kim, S.T.; Kang, J.H.; Lee, J.; Lee, H.W.; Oh, S.Y.; Jang, J.S.; Lee, M.A.; Sohn, B.S.; Yoon, S.Y.; Choi, H.J.; et al. Capecitabine plus oxaliplatin versus gemcitabine plus oxaliplatin as first-line therapy for advanced biliary tract cancers: A multicenter, open-label, randomized, phase III, noninferiority trial. *Ann. Oncol.* **2019**, *30*, 788–795. [CrossRef]
21. Phelip, J.M.; Desrame, J.; Edeline, J.; Barbier, E.; Terrebonne, E.; Michel, P.; Perrier, H.; Dahan, L.; Bourgeois, V.; Khemissa Akouz, F.; et al. Modified FOLFIRINOX versus CISGEM first-line chemotherapy for locally advanced, non resectable and/or metastatic biliary tract cancer: Results of AMEBICA PRODIGE 38 Phase II trial. *Ann. Oncol.* **2020**, *31* (Suppl. 4), S260–S273. [CrossRef]
22. Kang, M.J.; Lee, J.; Kim, T.W.; Lee, S.S.; Ahn, S.; Park, D.H.; Lee, S.S.; Seo, D.W.; Lee, S.K.; Kim, M. Randomized phase II trial of S-1 and cisplatin versus gemcitabine and cisplatin in patients with advanced biliary tract cancer. *Acta Oncol.* **2012**, *7*, 860–866. [CrossRef]

23. Lee, J.; Hong, T.H.; Lee, I.S.; You, Y.K.; Lee, M.A. Comparison of the Efficacy between Gemcitabine-Cisplatin and Capecitabine-Cisplatin Combination Chemotherapy for Advanced Biliary Tract Cancer. *Cancer Res. Treat.* **2015**, *47*, 259–265. [CrossRef]
24. Malka, D.; Cervera, P.; Foulon, S.; Trarbach, T.; de la Fouchardière, C.; Boucher, E.; Fartoux, L.; Faivre, S.; Blanc, J.F.; Viret, F.; et al. Gemcitabine and oxaliplatin with or without cetuximab in advanced biliary-tract cancer (BINGO): A randomised, open-label, non-comparative phase 2 trial. *Lancet Oncol.* **2014**, *15*, 819–828. [CrossRef]
25. Chen, J.S.; Hsu, C.; Chiang, N.J.; Tsai, C.S.; Tsou, H.H.; Huang, S.F.; Bai, L.Y.; Chang, I.C.; Shiah, H.S.; Ho, C.L.; et al. A KRAS mutation status-stratified randomized phase II trial of gemcitabine and oxaliplatin alone or in combination with cetuximab in advanced biliary tract cancer. *Ann. Oncol.* **2015**, *26*, 943–949. [CrossRef]
26. Leone, F.; Marino, D.; Cereda, S.; Filippi, R.; Belli, C.; Spadi, R.; Nasti, G.; Montano, M.; Amatu, A.; Aprile, G.; et al. Panitumumab in combination with gemcitabine and oxaliplatin does not prolong survival in wild-type KRAS advanced biliary tract cancer: A randomized phase 2 trial (Vecti-BIL study). *Cancer* **2016**, *122*, 574–581. [CrossRef] [PubMed]
27. Vogel, A.; Kasper, S.; Bitzer, M.; Block, A.; Sinn, M.; Schulze-Bergkamen, H.; Moehler, M.; Pfarr, N.; Endris, V.; Goeppert, B.; et al. PICCA study: Panitumumab in combination with cisplatin/gemcitabine chemotherapy in KRAS wild-type patients with biliary cancer-a randomised biomarker-driven clinical phase II AIO study. *Eur. J. Cancer* **2018**, *92*, 11–19. [CrossRef]
28. Valle, J.W.; Wasan, H.; Lopes, A.; Backen, A.C.; Palmer, D.H.; Morris, K.; Duggan, M.; Cunningham, D.; Anthoney, D.A.; Corrie, P.; et al. Cediranib or placebo in combination with cisplatin and gemcitabine chemotherapy for patients with advanced biliary tract cancer (ABC-03): A randomised phase 2 trial. *Lancet Oncol.* **2015**, *16*, 967–978. [CrossRef]
29. Moehler, M.; Maderer, A.; Schimanski, C.; Kanzler, S.; Denzer, U.; Kolligs, F.T.; Ebert, M.P.; Distelrath, A.; Geissler, M.; Trojan, J.; et al. Gemcitabine plus sorafenib versus gemcitabine alone in advanced biliary tract cancer: A double-blind placebo-controlled multicentre phase II AIO study with biomarker and serum programme. *Eur. J. Cancer* **2014**, *50*, 3125–3135. [CrossRef]
30. Santoro, A.; Gebbia, V.; Pressiani, T.; Testa, A.; Personeni, N.; Arrivas Bajardi, E.; Foa, P.; Buonadonna, A.; Bencardino, K.; Barone, C.; et al. A randomized, multicenter, phase II study of vandetanib monotherapy versus vandetanib in combination with gemcitabine versus gemcitabine plus placebo in subjects with advanced biliary tract cancer: The VanGogh study. *Ann. Oncol.* **2015**, *26*, 542–547. [CrossRef] [PubMed]
31. Schinzari, G.; Rossi, E.; Mambella, G.; Strippoli, A.; Cangiano, R.; Mutignani, M.; Basso, M.; Cassano, A.; Barone, C. First-line Treatment of Advanced Biliary Ducts Carcinoma: A Randomized Phase II Study Evaluating 5-FU/LV Plus Oxaliplatin (Folfox 4) Versus 5-FU/LV (de Gramont Regimen). *Anticancer Res.* **2017**, *37*, 5193–5197. [PubMed]
32. Markussen, A.; Jensen, L.H.; Diness, L.V.; Larsen, F.O. Treatment of Patients with Advanced Biliary Tract Cancer with Either Oxaliplatin, Gemcitabine, and Capecitabine or Cisplatin and Gemcitabine-A Randomized Phase II Trial. *Cancers* **2020**, *12*, 1975. [CrossRef]
33. dos Santos, L.V.; Pinto, G.S.F.; Ferraz, M.W.S.; Bragagnoli, A.; Santos, F.; Haddad, S.; Barros, A.; Dias, I.C.C.; Lima, J.P.S.; Abdalla, K.C. Cisplatin plus irinotecan versus cisplatin plus gemcitabine in the treatment of advanced or metastatic gallbladder or biliary tract cancer: Results of a randomized phase II trial (NCT01859728)–The Gambit trial. *J. Clin. Oncol.* **2020**, *38* (Suppl. 4), 529. [CrossRef]
34. Sasaki, T.; Isayama, H.; Nakai, Y.; Ito, Y.; Kogure, H.; Togawa, O.; Toda, N.; Yasuda, I.; Hasebe, O.; Maetani, I.; et al. Multicenter, phase II study of gemcitabine and S-1 combination chemotherapy in patients with advanced biliary tract cancer. *Cancer Chemother. Pharmacol.* **2010**, *65*, 1101–1107. [CrossRef]
35. Kanai, M.; Yoshimura, K.; Tsumura, T.; Asada, M.; Suzuki, C.; Niimi, M.; Matsumoto, S.; Nishimura, T.; Nitta, T.; Yasuchika, K.; et al. A multi-institution phase II study of gemcitabine/S-1 combination chemotherapy for patients with advanced biliary tract cancer. *Cancer Chemother. Pharmacol.* **2011**, *67*, 1429–1434. [CrossRef]
36. Sasaki, T.; Isayama, H.; Nakai, Y.; Ito, Y.; Yasuda, I.; Toda, N.; Kogure, H.; Hanada, K.; Maguchi, H.; Sasahira, N.; et al. A randomized phase II study of gemcitabine and S-1 combination therapy versus gemcitabine monotherapy for advanced biliary tract cancer. *Cancer Chemother. Pharmacol.* **2013**, *71*, 973–979. [CrossRef] [PubMed]
37. Morizane, C.; Okusaka, T.; Mizusawa, J.; Takashima, A.; Ueno, M.; Ikeda, M.; Hamamoto, Y.; Ishii, H.; Boku, N.; Furuse, J. Randomized phase II study of gemcitabine plus S-1 versus S-1 in advanced biliary tract cancer: A Japan Clinical Oncology Group trial (JCOG 0805). *Cancer Sci.* **2013**, *104*, 1211–1216. [CrossRef] [PubMed]
38. Kanai, M.; Hatano, E.; Kobayashi, S.; Fujiwara, Y.; Marubashi, S.; Miyamoto, A.; Shiomi, H.; Kubo, S.; Ikuta, S.; Yanagimoto, H.; et al. A multi-institution phase II study of gemcitabine/cisplatin/S-1 (GCS) combination chemotherapy for patients with advanced biliary tract cancer (KHBO 1002). *Cancer Chemother. Pharmacol.* **2015**, *75*, 293–300. [CrossRef] [PubMed]
39. Walter, T.; Horgan, A.M.; McNamara, M.; McKeever, L.; Min, T.; Hedley, D.; Serra, S.; Krzyzanowska, M.K.; Chen, E.; Mackay, H.; et al. Feasibility and benefits of second-line chemotherapy in advanced biliary tract cancer: A large retrospective study. *Eur. J. Cancer* **2013**, *49*, 329–335. [CrossRef]
40. Bridgewater, J.; Palmer, D.; Cunningham, D.; Iveson, T.; Gillmore, R.; Waters, J.; Harrison, M.; Wasan, H.; Corrie, P.; Valle, J. Outcome of second-line chemotherapy for biliary tract cancer. *Eur. J. Cancer* **2013**, *49*, 1511. [CrossRef]
41. Lamarca, A.; Hubner, R.A.; David Ryder, W.; Valle, J.W. Second-line chemotherapy in advanced biliary cancer: A systematic review. *Ann. Oncol.* **2014**, *25*, 2328–2338. [CrossRef]
42. Brieau, B.; Dahan, L.; De Rycke, Y.; Boussaha, T.; Vasseur, P.; Tougeron, D.; Lecomte, T.; Coriat, R.; Bachet, J.B.; Claudez, P.; et al. Second-line chemotherapy for advanced biliary tract cancer after failure of the gemcitabine-platinum combination: A large multicenter study by the Association des Gastro-Entérologues Oncologues. *Cancer* **2015**, *121*, 3290–3297. [CrossRef]

43. Takahara, N.; Nakai, Y.; Isayama, H.; Sasaki, T.; Saito, K.; Oyama, H.; Kanai, S.; Suzuki, T.; Sato, T.; Hakuta, R.; et al. Second-line chemotherapy in patients with advanced or recurrent biliary tract cancer: A single center, retrospective analysis of 294 cases. *Investig. New Drugs* **2018**, *36*, 1093–1102. [CrossRef] [PubMed]
44. Lowery, M.A.; Goff, L.W.; Keenan, B.P.; Jordan, E.; Wang, R.; Bocobo, A.G.; Chou, J.F.; O'Reilly, E.M.; Harding, J.J.; Kemeny, N.; et al. Second-line chemotherapy in advanced biliary cancers: A retrospective, multicenter analysis of outcomes. *Cancer* **2019**, *125*, 4426–4434. [CrossRef] [PubMed]
45. Zaidi, A.; Chandna, N.; Narasimhan, G.; Moser, M.; Haider, K.; Chalchal, H.; Shaw, J.; Ahmed, S. Second-line Chemotherapy Prolongs Survival in Real World Patients with Advanced Biliary Tract and Gallbladder Cancers: A Multicenter Retrospective Population-based Cohort Study. *Am. J. Clin. Oncol.* **2021**, *44*, 93–98. [CrossRef] [PubMed]
46. Sasaki, T.; Isayama, H.; Nakai, Y.; Mizuno, S.; Yamamoto, K.; Yagioka, H.; Yashima, Y.; Kawakubo, K.; Kogure, H.; Togawa, O.; et al. Multicenter phase II study of S-1 monotherapy as second-line chemotherapy for advanced biliary tract cancer refractory to gemcitabine. *Investig. New Drugs* **2012**, *30*, 708–713. [CrossRef]
47. Suzuki, E.; Ikeda, M.; Okusaka, T.; Nakamori, S.; Ohkawa, S.; Nagakawa, Y.; Boku, N.; Yanagimoto, H.; Sato, T.; Furuse, J. A multicenter phase II study of S-1 for gemcitabine-refractory biliary tract cancer. *Cancer Chemother. Pharmacol.* **2013**, *71*, 1141–1146. [CrossRef]
48. Tella, S.H.; Kommalapati, A.; Borad, M.J.; Mahipal, A. Second-line therapies in advanced biliary cancers. *Lancet Oncol.* **2020**, *21*, e29–e41. [CrossRef]
49. Abou-Alfa, G.K.; Macarulla, T.; Javle, M.M.; Kelley, R.K.; Lubner, S.J.; Adeva, J.; Cleary, J.M.; Catenacci, D.V.; Borad, M.J.; Bridgewater, J.; et al. Ivosidenib in IDH1-mutant, chemotherapy-refractory cholangiocarcinoma (ClarIDHy): A multicentre, randomised, double-blind, placebo-controlled, phase 3 study. *Lancet Oncol.* **2020**, *21*, 796–807. [CrossRef]
50. Lamarca, A.; Palmer, D.H.; Wasan, H.S.; Ross, P.J.; Ma, Y.T.; Arora, A.; Falk, S.; Gillmore, R.; Wadsley, J.; Patel, K.; et al. Second-line FOLFOX chemotherapy versus active symptom control for advanced biliary tract cancer (ABC-06): A phase 3, open-label, randomised, controlled trial. *Lancet Oncol.* **2021**, *22*, 690–701. [CrossRef]
51. Jalve, M.M.; Oh, D.Y.; Ikeda, M.; Yong, W.P.; McIntyre, N.; Lindmark, B.; McHale, M. Results from TreeTopp: A randomized phase II study of the efficacy and safety of varlitinib plus capecitabine versus placebo in second-line (2L) advanced or metastatic biliary tract cancer (BTC). *J. Clin. Oncol.* **2020**, *38* (Suppl. 15), 4597.
52. Cereda, S.; Milella, M.; Cordio, S.; Leone, F.; Aprile, G.; Galiano, A.; Mosconi, S.; Vasile, E.; Santini, D.; Belli, C.; et al. Capecitabine with/without mitomycin C: Results of a randomized phase II trial of second-line therapy in advanced biliary tract adenocarcinoma. *Cancer Chemother. Pharmacol.* **2016**, *77*, 109–114. [CrossRef] [PubMed]
53. Zheng, Y.; Tu, X.; Zhao, P.; Jiang, W.; Liu, L.; Tong, Z.; Zhang, H.; Yan, C.; Fang, W.; Wang, W. A randomised phase II study of second-line XELIRI regimen versus irinotecan monotherapy in advanced biliary tract cancer patients progressed on gemcitabine and cisplatin. *Br. J. Cancer* **2018**, *119*, 291–295. [CrossRef] [PubMed]
54. Kim, R.D.; McDonough, S.; El-Khoueiry, A.B.; Bekaii-Saab, T.S.; Stein, S.M.; Sahai, V.; Keogh, G.P.; Kim, E.J.; Baron, A.D.; Siegel, A.B.; et al. Randomised phase II study (SWOG S1310) of single agent MEK inhibitor trametinib Versus 5-fluorouracil or capecitabine in refractory advanced biliary cancer. *Eur. J. Cancer* **2020**, *130*, 219–227. [CrossRef] [PubMed]
55. Demols, A.; Borbath, I.; Van den Eynde, M.; Houbiers, G.; Peeters, M.; Marechal, R.; Delaunoit, T.; Goemine, J.C.; Laurent, S.; Holbrechts, S.; et al. Regorafenib after failure of gemcitabine and platinum-based chemotherapy for locally advanced/metastatic biliary tumors: REACHIN, a randomized, double-blind, phase II trial. *Ann. Oncol.* **2020**, *31*, 1169–1177. [CrossRef] [PubMed]
56. Ramaswamy, A.; Ostwal, V.; Sharma, A.; Bhargava, P.; Srinivas, S.; Goel, M.; Patkar, S.; Mandavkar, S.; Jadhav, P.; Parulekar, M.; et al. Efficacy of Capecitabine Plus Irinotecan vs Irinotecan Monotherapy as Second-Line Treatment in Patients With Advanced Gallbladder Cancer: A Multicenter Phase 2 Randomized Clinical Trial (GB-SELECT). *JAMA Oncol.* **2021**, *7*, 436–439. [CrossRef]
57. Ueno, M.; Morizane, C.; Furukawa, M.; Sakai, D.; Komatsu, Y.; Nakai, Y.; Tsuda, M.; Ozaka, M.; Mizuno, N.; Muto, M.; et al. A randomized, double-blind, phase II study of oral histone deacetylase inhibitor resminostat plus S-1 versus placebo plus S-1 in biliary tract cancers previously treated with gemcitabine plus platinum-based chemotherapy. *Cancer Med.* **2021**, *10*, 2088–2099. [CrossRef] [PubMed]
58. Yoo, C.; Kim, K.P.; Kim, I.; Kang, M.J.; Cheon, J.; Kang, B.W.; Ryu, H.; Jeong, J.H.; Lee, J.S.; Kim, K.W.; et al. Liposomal Irinotecan (nal-IRI) in combination with Fluorouracil (5-FU) and Leucovorin (LV) for Patients (pts) with Metastatic Biliary Tract Cancer (BTC) after Progression on Gemcitabine plus Cisplatin (GemCis): Multicenter Comparative Randomized Phase 2B study (NIFTY). *J. Clin. Oncol.* **2021**, *39* (Suppl. 15), 4006.
59. Nakamura, H.; Arai, Y.; Totoki, Y.; Shirota, T.; Elzawahry, A.; Kato, M.; Hama, N.; Hosoda, F.; Urushidate, T.; Ohashi, S.; et al. Genomic spectra of biliary tract cancer. *Nat. Genet.* **2015**, *47*, 1003–1010. [CrossRef]
60. Valle, J.W.; Lamarca, A.; Goyal, L.; Barriuso, J.; Zhu, A.X. New Horizons for Precision Medicine in Biliary Tract Cancers. *Cancer Discov.* **2017**, *7*, 943–962. [CrossRef]
61. Jusakul, A.; Cutcutache, I.; Yong, C.H.; Lim, J.Q.; Huang, M.N.; Padmanabhan, N.; Nellore, V.; Kongpetch, S.; Ng, A.W.T.; Ng, L.M.; et al. Whole-Genome and Epigenomic Landscapes of Etiologically Distinct Subtypes of Cholangiocarcinoma. *Cancer Discov.* **2017**, *7*, 1116–1135. [CrossRef]
62. Silverman, I.M.; Hollebecque, A.; Friboulet, L.; Owens, S.; Newton, R.C.; Zhen, H.; Féliz, L.; Zecchetto, C.; Melisi, D.; Burn, T.C. Clinicogenomic Analysis of FGFR2-Rearranged Cholangiocarcinoma Identifies Correlates of Response and Mechanisms of Resistance to Pemigatinib. *Cancer Discov.* **2021**, *11*, 326–339. [CrossRef]

3. Javle, M.; Lowery, M.; Shroff, R.T.; Weiss, K.H.; Springfeld, C.; Borad, M.J.; Ramanathan, R.K.; Goyal, L.; Sadeghi, S.; Macarulla, T.; et al. Phase II Study of BGJ398 in Patients With FGFR-Altered Advanced Cholangiocarcinoma. *J. Clin. Oncol.* **2018**, *36*, 276–282. [CrossRef]
4. Mazzaferro, V.; El-Rayes, B.F.; Droz Dit Busset, M.; Cotsoglou, C.; Harris, W.P.; Damjanov, N.; Masi, G.; Rimassa, L.; Personeni, N.; Braiteh, F.; et al. Derazantinib (ARQ 087) in advanced or inoperable FGFR2 gene fusion-positive intrahepatic cholangiocarcinoma. *Br. J. Cancer* **2019**, *120*, 165–171. [CrossRef]
5. Abou-Alfa, G.K.; Sahai, V.; Hollebecque, A.; Vaccaro, G.; Melisi, D.; Al-Rajabi, R.; Paulson, A.S.; Borad, M.J.; Gallinson, D.; Murphy, A.G.; et al. Pemigatinib for previously treated, locally advanced or metastatic cholangiocarcinoma: A multicentre, open-label, phase 2 study. *Lancet Oncol.* **2020**, *21*, 671–685. [CrossRef]
6. Goyal, L.; Meric-Bernstam, F.; Hollebecque, A.; Morizane, C.; Valle, J.W.; Karasic, T.B.; Abrams, T.A.; Kelley, R.B.; Cassier, P.; Furuse, J.; et al. Primary results of phase 2 FOENIX-CCA2: The irreversible FGFR1-4 inhibitor futibatinib in intrahepatic cholangiocarcinoma (iCCA) with FGFR2 fusions/rearrangements. In Proceedings of the AACR Annual Meeting, Virtual Meeting, Philadelphia, PA, USA, 10–15 April/17–21 May 2021. Abstract CT-010.
7. Maruki, Y.; Morizane, C.; Arai, Y.; Ikeda, M.; Ueno, M.; Ioka, T.; Naganuma, A.; Furukawa, M.; Mizuno, N.; Uwagawa, T.; et al. Molecular detection and clinicopathological characteristics of advanced/recurrent biliary tract carcinomas harboring the FGFR2 rearrangements: A prospective observational study (PRELUDE Study). *J. Gastroenterol.* **2021**, *56*, 250–260. [CrossRef]
8. Le, D.T.; Durham, J.N.; Smith, K.N.; Wang, H.; Bartlett, B.R.; Aulakh, L.K.; Lu, S.; Kemberling, H.; Wilt, C.; Luber, B.S.; et al. Mismatch repair deficiency predicts response of solid tumors of PD-1 blockade. *Science* **2017**, *357*, 409–413. [CrossRef]
9. Doebele, R.C.; Drilon, A.; Paz-Ares, L.; Siena, S.; Shaw, A.T.; Farago, A.F.; Blakely, C.M.; Seto, T.; Cho, B.C.; Tosi, D.; et al. Entrectinib in patients with advanced or metastatic NTRK fusion-positive solid tumours: Integrated analysis of three phase 1-2 trials. *Lancet Oncol.* **2020**, *21*, 271–282. [CrossRef]
10. Drilon, A.; Laetsch, T.W.; Kummar, S.; DuBois, S.G.; Lassen, U.N.; Demetri, G.D.; Natheson, M.; Doebele, R.C.; Fargo, A.F.; Pappo, A.S.; et al. Efficacy of Larotrectinib in TRK Fusion-Positive Cancers in Adults and Children. *N. Engl. J. Med.* **2018**, *378*, 731–739. [CrossRef]
11. Akagi, K.; Oki, E.; Taniguchi, H.; Nakatani, K.; Aoki, D.; Kuwata, T.; Yoshino, T. The real-world data on microsatellite instability status in various unresectable or metastatic solid tumors. *Cancer Sci.* **2021**, *112*, 1105. [CrossRef] [PubMed]
12. Yoshino, T.; Pentheroudakis, G.; Mishima, S.; Overman, M.J.; Yeh, K.H.; Baba, E.; Naito, Y.; Calvo, F.; Saxena, A.; Chen, L.T.; et al. JSCO-ESMO-ASCO-JSMO-TOS: International expert consensus recommendations for tumour-agnostic treatments in patients with solid tumours with microsatellite instability or NTRK fusions. *Ann. Oncol.* **2020**, *31*, 861–872. [CrossRef]
13. Piha-Paul, S.A.; Oh, D.Y.; Ueno, M.; Malka, D.; Chung, H.C.; Nagrial, A.; Kelley, R.K.; Ros, W.; Italiano, A.; Nakagawa, K.; et al. Efficacy and safety of pembrolizumab for the treatment of advanced biliary cancer: Results from the KEYNOTE-158 and KEYNOTE-028 studies. *Int. J. Cancer* **2020**, *147*, 2190–2198. [CrossRef]
14. Ueno, M.; Ikeda, M.; Morizane, C.; Kobayashi, S.; Ohno, I.; Kondo, S.; Okano, N.; Kimura, K.; Asada, S.; Namba, Y.; et al. Nivolumab alone or in combination with cisplatin plus gemcitabine in Japanese patients with unresectable or recurrent biliary tract cancer: A non-randomised, multicentre, open-label, phase 1 study. *Lancet Gastroenterol. Hepatol.* **2019**, *4*, 611–621.
15. Kim, R.D.; Chung, V.; Alese, O.B.; El-Rayes, B.F.; Li, D.; Al-Toubah, T.E.; Schell, M.J.; Zhou, J.M.; Mahipal, A.; Kim, B.H.; et al. A Phase 2 Multi-institutional Study of Nivolumab for Patients With Advanced Refractory Biliary Tract Cancer. *JAMA Oncol.* **2020**, *6*, 888–894. [CrossRef]
16. Feng, K.; Liu, Y.; Zhao, Y.; Yang, Q.; Dong, L.; Liu, J.; Li, X.; Zhao, Z.; Mei, Q.; Han, W. Efficacy and biomarker analysis of nivolumab plus gemcitabine and cisplatin in patients with unresectable or metastatic biliary tract cancers: Results from a phase II study. *J. Immunother. Cancer* **2020**, *8*, e000367. [CrossRef] [PubMed]
17. Klein, O.; Kee, D.; Nagrial, A.; Markman, B.; Underhill, C.; Michael, M.; Jackett, L.; Lum, C.; Behren, A.; Palmer, J.; et al. Evaluation of Combination Nivolumab and Ipilimumab Immunotherapy in Patients With Advanced Biliary Tract Cancers: Subgroup Analysis of a Phase 2 Nonrandomized Clinical Trial. *JAMA Oncol.* **2020**, *6*, 1405–1409. [CrossRef]
18. Chen, X.; Wu, X.; Wu, H.; Gu, Y.; Shao, Y.; Shao, Q.; Zhu, F.; Li, X.; Qian, X.; Hu, J.; et al. Camrelizumab plus gemcitabine and oxaliplatin (GEMOX) in patients with advanced biliary tract cancer: A single-arm, open-label, phase II trial. *J. Immunother. Cancer* **2020**, *8*, e001240. [CrossRef] [PubMed]
19. Villanueva, L.; Lwin, Z.; Chung, H.C.; Gomez-Roca, C.A.; Longo, F.; Yanez, E.; Senellart, H.; Doherty, M.; Garcia-Corbacho, J.; Hendifar, A.E.; et al. Lenvatinib plus pembrolizumab for patients with previously treated biliary tract cancers in the multicohort phase 2 LEAP-005 study. *J. Clin. Oncol.* **2021**, *39* (Suppl. 15), 4080. [CrossRef]
20. Takada, T.; Amano, H.; Yasuda, H.; Nimura, Y.; Matsushiro, T.; Kato, H.; Nagakawa, T.; Nakayama, T.; Study Group of Surgical Adjuvant Therapy for Carcinomas of the Pancreas and Biliary Tract. Is postoperative adjuvant chemotherapy useful for gallbladder carcinoma? A phase III multicenter prospective randomized controlled trial in patients with resected pancreaticobiliary carcinoma. *Cancer* **2002**, *95*, 1685–1695.
21. Neoptolemos, J.P.; Moore, M.J.; Cox, T.F.; Valle, J.W.; Palmer, D.H.; McDonald, A.C.; Carter, R.; Tebbutt, N.C.; Dervenis, C.; Smith, D.; et al. Effect of adjuvant chemotherapy with fluorouracil plus folinic acid or gemcitabine vs observation on survival in patients with resected periampullary adenocarcinoma. *JAMA* **2012**, *308*, 147–156. [CrossRef]

82. Ebata, T.; Hirano, S.; Konishi, M.; Uesaka, K.; Tsuchiya, Y.; Ohtsuka, M.; Kaneoka, Y.; Yamamoto, M.; Ambo, Y.; Shimizu, Y.; et al. Randomized clinical trial of adjuvant gemcitabine chemotherapy versus observation in resected bile duct cancer. *Br. J. Surg.* **2018**, *105*, 192–202. [CrossRef]
83. Edeline, J.; Benabdelghani, M.; Bertaut, A.; Watelet, J.; Hammel, P.; Joly, J.P.; Boudjema, K.; Fartoux, L.; Bouhier-Leporrier, K.; Jouve, J.L.; et al. Gemcitabine and Oxaliplatin Chemotherapy or Surveillance in Resected Biliary Tract Cancer (PRODIGE 12-ACCORD 18-UNICANCER GI): A Randomized Phase III Study. *J. Clin. Oncol.* **2019**, *37*, 658–667. [CrossRef]
84. Primrose, J.N.; Fox, R.P.; Palmer, D.H.; Malik, H.Z.; Prasad, R.; Mirza, D.; Anthony, A.; Corrie, P.; Falk, S.; Finch-Jones, M.; et al. Capecitabine compared with observation in resected biliary tract cancer (BILCAP): A randomised, controlled, multicentre, phase 3 study. *Lancet Oncol.* **2019**, *20*, 663–673. [CrossRef]
85. Shroff, R.T.; Kennedy, E.B.; Bachini, M.; Bekaii-Saab, T.; Crane, C.; Edeline, J.; El-Khoueiry, A.; Feng, M.; Katz, M.H.G.; Primrose, J.; et al. Adjuvant Therapy for Resected Biliary Tract Cancer: ASCO Clinical Practice Guideline. *J. Clin. Oncol.* **2019**, *37*, 1015–1027. [CrossRef]
86. McNamara, M.G.; Goyal, L.; Doherty, M.; Springfeld, C.; Cosgrove, D.; Sjoquist, K.M.; Park, J.O.; Verdaguer, H.; Braconi, C.; Ross, P.J.; et al. NUC-1031/cisplatin versus gemcitabine/cisplatin in untreated locally advanced/metastatic biliary tract cancer (NuTide:121). *Future Oncol.* **2020**, *16*, 1069–1081. [CrossRef]
87. Bekaii-Saab, T.S.; Valle, J.W.; Van Cutsem, E.; Rimassa, L.; Furuse, J.; Ioka, T.; Melisi, D.; Macarulla, T.; Bridgewater, J.; Wasan, H.; et al. FIGHT-302: First-line pemigatinib vs gemcitabine plus cisplatin for advanced cholangiocarcinoma with FGFR2 rearrangements. *Future Oncol.* **2020**, *16*, 2385–2399. [CrossRef]
88. Makawita, S.; Abou-Alfa, G.K.; Roychowdhury, S.; Sadeghi, S.; Borbath, I.; Goyal, L.; Cohn, A.; Lamarca, A.; Oh, D.Y.; Macarulla, T.; et al. Infigratinib in patients with advanced cholangiocarcinoma with FGFR2 gene fusions/translocations: The PROOF 301 trial. *Future Oncol.* **2020**, *16*, 2375–2384. [CrossRef]
89. Stein, A.; Arnold, D.; Bridgewater, J.; Goldstein, D.; Jensen, L.H.; Klümpen, H.J.; Lohse, A.W.; Nashan, B.; Primrose, J.; Schrum, S.; et al. Adjuvant chemotherapy with gemcitabine and cisplatin compared to observation after curative intent resection of cholangiocarcinoma and muscle invasive gallbladder carcinoma (ACTICCA-1 trial)—A randomized, multidisciplinary, multinational phase III trial. *BMC Cancer* **2015**, *15*, 564. [CrossRef]
90. Nakachi, K.; Konishi, M.; Ikeda, M.; Mizusawa, J.; Eba, J.; Okusaka, T.; Ishii, H.; Fukuda, H.; Furuse, J.; Hepatobiliary and Pancreatic Oncology Group of the Japan Clinical Oncology Group. A randomized Phase III trial of adjuvant S-1 therapy vs. observation alone in resected biliary tract cancer: Japan Clinical Oncology Group Study (JCOG1202, ASCOT). *Jpn. J. Clin. Oncol.* **2018**, *48*, 392–395. [CrossRef]
91. Goetze, T.O.; Bechstein, W.O.; Bankstahl, U.S.; Keck, T.; Königsrainer, A.; Lang, S.A.; Pauligk, C.; Piso, P.; Vogel, A.; Al-Batran, S.E. Neoadjuvant chemotherapy with gemcitabine plus cisplatin followed by radical liver resection versus immediate radical liver resection alone with or without adjuvant chemotherapy in incidentally detected gallbladder carcinoma after simple cholecystectomy or in front of radical resection of BTC (ICC/ECC)—A phase III study of the German registry of incidental gallbladder carcinoma platform (GR)- the AIO/ CALGP/ ACO- GAIN-trial. *BMC Cancer* **2020**, *20*, 122.
92. Shroff, R.T.; Javle, M.M.; Xiao, L.; Kaseb, A.O.; Varadhachary, G.R.; Wolff, R.A.; Raghav, K.P.S.; Iwasaki, M.; Masci, P.; Ramanathan, R.K.; et al. Gemcitabine, Cisplatin, and nab-Paclitaxel for the Treatment of Advanced Biliary Tract Cancers. A Phase 2 Clinical Trial. *JAMA Oncol.* **2019**, *5*, 824–830. [CrossRef]
93. Yoo, C.; Oh, D.Y.; Choi, H.J.; Kudo, M.; Ueno, M.; Kondo, S.; Chen, L.T.; Osada, M.; Helwig, C.; Dussault, I.; et al. Phase I study of bintrafusp alfa, a bifunctional fusion protein targeting TGF-β and PD-L1, in patients with pretreated biliary tract cancer. *J. Immunother. Cancer* **2020**, *8*, e000564. [CrossRef] [PubMed]
94. Boilève, A.; Hilmi, M.; Gougis, P.; Cohen, R.; Rousseau, B.; Blanc, J.F.; Ben Abdelghani, M.; Castanié, H.; Dahan, L.; Tougeron, D.; et al. Triplet combination of durvalumab, tremelimumab, and paclitaxel in biliary tract carcinomas: Safety run-in results of the randomized IMMUNOBIL PRODIGE 57 phase II trial. *Eur. J. Cancer* **2021**, *143*, 55–63. [CrossRef] [PubMed]

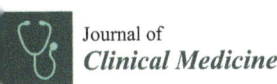

Article

Balloon Enteroscopy-Assisted Endoscopic Retrograde Cholangiopancreatography for the Treatment of Common Bile Duct Stones in Patients with Roux-en-Y Gastrectomy: Outcomes and Factors Affecting Complete Stone Extraction

Taisuke Obata [1], Koichiro Tsutsumi [1,*], Hironari Kato [1], Toru Ueki [2], Kazuya Miyamoto [3], Tatsuhiro Yamazaki [1], Akihiro Matsumi [1], Yuki Fujii [1], Kazuyuki Matsumoto [1], Shigeru Horiguchi [1], Kengo Yasugi [2], Tsuneyoshi Ogawa [2], Ryuta Takenaka [3] and Hiroyuki Okada [1]

1. Department of Gastroenterology, Okayama University Hospital, Okayama 7008558, Japan; p47691mh@s.okayama-u.ac.jp (T.O.); katou-h@cc.okayama-u.ac.jp (H.K.); ty1114db@gmail.com (T.Y.); akihiro.matsumi.gastro@gmail.com (A.M.); y_f1105@yahoo.co.jp (Y.F.); matsumotokazuyuki0227@yahoo.co.jp (K.M.); horiguchis@gmail.com (S.H.); hiro@md.okayama-u.ac.jp (H.O.)
2. Department of Internal Medicine, Fukuyama City Hospital, Fukuyama 7218511, Japan; ueki0041@fchp.jp (T.U.); ppur0jyn@s.okayama-u.ac.jp (K.Y.); t-ogawa@xa3.so-net.ne.jp (T.O.)
3. Department of Internal Medicine, Tsuyama Chuo Hospital, Okayama 7080841, Japan; ttpcx442@yahoo.co.jp (K.M.); rtakenak@gmail.com (R.T.)
* Correspondence: tsutsumi@okayama-u.ac.jp; Tel.: +81-86-235-7219

Abstract: Background: Endoscopic retrograde cholangiopancreatography (ERCP) for extraction of common bile duct (CBD) stones in patients with Roux-en-Y gastrectomy (RYG) remains technically challenging. Methods: Seventy-nine RYG patients (median 79 years old) underwent short-type double-balloon enteroscopy-assisted ERCP (sDBE-ERCP) for CBD stones at three referral hospitals from 2011–2020. We retrospectively investigated the treatment outcomes and potential factors affecting complete stone extraction. Results: The initial success rates of reaching the papilla of Vater, biliary cannulation, and biliary intervention, including complete stone extraction or biliary stent placement, were 92%, 81%, and 78%, respectively. Of 57 patients with attempted stone extraction, complete stone extraction was successful in 74% for the first session and ultimately in 88%. The adverse events rate was 5%. The multivariate analysis indicated that the largest CBD diameter ≥ 14 mm (odds ratio (OR), 0.04; 95% confidence interval (CI), 0.01–0.58; p = 0.018) and retroflex position (OR, 6.43; 95% CI, 1.12–36.81; p = 0.037) were independent predictive factors affecting complete stone extraction achievement. Conclusions: Therapeutic sDBE-ERCP for CBD stones in a relatively elderly RYG cohort, was effective and safe. A larger CBD diameter negatively affected complete stone extraction, but using the retroflex position may be useful for achieving complete stone clearance.

Keywords: bile duct stone; endoscopic retrograde cholangiography; Roux-en-Y anastomosis; short-type balloon enteroscopy; complete stone removal; gastrectomy

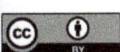

1. Introduction

Cholelithiasis is an adverse event in patients with surgically altered anatomies due to a history of gastrectomies, such as Billroth-II reconstruction and Roux-en-Y (R-Y) anastomosis [1–3]. Since common bile duct (CBD) stones often cause patients life-threatening severe cholangitis and pancreatitis, biliary intervention, such as stone extraction or biliary drainage, is required [4,5]. However, endoscopic treatment of CBD stones via the papilla of Vater is technically challenging, especially in patients who have undergone R-Y gastrectomy (RYG), due to the difficulty of not only reaching the papilla but also performing biliary cannulation or ampullary procedures or stone extraction [6–10], compared to those with normal anatomy. Thus, percutaneous transhepatic intervention or surgery is often performed as an alternative treatment [11–14].

Recently, balloon enteroscopy-assisted endoscopic retrograde cholangiopancreatography (BE-ERCP) has been reported to be a useful method for post-operative biliary or pancreatic diseases in patients with such surgically altered anatomies [15–23]. Owing to the improvement of reachability up to the papilla, the extraction of CBD stones as well as biliary stent placement have been facilitated using this innovative enteroscopy procedure. However, little is known about the detailed outcomes of this treatment in RYG patients, and the factors affecting CBD stone clearance have not been investigated.

In the present study, we clarified the efficacy and safety of BE-ERCP for the treatment of CBD stones in patients with RYG and identified the predictive factors for complete stone extraction.

2. Materials and Methods

2.1. Study Design

This was a multi-center retrospective study conducted in three tertiary hospitals. This study was approved by the ethics committee at each institution.

2.2. Patients

Among the total of 699 patients (1846 sessions) who underwent BE-ERCP between January 2010 and December 2020 at Okayama University Hospital, Fukuyama City Hospital or Tsuyama Chuo Hospital, 79 (11%) who had previously undergone total gastrectomy or subtotal gastrectomy with R-Y anastomosis and had received initial BE-ERCP for the treatment of CBD stones were included in this study. Before BE-ERCP, all patients received blood tests and underwent imaging examinations, such as abdominal ultrasonography, computed tomography, or magnetic resonance cholangiopancreatography, to investigate the suspected CBD stones. Written informed consent was obtained from all patients.

2.3. BE-ERCP Procedure

All BE-ERCP procedures were performed using a short-type double-balloon enteroscope (DBE; EI-530B or EI-580BT; Fujifilm, Tokyo, Japan) with a 2.8- or 3.2-mm working channel and a 152-cm working length and a transparent cap attached to its tip, by skilled endoscopists with extensive experience in performing ERCP for patients with normal anatomy. All patients were admitted to each hospital and were in the prone position under conscious sedation with propofol, midazolam, diazepam, or pethidine hydrochloride during the procedure. In addition, all of these procedures were performed under CO_2 insufflation.

The scope was perorally advanced toward the papilla of Vater beyond the R-Y anastomosis [24]. After reaching the papilla, biliary cannulation and cholangiography were generally attempted using a catheter (PR-V220Q; Olympus Medical Systems, Tokyo, Japan or MTW ERCP catheter; Medizin-Technische-Werkstätte, Wesel, Germany) with a 0.025-inch guidewire (VisiGlide2; Olympus Medical Systems or RevoWave; Piolax Medical Devices, Kanagawa, Japan). Following confirmation of filling defect suspected of being CBD stones, endoscopic sphincterotomy (EST), precutting, endoscopic papillary balloon dilation (EPBD), and/or endoscopic papillary large balloon dilation (EPLBD; ≥ 12 mm) [4,16,17,25–29] was performed using a sphincterotome (RotacutII; Medi-Globe GmbH, Achenmühle, Germany or TRUEtome; Boston Scientific, MA, USA), a needle-knife (KD-10Q-1; Olympus Medical Systems) and/or a balloon dilation catheter (ZARA; Century Medical Inc., Tokyo, Japan or GIGA2; Century Medical Inc., Tokyo, Japan). For stone extraction, a retrieval balloon catheter (Tri-Ex; Cook Medical, Tokyo, Japan), basket catheter (Flower Basket V 8-wire type; Olympus Medical Systems), and mechanical lithotripter (ML) (Crusher Catheter; Xemex, Tokyo, Japan or LithoCrushV BML-V437QR-30; Olympus Medical Systems) were usually used. Prophylactic administration of ulinastatin was performed for the prevention of post-ERCP pancreatitis in all patients.

In patients in whom scope insertion to the papilla or biliary cannulation failed, the second BE-ERCP or alternative approach, including surgery, endoscopic ultrasound-guided biliary drainage (EUS-BD) [5,30–33], percutaneous transhepatic biliary drainage (PTBD), and conservative therapy, was carried out. In some patients with a serious condition or incomplete extraction of CBD stones, endoscopic biliary stenting (EBS) using a 5- to 7-Fr plastic stent was performed for treatment of cholangitis in an initial session; thereafter, complete stone extraction was attempted on readmission.

2.4. Definitions

The primary outcome of this study was to reveal the factors affecting complete stone extraction using variables associated with both patient characteristics and procedural contents. The patient-related factors were age, sexuality, the American Society of Anesthesiologists physical status (ASA-PS) classification, diameter of the largest CBD, size of the largest CBD stone, number of stones, and time from RYG to BE-ERCP. Furthermore, the procedure-related factors were initial BE-ERCP, EST/precutting or EPBD/EPLBD, and retroflex position, which was able to provide a better view of the papilla with a J-turn form of the scope at the inferior duodenal angle (IDA) [20] (Figure 1). The secondary outcomes were the technical success rates of initial BE-ERCP, including the rate of reaching the papilla, rate of biliary cannulation, and rate of biliary intervention, such as complete stone extraction and biliary stent placement, as well as adverse events. Complete stone extraction was defined as no detection of residual stones by a cholangiogram. The time to reach the papilla was the duration from the scope insertion to when the papilla was reached. The time to biliary cannulation was the duration from when the papilla was reached to the achievement of biliary cannulation. The total procedural time was defined as the time from scope insertion until withdrawal. Adverse events were defined according to the ASGE guidelines [34].

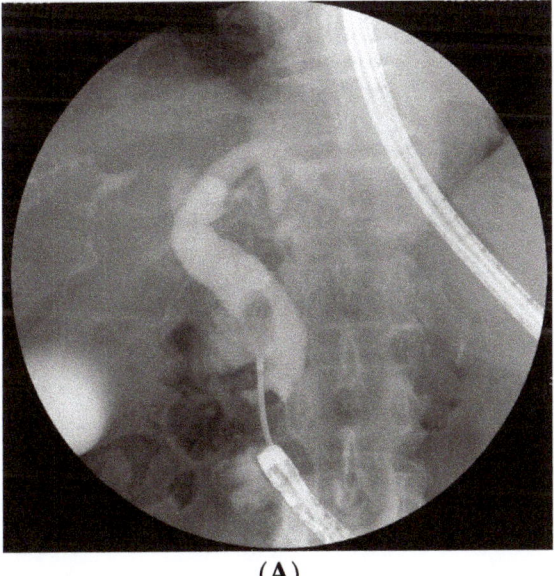

(A)

Figure 1. *Cont.*

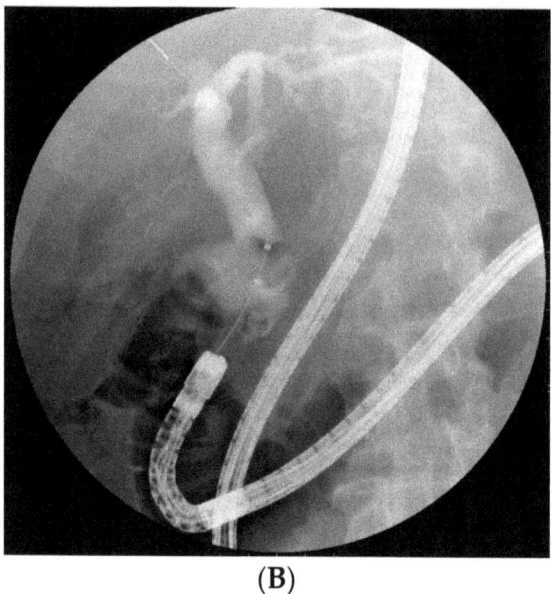

(B)

Figure 1. A useful "retroflex position" for stone extraction in a Roux-en-Y gastrectomy patient. (**A**) At the initial session, the scope was stretched after reaching the papilla (not formed the retroflex position). Following successful biliary cannulation, precutting, and endoscopic papillary large balloon dilation, a stone was able to be grabbed with a mechanical lithotripter. However, complete stone extraction was not able to be conducted using any devices, including a basket catheter or balloon catheter, as the axis of the devices did not align with the distal bile duct during the extraction. (**B**) In the second session, the retroflex position was obtained by forming a looped-scope shape. In this manner, the coaxial relationship between the devices and the distal bile duct and a proper distance from the tip of the scope to the papilla of Vater with a better view of the papilla could thus be successfully obtained. This situation allowed stones to be easily removed along the axis of the distal bile duct.

2.5. Statistical Analyses

Continuous variables were expressed as the median and interquartile range (IQR). To identify predictive factors for complete stone extraction, continuous variables were categorized into two groups by the median value, and several factors described above were analyzed in a univariate and multivariate Cox proportional hazard model, along with the odds ratio (OR) and confidence intervals (CIs). The multivariate model included variables with a p-value of <0.10 in the univariate model. Statistical significance was considered to be indicated by a p-value of <0.05. All analyses were carried out using the JMP (version 15.1.0, SAS Institute Inc., Cary, NC, USA) software program.

3. Results

3.1. Patients' Characteristics

All enrolled 79 patients had undergone BE-ERCP for the treatment of CBD stones over a total of 90 sessions. The patient characteristics are shown in Table 1.

Table 1. Patients' characteristics.

Patients/sessions, n	79/90
Age, years, median (IQR)	79 (73–84)
Sex, male/female, n	62/17
ASA-PS, 2/3/4, n	57/19/3
Reasons for gastrectomy, n (%)	
Gastric cancer	72 (91)
Esophageal cancer	1 (1)
Malignant lymphoma	1 (1)
Gastric ulcer	2 (3)
Unknown	3 (4)
Diameter of the largest CBD, mm, median (IQR)	14 (11–16)
Size of the largest CBD stone, mm, median (IQR)	10 (6–14)
Number of CBD stones, n (%)	
Debris	2 (3)
1	40 (51)
2	15 (19)
≥3	22 (28)

IQR, interquartile range; ASA-PS, American Society of Anesthesiologists physical status; CBD, common bile duct.

The median age was 79 years old, which was considered relatively elderly, and 78% of patients were male. The most common reason for gastrectomy was gastric cancer (91%). Regarding the ASA-PS classification, 57 patients (72%) were classified as ASA-PS 2, while the remaining 22 were ASA-PS 3 or 4. The median diameter of the largest CBD was 14 mm, the median size of the largest CBD stone was 10 mm, and the median number of stones was 2.

3.2. Scope Insertion and Biliary Cannulation in an Initial BE-ERCP

Outcomes of initial BE-ERCP for treatment of CBD stones are shown in Table 2. Of the 79 patients, successful scope insertion to the papilla of Vater was obtained in 73 (92%). The reason of unsuccessful scope insertion was the bowel adhesion or long length of R-Y limb, and it took median 64 (IQR, 46–80) mins to discontinue. Subsequent selective biliary cannulation was successfully performed in 64 patients (81%). Of the 15 patients in whom these biliary approaches had failed, surgery was performed in 3 patients, PTBD in 3 patients, and EUS-guided antegrade therapy for stone extraction in 2 patients, while 6 patients were treated with conservative therapy. The remaining patient who had failed biliary cannulation achieved successful cannulation in the second session.

Table 2. Results of initial BE-ERCP (n = 79).

Reaching the papilla of Vatar, n (%)		73 (92)
Successful biliary cannulation, n (%)		64 (81)
Detection of stones by cholangiogram, n (%)		63 (80)
Overall procedure success, n (%)		62 (78)
Complete stone extraction, n (%)		42 (53)
Biliary stenting, n (%)		20 (25)
Time to reaching the papilla, min, median (IQR)		25 (11–40)
Time to biliary cannulation, min, median (IQR)		25 (6–33)
Total procedural time, min, median (IQR)		90 (67–120)
Adverse events, n (%)		4 (5)
Perforation	moderate/severe	1/1 (3)
Pancreatitis	mild	1 (1)
Hypoxia	mild	1 (1)

BE-ERCP, balloon enteroscopy-assisted endoscopic retrograde cholangiopancreatography; IQR, interquartile range.

3.3. Ampullary Procedure for Stone Extraction at Initial BE-ERCP

Among the 63 patients who achieved a successful cholangiogram, excluding 1 patient in whom the stone had spontaneously passed through the papilla, ampullary procedures were performed for biliary interventions, as shown in Table 3. For stone extraction, EPBD or EPLBD was conducted in 87% (48/55), while EST or precutting alone was performed in 13% (7/55). Of the remaining 8 patients who underwent EBS without stone extraction, 3 (38%) underwent precutting alone, and 5 underwent no ampullary procedure.

Table 3. Details of ampullary procedure and biliary intervention in initial BE-ERCP ($n = 63$).

Ampullary Procedure	n (%)
Precut alone	4 (6)
EST alone	6 (10)
EPBD alone	9 (14)
EPLBD alone	5 (8)
Precut + EPBD	12 (19)
Precut + EPLBD	5 (8)
EST + EPBD	12 (19)
EST + EPLBD	5 (8)
None	5 (8)
Biliary Intervention	**n(%)**
Balloon catheter	46 (73)
Basket catheter	21 (29)
ML	22 (30)
Plastic stent	20 (27)
ENBD	2 (3)

EST, endoscopic sphincterotomy; EPBD, endoscopic papillary balloon dilation; EPLBD, endoscopic papillary large balloon dilation; ML, mechanical lithotripsy; ENBD, endoscopic nasobiliary drainage.

3.4. Biliary Intervention and Complete CBD Stone Extraction in an Initial BE-ERCP

Of the 63 patients, 42 (53%) received complete stone extraction in a single session. Of the remaining 21 patients, 20 had EBS for drainage due to incomplete CBD stone extraction ($n = 12$), poor maneuverability ($n = 4$), or a poor patient condition ($n = 4$). Another patient failed biliary intervention due to edema of the papilla of Vater and was treated conservatively. Thus, the overall success rate of biliary intervention was 78% (62/79) at the initial BE-ERCP procedure.

3.5. Potential Factors Affecting Complete CBD Stone Extraction

CBD stone extraction was ultimately attempted in 66 sessions for 57 patients, including 9 who underwent BE-ERCP twice, due to incomplete extraction at the initial session in 7 and recurrent CBD stone in 2. As a result, complete stone extraction was achieved in 52 sessions (79%). Among the 11 variables examined, the largest CBD diameter ≥ 14 mm ($p = 0.002$) and the largest CBD stone size ≥ 10 mm ($p = 0.031$) were associated with complete stone extraction according to the univariate analysis. In the multivariate analysis, the largest CBD diameter ≥ 14 mm (OR 0.04; 95% CI 0.01–0.58; $p = 0.018$) and retroflex position (OR 6.43; 95% CI 1.12–36.81; $p = 0.037$) were identified as independent relevant factors for complete stone extraction (Table 4).

Table 4. Potential factors affecting complete stone extraction (n = 66, overall).

Variable	Complete Stone Extraction		Univariate		Multivariates	
	n	%	OR (95% CI)	p Value	OR (95% CI)	p Value
Age > 78 years old	28/34	82	1.56 (0.47–5.12)	0.55		
Male	46/57	81	2.09 (0.45–9.67)	0.39		
ASA-PS 3 or 4	13/16	81	1.22 (0.30–5.07)	>0.99		
Initial BE-ERCP	40/50	80	1.33 (0.35–5.03)	0.73		
Largest CBD diameter ≥ 14 mm	23/36	64	0.06 (0.01–0.50)	0.002	0.04 (0.003–0.58)	0.018
Retroflex position	26/29	90	3.67 (0.92–14.69)	0.073	6.43 (1.12–36.81)	0.037
Largest CBD stone size ≥ 10 mm	27/39	69	0.18 (0.04–0.89)	0.031	0.94 (0.11–8.15)	0.96
Number of CBD stones ≥ 3	13/19	68	0.44 (0.13–1.52)	0.20		
EST/Precut	36/43	84	2.25 (0.68–7.48)	0.21		
EPBD/EPLBD	46/59	78	0.59 (0.07–5.35)	>0.99		
Time from RYG to BE-ERCP > 4.9 years	26/33	79	1.00 (0.31–3.26)	>0.99		

ASA-PS, the American Society of Anesthesiologists physical status classification system; BE-ERCP, balloon enteroscope assisted-endoscopic retrograde cholangiopancreatography; CBD, common bile duct; EST, endoscopic sphincterotomy; EPBD, endoscopic papillary balloon dilation; EPLBD, endoscopic papillary large balloon dilation; RYG, Roux-en-Y gastrectomy; OR, odds ratio; CI, confidence interval.

Furthermore, among 36 patients with a large CBD diameter (≥14 mm), the retroflex position ($p = 0.035$) was the only potential factor affecting complete stone extraction in univariate analysis (Table 5). Among 39 patients with a large CBD stone size (≥10 mm), the largest CBD diameter ≥ 14 mm ($p = 0.017$) and retroflex position ($p = 0.037$) were significant factors associated with complete stone extraction (Table 6).

Table 5. Potential factors associated with complete stone extraction (n = 36, Largest CBD diameter ≥14 mm).

Variable	Complete Stone Extraction		Univariate	
	n	%	OR (95% CI)	p Value
Age > 78 years old	9/15	60	0.75 (0.19–2.97)	0.74
Male	21/31	68	3.15 (0.45–21.95)	0.33
ASA-PS 3 or 4	4/7	57	0.70 (0.13–3.77)	0.69
Initial BE-ERCP	18/27	67	1.60 (0.34–7.46)	0.69
Retroflex position	15/18	83	6.25 (1.33–29.43)	0.035
Largest CBD stone size ≥ 10 mm	16/28	57	0.24 (0.03–2.22)	0.21
Number of CBD stones ≥ 3	10/16	63	0.90 (0.23–3.52)	>0.99
EST/Precut	16/22	73	2.67 (0.65–10.88)	0.29
EPBD/EPLBD	20/32	63	0.56 (0.05–5.97)	>0.99
Time from RYG to BE-ERCP > 4.9 years	14/21	67	1.33 (0.34–5.27)	0.74

ASA-PS, the American Society of Anesthesiologists physical status classification system; BE-ERCP, balloon enteroscope assisted-endoscopic retrograde cholangiopancreatography; CBD, common bile duct; EST, endoscopic sphincterotomy; EPBD, endoscopic papillary balloon dilation; EPLBD, endoscopic papillary large balloon dilation; RYG, Roux-en-Y gastrectomy; OR, odds ratio; CI, confidence interval.

Table 6. Potential factors associated with complete stone extraction ($n = 39$, largest CBD stone size ≥ 10 mm).

Variable	Complete Stone Extraction		Univariate	
	n	%	OR (95% CI)	p Value
Age > 78 years old	14/20	70	1.08 (0.28–4.20)	>0.99
Male	24/33	73	2.67 (0.45–15.72)	0.35
ASA-PS 3 or 4	8/11	73	1.26 (0.27–5.93)	>0.99
Initial BE-ERCP	20/28	71	1.43 (0.33–6.26)	0.71
Largest CBD diameter ≥ 14 mm	16/28	57	N.A.	0.017
Retroflex position	15/17	88	6.25 (1.15–34.12)	0.037
Number of CBD stones ≥ 3	9/15	60	0.50 (0.13–2.00)	0.48
EST/Precut	19/25	76	2.38 (0.59–9.64)	0.29
EPBD/EPLBD	25/36	69	1.14 (0.09–13.89)	>0.99
Time from RYG to BE-ERCP > 4.9 years	14/21	67	0.89 (0.23–3.54)	0.74

ASA-PS, the American Society of Anesthesiologists physical status classification system; BE-ERCP, balloon enteroscope assisted-endoscopic retrograde cholangiopancreatography; CBD, common bile duct; EST, endoscopic sphincterotomy; EPBD, endoscopic papillary balloon dilation; EPLBD, endoscopic papillary large balloon dilation; RYG, Roux-en-Y gastrectomy; OR, odds ratio; CI, confidence interval; N.A., not applicable.

3.6. Adverse Events

Adverse events were observed in 4 patients (5%; 4/79), including bowel perforation in 2, pancreatitis in 1, and hypoxia in 1 (Table 2). In a patient whose perforation was detected at the IDA after complete stone extraction, a naso-drainage tube was placed around the area, but a high fever with retroperitoneal free air was observed two days later, so laparotomy drainage was performed. The condition gradually improved, but it took 28 days after BE-ERCP before the patient could leave the hospital. The other patient who had small intestinal perforation during scope insertion was able to be treated with double naso-drainage tubes. The mild pancreatitis improved conservatively, with dietary intake delayed one day. Hypoxia occurred in an 83-year-old patient with sepsis (ASA-PS 3) but improved immediately by oxygenation and scope withdrawal after EBS. There were no procedure-related mortalities.

4. Discussion

In this study, we retrospectively analyzed the outcomes of therapeutic BE-ERCP for CBD stones in RYG patients treated at three tertiary institutions. Initial biliary intervention, including complete stone extraction or biliary stent placement, was successful in 78% (62/79), complete stone extraction was initially achieved in 53% (42/79) and ultimately in 63% (50/79), and adverse events occurred in 5% (5/79). In addition, we identified two independent factors affecting complete stone extraction: the largest CBD diameter ≥ 14 mm was a negative factor, and the retroflex position was a positive factor, especially in difficult cases with a large CBD diameter or stone size. Thus, this study was the first to clarify the efficacy and safety of therapeutic BE-ERCP for CBD stones in RYG patients and identify the factors affecting complete stone clearance.

To achieve successful endoscopic extraction of CBD stones in patients who had had surgically altered anatomies due to having undergone gastrectomy, such as Billroth-II reconstruction or R-Y anastomosis, four processes needed to be carried out: reaching the papilla of Vater endoscopically, performing selective biliary cannulation, conducting an ampullary procedure (e.g., sphincterotomy or balloon dilation) and performing stone extraction. The first step was considered the most challenging in ERCP for RYG patients due to the excessive length or rigid adhesion of the R-Y limb, especially when using a conventional side-viewing duodenoscope [6] or a forward-viewing colonoscope [7–9]. Indeed, successfully reaching the papilla has been reported in 92% (54/59) of Billroth-II patients but only 33–67% of RYG patients. However, due to recent advances in enteroscopes, such as the advent of single-balloon enteroscopy (SBE) as well as DBE, the successful approach rate has remarkably improved to 91–96% in RYG patients with short-type SBE [18,20,22] and 95–98% with short-type DBE [15,19,21]. Similarly, successful scope insertion to the papilla of Vater was obtained in 92% (73/79) of RYG patients using short-type DBE in this study.

Selective biliary cannulation was also challenging due to the difficulty of positioning the scope from a front view of the papilla of Vater and the limited controllability of the catheter through elevator-unequipped enteroscopes, in contrast to standard duodenoscopes. Previous studies reported the success rate of biliary cannulation in RYG patients to be 74–95% [15,18–22]. One of the tips for biliary cannulation is to perform the procedure using the retroflex position, which can facilitate direct visualization of the papilla from the front [20]. Recently, the position was reported to be a potential favorable factor for successful biliary cannulation [22]. In the present study, 12% (9/73) of patients had failed biliary cannulation, but alternative approaches, such as PTBD which might induce pain and discomfort associated with the external transhepatic catheter [11–14], EUS-BD (including EUS-guided antegrade intervention) which required complicated process for stone extraction and had a risk of biliary peritonitis [5,30–33], surgery or conservative therapy, improved the situation. Depending on the patient condition and capabilities of the institution, an immediate decision to alter the treatment plan may also be crucial.

The basic strategy for an ampullary procedure and subsequent stone extraction is considered to be the same as for managing patients with normal anatomy. In the present study, several combinations of an ampullary procedure were performed, as shown in Table 3. Given the difficulty of sphincterotomy and the precutting method due to the inverted view, EPBD or EPLBD alone may be acceptable for RYG patients [35], as it is for normal anatomies [36,37] and Billroth-II gastrectomy patients [27]. Regarding stone extraction, the latest enteroscope with a 3.2 mm working channel can utilize most devices, including an ML, and complete stone extraction was ultimately achieved in 88% of patients in the present study in whom such a procedure was attempted. For difficult cases, stone extraction in two sessions following drainage was recommended [4,5]. In addition, in some cases with large CBD stones, electrohydraulic lithotripsy (EHL) using cholangioscopy [4,38–40], percutaneous transhepatic cholangioscopy (PTCS) [14], or EUS-guided antegrade cholangioscopy [31–33] might need to be considered for complete extraction.

This was the first study to reveal the factors affecting complete stone extraction in RYG patients who underwent BE-ERCP. First, we identified an interesting risk factor for incomplete stone extraction: the largest CBD diameter ≥ 14 mm. Dilation of the CBD in RYG patients is often seen post-cholecystectomy [41]. In patients with a large CBD stone size and large CBD diameter, sufficient papillary dilation by EPLBD with or without crushing stones using an ML was usually required for successful stone extraction [4,16,17,25–29,36,37,42], but achieving stone clearance is not easy. A previous study reported that a large stone size was a risk factor for incomplete stone extraction by ERCP, in patients with a history of Billroth-II [42] as well as those with normal anatomy [43]. In contrast, small stones floating into larger diameter CBD are often difficult to grasp, even when using available devices, such as a basket or retrieval balloon catheter. This was also an issue when large stones were crushed with an ML. Thus, regardless of the CBD stone size, a large CBD diameter can make complete stone extraction difficult. Dedicated devices that can easily catch small stones floating in large diameter CBDs are desired.

In addition, a retroflex position was identified as a positive factor affecting complete stone extraction. As mentioned above, this position was reported to be useful for successful biliary cannulation in RYG patients [20,22]. The retroflex position can be obtained by advancing the endoscope without releasing the looped scope and forming a J-turn at the IDA. Thereby, a coaxial relationship between the devices and distal CBD and maintaining a proper distance from the tip of the scope to the papilla of Vater with a better view of the papilla can thus be obtained. Such a situation can facilitate stones to be removed along the axis of the CBD. In the present study, in a sub-analysis of the difficult-to-manage cohorts—i.e., those with a large CBD diameter (≥ 14 mm) or stone size (≥ 10 mm)—the retroflex position was also a significant factor affecting successful complete stone extraction. In fact, we experienced several cases where stone extraction could not be completed initially in the non-retroflex position, whereas the retroflex position allowed complete stone extraction to be easily performed in the second session, as shown in Figure 1. Taken together, these findings suggest that the retroflex position may be recommended for complete stone extraction as well as successful biliary cannulation in RYG patients. However, this technique should be performed carefully due to the risk of perforation at the IDA.

Adverse events occur in 5–18% of patients treated with this procedure [15,20,22,44], and the incidence rate was 5% in the present study. In contrast to conventional ERCP, perforation is one of the most common adverse events for this procedure [45] and occurs mainly during scope insertion or stone extraction. Immediately noticing the issue and thoroughly performing intraluminal drainage is important, as the situation can sometimes be managed if minor perforation occurs, as shown in one of our cases. Acute pancreatitis occurred in a patient who had a 15 mm diameter CBD stone in an 18 mm diameter CBD and was treated with precutting, a 10 mm diameter EPBD, and an ML. In a systematic review, EPLBD with EST is reported to carry a low risk of pancreatitis compared with EST or EPBD alone (2.4%, 4.3%, and 8.6%, respectively; $p < 0.001$) [46], therefore, a sufficient EPLBD for a dilated CBD may be important to avoid a risk of procedure-related pancreatitis, but further prospective studies will be needed, as described above.

In addition, patients enrolled in this study were relatively elderly, showing a median age of 79 years old. A previous study also reported that both technical success rates and the rates of adverse events were similar between elderly ($\geq$75 years old) and non-elderly groups (<75 years old), suggesting that BE-ERCP is a feasible procedure for elderly individuals with a surgically altered anatomy [44]. Repeated BE-ERCP may carry a risk for elderly patients, so middle-term stent placement may be an option for the treatment of cases of complicated CBD stones, although caution against life-threatening cholangitis should be practiced [4,47].

Several limitations associated with the present study warrant mention. First, this was a retrospective study with a relatively small cohort, but three tertiary hospitals participated in it. Further prospective studies are needed to validate the present findings. Second, most of the patients were unable to be followed at the hospital, instead visiting family doctors. Therefore, an analysis based on long-term follow-up data, such as the stone recurrence rate, was not conducted.

In conclusion, therapeutic BE-ERCP for CBD stones in RYG patients, with a relatively elderly cohort, was effective and safe using short-type DBE. The largest CBD diameter $\geq$ 14 mm was an independent risk factor for failed complete stone extraction, but the use of a retroflex position may be considered as a recommended technique to achieve complete stone clearance.

Author Contributions: Conception and design of the study, analysis and interpretation of the data, and drafting of the article, T.O. (Taisuke Obata) and K.T.; collection and interpretation of the data, H.K., T.U., K.M. (Kazuya Miyamoto), T.Y., A.M., Y.F., K.M. (Kazuyuki Matsumoto), S.H., K.Y., T.O. (Tsuneyoshi Ogawa), R.T. and H.O.; final approval of the article, all authors. All authors have read and agreed to the published version of the manuscript.

Funding: This research received no external funding.

Institutional Review Board Statement: This study was approved by the Okayama University Human Ethics Committee (Approval number: 2104-041).

Informed Consent Statement: Informed consent was obtained from all subjects involved in the study.

Data Availability Statement: Data sharing is not applicable.

Conflicts of Interest: The authors declare no conflict of interest.

References

1. Hauters, P.; de Roden, A.d.N.; Pourbaix, A.; Aupaix, F.; Coumans, P.; Therasse, G. Cholelithiasis: A serious complication after total gastrectomy. *Br. J. Surg.* **1988**, *75*, 899–900. [CrossRef]
2. Inoue, K.; Fuchigami, A.; Higashide, S.; Sumi, S.; Kogire, M.; Suzuki, T.; Tobe, T. Gallbladder sludge and stone formation in relation to contractile function after gastrectomy. A prospective study. *Ann. Surg.* **1992**, *215*, 19–26. [CrossRef]
3. Pezzolla, F.; Lantone, G.; Guerra, V.; Misciagna, G.; Prete, F.; Giorgio, I.; Lorusso, D. Influence of the method of digestive tract reconstruction on gallstone development after total gastrectomy for gastric cancer. *Am. J. Surg.* **1993**, *166*, 6–10. [CrossRef]
4. Manes, G.; Paspatis, G.; Aabakken, L.; Anderloni, A.; Arvanitakis, M.; Ah-Soune, P.; Barthet, M.; Domagk, D.; Dumonceau, J.M.; Gigot, J.F.; et al. Endoscopic management of common bile duct stones: European Society of Gastrointestinal Endoscopy (ESGE) guideline. *Endoscopy* **2019**, *51*, 472–491. [CrossRef]
5. Mukai, S.; Itoi, T.; Baron, T.H.; Takada, T.; Strasberg, S.M.; Pitt, H.A.; Ukai, T.; Shikata, S.; Teoh, A.Y.B.; Kim, M.H.; et al. Indications and techniques of biliary drainage for acute cholangitis in updated Tokyo Guidelines 2018. *J. Hepatobiliary Pancreat Sci.* **2017**, *24*, 537–549. [CrossRef]
6. Hintze, R.E.; Adler, A.; Veltzke, W.; Abou-Rebyeh, H. Endoscopic access to the papilla of Vater for endoscopic retrograde cholangiopancreatography in patients with Billroth II or roux-en-Y gastrojejunostomy. *Endoscopy* **1997**, *29*, 69–73. [CrossRef]
7. Wright, B.E.; Cass, O.W.; Freeman, M.L. ERCP in patients with long-limb Roux-en-Y gastrojejunostomy and intact papilla. *Gastrointest. Endosc.* **2002**, *56*, 225–232. [CrossRef]
8. Gostout, C.J.; Bender, C.E. Cholangiopancreatography, sphincterotomy, and common duct stone removal via Roux-en-Y limb enteroscopy. *Gastroenterology* **1988**, *95*, 156–163. [CrossRef]
9. Nakaji, S.; Hirata, N.; Yamauchi, K.; Shiratori, T.; Kobayashi, M.; Fujii, H.; Ishii, E. Endoscopic retrograde cholangiopancreatography using a cap-assisted highly flexible colonoscope in patients with Roux-en-Y anastomosis. *Endoscopy* **2014**, *46*, 529–532. [CrossRef] [PubMed]
10. Uchida, D.; Tsutsumi, K.; Kato, H.; Matsumi, A.; Saragai, Y.; Tomoda, T.; Matsumoto, K.; Horiguchi, S.; Okada, H. Potential Factors Affecting Results of Short-Type Double-Balloon Endoscope-Assisted Endoscopic Retrograde Cholangiopancreatography. *Dig. Dis. Sci.* **2020**, *65*, 1460–1470. [CrossRef] [PubMed]
11. Clouse, M.; Stokes, K.; Lee, R.; Falchuk, K. Bile duct stones: Percutaneous transhepatic removal. *Radiology* **1986**, *160*, 525–529. [CrossRef]
12. van der Velden, J.J.; Berger, M.Y.; Bonjer, H.J.; Brakel, K.; Laméris, J.S. Percutaneous treatment of bile duct stones in patients treated unsuccessfully with endoscopic retrograde procedures. *Gastrointest. Endosc.* **2000**, *51*, 418–422. [CrossRef]
13. Jeong, E.J.; Kang, D.H.; Kim, D.U.; Choi, C.W.; Eum, J.S.; Jung, W.J.; Kim, P.J.; Kim, Y.W.; Jung, K.S.; Bae, Y.M.; et al. Percutaneous transhepatic choledochoscopic lithotomy as a rescue therapy for removal of bile duct stones in Billroth II gastrectomy patients who are difficult to perform ERCP. *Eur. J. Gastroenterol. Hepatol.* **2009**, *21*, 1358–1362. [CrossRef] [PubMed]
14. Tsutsumi, K.; Kato, H.; Yabe, S.; Mizukawa, S.; Seki, H.; Akimoto, Y.; Uchida, D.; Matsumoto, K.; Tomoda, T.; Yamamoto, N.; et al. A comparative evaluation of treatment methods for bile duct stones after hepaticojejunostomy between percutaneous transhepatic cholangioscopy and peroral, short double-balloon enteroscopy. *Therap. Adv. Gastroenterol.* **2017**, *10*, 54–67. [CrossRef]
15. Shimatani, M.; Matsushita, M.; Takaoka, M.; Koyabu, M.; Ikeura, T.; Kato, K.; Fukui, T.; Uchida, K.; Okazaki, K. Effective "short" double-balloon enteroscope for diagnostic and therapeutic ERCP in patients with altered gastrointestinal anatomy: A large case series. *Endoscopy* **2009**, *41*, 849–854. [CrossRef]
16. Oana, S.; Shibata, S.; Matsuda, N.; Matsumoto, T. Efficacy and safety of double-balloon endoscopy-assisted endoscopic papillary large-balloon dilatation for common bile duct stone removal. *Dig. Liver Dis.* **2015**, *47*, 401–404. [CrossRef] [PubMed]
17. Itoi, T.; Ishii, K.; Sofuni, A.; Itokawa, F.; Kurihara, T.; Tsuchiya, T.; Tsuji, S.; Ikeuchi, N.; Umeda, J.; Tanaka, R.; et al. Large balloon dilatation following endoscopic sphincterotomy using a balloon enteroscope for the bile duct stone extractions in patients with Roux-en-Y anastomosis. *Dig. Liver Dis.* **2011**, *43*, 237–241. [CrossRef]
18. Yamauchi, H.; Kida, M.; Okuwaki, K.; Miyazawa, S.; Iwai, T.; Takezawa, M.; Kikuchi, H.; Watanabe, M.; Imaizumi, H.; Koizumi, W. Short-type single balloon enteroscope for endoscopic retrograde cholangiopancreatography with altered gastrointestinal anatomy. *World J. Gastroenterol.* **2013**, *19*, 1728–1735. [CrossRef] [PubMed]
19. Osoegawa, T.; Motomura, Y.; Akahoshi, K.; Higuchi, N.; Tanaka, Y.; Hisano, T.; Itaba, S.; Gibo, J.; Yamada, M.; Kubokawa, M.; et al. Improved techniques for double-balloon-enteroscopy-assisted endoscopic retrograde cholangiopancreatography. *World J. Gastroenterol.* **2012**, *18*, 6843–6849. [CrossRef] [PubMed]
20. Ishii, K.; Itoi, T.; Tonozuka, R.; Itokawa, F.; Sofuni, A.; Tsuchiya, T.; Tsuji, S.; Ikeuchi, N.; Kamada, K.; Umeda, J.; et al. Balloon enteroscopy-assisted ERCP in patients with Roux-en-Y gastrectomy and intact papillae (with videos). *Gastrointest. Endosc.* **2016**, *83*, 377–386. [CrossRef]
21. Shimatani, M.; Hatanaka, H.; Kogure, H.; Tsutsumi, K.; Kawashima, H.; Hanada, K.; Matsuda, T.; Fujita, T.; Takaoka, M.; Yano, T.; et al. Diagnostic and Therapeutic Endoscopic Retrograde Cholangiography Using a Short-Type Double-Balloon Endoscope in Patients With Altered Gastrointestinal Anatomy: A Multicenter Prospective Study in Japan. *Am. J. Gastroenterol.* **2016**, *111*, 1750–1758. [CrossRef]
22. Tanisaka, Y.; Ryozawa, S.; Mizuide, M.; Fujita, A.; Ogawa, T.; Harada, M.; Noguchi, T.; Suzuki, M.; Araki, R. Biliary Cannulation in Patients with Roux-en-Y Gastrectomy: An Analysis of the Factors Associated with Successful Cannulation. *Intern. Med.* **2020**, *59*, 1687–1693. [CrossRef] [PubMed]

23. Anvari, S.; Lee, Y.; Patro, N.; Soon, M.S.; Doumouras, A.G.; Hong, D. Double-balloon enteroscopy for diagnostic and therapeutic ERCP in patients with surgically altered gastrointestinal anatomy: A systematic review and meta-analysis. *Surg. Endosc.* **2021**, *35*, 18–36. [CrossRef]
24. Tsutsumi, K.; Kato, H.; Okada, H. Side-to-side jejunojejunostomy is favorable for scope insertion during endoscopic retrograde cholangiopancreatography in patients with Roux-en-Y hepaticojejunostomy. *Dig. Endosc.* **2015**, *27*, 708. [CrossRef]
25. Kim, G.H.; Kang, D.H.; Song, G.A.; Heo, J.; Park, C.H.; Ha, T.I.; Kim, K.Y.; Lee, H.J.; Kim, I.D.; Choi, S.H.; et al. Endoscopic removal of bile-duct stones by using a rotatable papillotome and a large-balloon dilator in patients with a Billroth II gastrectomy (with video). *Gastrointest. Endosc.* **2008**, *67*, 1134–1138. [CrossRef]
26. Itoi, T.; Ishii, K.; Itokawa, F.; Kurihara, T.; Sofuni, A. Large balloon papillary dilation for removal of bile duct stones in patients who have undergone a billroth II gastrectomy. *Dig. Endosc.* **2010**, *22*, S98–S102. [CrossRef] [PubMed]
27. Jang, H.W.; Lee, K.J.; Jung, M.J.; Jung, J.W.; Park, J.Y.; Park, S.W.; Song, S.Y.; Chung, J.B.; Bang, S. Endoscopic papillary large balloon dilatation alone is safe and effective for the treatment of difficult choledocholithiasis in cases of Billroth II gastrectomy: A single center experience. *Dig. Dis. Sci.* **2013**, *58*, 1737–1743. [CrossRef]
28. Kim, T.H.; Kim, J.H.; Seo, D.W.; Lee, D.K.; Reddy, N.D.; Rerknimitr, R.; Ratanachu-Ek, T.; Khor, C.J.; Itoi, T.; Yasuda, I.; et al. International consensus guidelines for endoscopic papillary large-balloon dilation. *Gastrointest. Endosc.* **2016**, *83*, 37–47. [CrossRef]
29. Itoi, T.; Ryozawa, S.; Katanuma, A.; Okabe, Y.; Kato, H.; Horaguchi, J.; Tsuchiya, T.; Gotoda, T.; Fujita, N.; Yasuda, K.; et al. Japan Gastroenterological Endoscopy Society guidelines for endoscopic papillary large balloon dilation. *Dig. Endosc.* **2018**, *30*, 293–309. [CrossRef]
30. Iwashita, T.; Nakai, Y.; Hara, K.; Isayama, H.; Itoi, T.; Park, D.H. Endoscopic ultrasound-guided antegrade treatment of bile duct stone in patients with surgically altered anatomy: A multicenter retrospective cohort study. *J. Hepatobiliary Pancreat Sci.* **2016**, *23*, 227–233. [CrossRef]
31. James, T.W.; Fan, Y.C.; Baron, T.H. EUS-guided hepaticoenterostomy as a portal to allow definitive antegrade treatment of benign biliary diseases in patients with surgically altered anatomy. *Gastrointest. Endosc.* **2018**, *88*, 547–554. [CrossRef]
32. Hosmer, A.; Abdelfatah, M.M.; Law, R.; Baron, T.H. Endoscopic ultrasound-guided hepaticogastrostomy and antegrade clearance of biliary lithiasis in patients with surgically-altered anatomy. *Endosc. Int. Open* **2018**, *6*, E127–E130. [CrossRef]
33. Mukai, S.; Itoi, T.; Sofuni, A.; Tsuchiya, T.; Tanaka, R.; Tonozuka, R.; Honjo, M.; Fujita, M.; Yamamoto, K.; Nagakawa, Y. EUS-guided antegrade intervention for benign biliary diseases in patients with surgically altered anatomy (with videos). *Gastrointest. Endosc.* **2019**, *89*, 399–407. [CrossRef] [PubMed]
34. Cotton, P.B.; Eisen, G.M.; Aabakken, L.; Baron, T.H.; Hutter, M.M.; Jacobson, B.C.; Mergener, K.; Nemcek, A., Jr.; Petersen, B.T.; Petrini, J.L.; et al. A lexicon for endoscopic adverse events: Report of an ASGE workshop. *Gastrointest. Endosc.* **2010**, *71*, 446–454. [CrossRef]
35. Testoni, P.A.; Mariani, A.; Aabakken, L.; Arvanitakis, M.; Bories, E.; Costamagna, G.; Devière, J.; Dinis-Ribeiro, M.; Dumonceau, J.M.; Giovannini, M.; et al. Papillary cannulation and sphincterotomy techniques at ERCP: European Society of Gastrointestinal Endoscopy (ESGE) Clinical Guideline. *Endoscopy* **2016**, *48*, 657–683. [CrossRef] [PubMed]
36. Park, J.S.; Jeong, S.; Lee, D.K.; Jang, S.I.; Lee, T.H.; Park, S.H.; Hwang, J.C.; Kim, J.H.; Yoo, B.M.; Park, S.G.; et al. Comparison of endoscopic papillary large balloon dilation with or without endoscopic sphincterotomy for the treatment of large bile duct stones. *Endoscopy* **2019**, *51*, 125–132. [CrossRef]
37. Kogure, H.; Kawahata, S.; Mukai, T.; Doi, S.; Iwashita, T.; Ban, T.; Ito, Y.; Kawakami, H.; Hayashi, T.; Sasahira, N.; et al. Multicenter randomized trial of endoscopic papillary large balloon dilation without sphincterotomy versus endoscopic sphincterotomy for removal of bile duct stones: MARVELOUS trial. *Endoscopy* **2020**, *52*, 736–744. [CrossRef]
38. Binmoeller, K.; Brückner, M.; Thonke, F.; Soehendra, N. Treatment of difficult bile duct stones using mechanical, electrohydraulic and extracorporeal shock wave lithotripsy. *Endoscopy* **1993**, *25*, 201–206. [CrossRef]
39. Veld, J.V.; van Huijgevoort, N.C.M.; Boermeester, M.A.; Besselink, M.G.; van Delden, O.M.; Fockens, P.; van Hooft, J.E. A systematic review of advanced endoscopy-assisted lithotripsy for retained biliary tract stones: Laser, electrohydraulic or extracorporeal shock wave. *Endoscopy* **2018**, *50*, 896–909. [CrossRef]
40. Tonozuka, R.; Itoi, T.; Sofuni, A.; Tsuchiya, T.; Ishii, K.; Tanaka, R.; Honjo, M.; Mukai, S.; Yamamoto, K.; Fujita, M.; et al. Novel peroral direct digital cholangioscopy-assisted lithotripsy using a monorail technique through the overtube in patients with surgically altered anatomy (with video). *Dig. Endosc.* **2019**, *31*, 203–208. [CrossRef]
41. Holm, A.N.; Gerke, H. What should be done with a dilated bile duct? *Curr. Gastroenterol. Rep.* **2010**, *12*, 150–156. [CrossRef]
42. Li, J.S.; Zou, D.W.; Jin, Z.D.; Shi, X.G.; Chen, J.; Li, Z.S.; Liu, F. Predictive factors for extraction of common bile duct stones during endoscopic retrograde cholangiopancreatography in Billroth II anatomy patients. *Surg. Endosc.* **2020**, *34*, 2454–2459. [CrossRef]
43. Lee, S.H.; Park, J.K.; Yoon, W.J.; Lee, J.K.; Ryu, J.K.; Kim, Y.T.; Yoon, Y.B. How to predict the outcome of endoscopic mechanical lithotripsy in patients with difficult bile duct stones? *Scand. J. Gastroenterol.* **2007**, *42*, 1006–1010. [CrossRef]
44. Hakuta, R.; Kogure, H.; Nakai, Y.; Hamada, T.; Sato, T.; Suzuki, Y.; Inokuma, A.; Kanai, S.; Nakamura, T.; Noguchi, K.; et al. Feasibility of balloon endoscope-assisted endoscopic retrograde cholangiopancreatography for the elderly. *Endosc. Int. Open* **2020**, *8*, E1202–E1211. [CrossRef]

45. Tokuhara, M.; Shimatani, M.; Mitsuyama, T.; Masuda, M.; Ito, T.; Miyamoto, S.; Fukata, N.; Miyoshi, H.; Ikeura, T.; Takaoka, M.; et al. Evaluation of complications after endoscopic retrograde cholangiopancreatography using a short type double balloon endoscope in patients with altered gastrointestinal anatomy: A single-center retrospective study of 1,576 procedures. *J. Gastroenterol. Hepatol.* **2020**, *35*, 1387–1396. [CrossRef] [PubMed]
46. Kim, J.H.; Yang, M.J.; Hwang, J.C.; Yoo, B.M. Endoscopic papillary large balloon dilation for the removal of bile duct stones. *World J. Gastroenterol.* **2013**, *19*, 8580–8594. [CrossRef]
47. Bergman, J.J.; Rauws, E.A.; Tijssen, J.G.; Tytgat, G.N.; Huibregtse, K. Biliary endoprostheses in elderly patients with endoscopically irretrievable common bile duct stones: Report on 117 patients. *Gastrointest. Endosc.* **1995**, *42*, 195–201. [CrossRef]

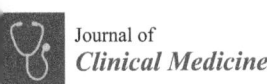

Review

Endoscopic Double Stenting for the Management of Combined Malignant Biliary and Duodenal Obstruction

Tsuyoshi Takeda, Takashi Sasaki *, Takeshi Okamoto and Naoki Sasahira

Department of Hepato-Biliary-Pancreatic Medicine, Cancer Institute Hospital of Japanese Foundation for Cancer Research, 3-8-31, Ariake, Koto-ku, Tokyo 135-8550, Japan; tsuyoshi.takeda@jfcr.or.jp (T.T.); takeshi.okamoto@jfcr.or.jp (T.O.); naoki.sasahira@jfcr.or.jp (N.S.)
* Correspondence: sasakit-tky@umin.ac.jp; Tel.: +81-3-3520-0111; Fax: +81-3-3520-0141

Abstract: Periampullary cancers are often diagnosed at advanced stages and can cause both biliary and duodenal obstruction. As these two obstructions reduce patients' performance status and quality of life, appropriate management of the disease is important. Combined malignant biliary and duodenal obstruction is classified according to the location and timing of the duodenal obstruction, which also affect treatment options. Traditionally, surgical bypass (gastrojejunostomy and hepaticojejunostomy) has been performed for the treatment of unresectable periampullary cancer. However, it has recently been substituted by less invasive endoscopic procedures due to its high morbidity and mortality. Thus, endoscopic double stenting (transpapillary stenting and enteral stenting) has become the current standard of care. Limitations of transpapillary stenting include its technical difficulty and the risk of duodenal-biliary reflux. Recently, endoscopic ultrasound-guided procedures have emerged as a novel platform and have been increasingly utilized in the management of biliary and duodenal obstruction. As the prognosis of periampullary cancer has improved due to recent advances in chemotherapy, treatment strategies for biliary and duodenal obstruction are becoming more important. In this article, we review the treatment strategies for combined malignant biliary and duodenal obstruction based on the latest evidence.

Keywords: biliary obstruction; duodenal obstruction; double stenting; anti-reflux metal stent; lumen-opposing metal stent

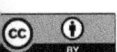

1. Introduction

Periampullary cancers, including pancreatic cancer, biliary tract cancer, duodenal cancer and ampullary cancer, are often diagnosed at advanced stages and can cause both biliary and duodenal obstruction. Biliary obstruction may lead to cholangitis or liver dysfunction, whereas duodenal obstruction may present with decreased oral intake, nausea and vomiting. These two obstructions reduce patients' performance status and quality of life and may deprive them of the opportunity to receive antitumor treatment. Therefore, appropriate treatment and management are very important.

Traditionally, double surgical bypass (gastrojejunostomy and hepaticojejunostomy) has been performed for the treatment of combined biliary and duodenal obstruction in patients with unresectable periampullary cancer [1–3]. Endoscopic double stenting (transpapillary stenting and enteral stenting) has become the standard treatment due to its lower invasiveness and shorter recovery time [4]. Percutaneous transhepatic biliary drainage (PTBD) has been widely used as an alternative treatment after failed endoscopic retrograde cholangiopancreatography (ERCP), but it has disadvantages such as skin infection, pain and decreased quality of life. Recently, endoscopic ultrasound (EUS)-guided procedures have emerged as a novel platform and have been increasingly utilized in the management of biliary and duodenal obstruction. As the prognosis of periampullary cancer has improved due to recent advances in chemotherapy, treatment strategies for biliary and duodenal obstruction are becoming more important. In this article, we review the treatment strategies for combined malignant biliary and duodenal obstruction based on the latest evidence.

2. Classification of Combined Malignant Biliary and Duodenal Obstruction

Combined malignant biliary and duodenal obstruction has been classified according to the location and timing of the duodenal obstruction (Table 1) [5]. First, duodenal obstruction can be categorized into three types based on the location relative to the major papilla: type I, duodenal obstruction proximal to the major papilla; type II, duodenal obstruction involving the major papilla; and type III, duodenal obstruction distal to the major papilla. Double stenting is most technically challenging in patients with type II obstruction because transpapillary biliary access is difficult, if not impossible [5]. Transpapillary biliary stenting may not be difficult in patients with type I obstruction if the scope can pass through the duodenal stricture after dilation of the duodenal stricture or placement of a duodenal stent [6,7]. Transpapillary biliary stenting in patients with type III obstruction may also be easy to manage because the major papilla is located proximal to the duodenal stricture. However, these types face a risk of duodenal-biliary reflux [8]. Such patients are good candidates for EUS-guided biliary drainage (EUS-BD) [9–12].

Table 1. Classification of combined malignant biliary and duodenal obstruction.

	Location
Type I	Duodenal obstruction proximal to the major papilla
Type II	Duodenal obstruction involving the major papilla
Type III	Duodenal obstruction distal to the major papilla

	Timing
Group 1	Biliary obstruction occurring before the onset of duodenal obstruction
Group 2	Biliary and duodenal obstruction occurring simultaneously
Group 3	Biliary obstruction occurring after the onset of duodenal obstruction

Second, biliary obstruction can be classified into three groups according to the timing of duodenal and biliary obstruction: group 1, biliary obstruction occurring before the onset of duodenal obstruction; group 2, biliary obstruction occurring simultaneously with duodenal obstruction; and group 3, biliary obstruction occurring after the onset of duodenal obstruction. Group 1 is the most common, followed by group 3 and group 2. In group 1, the type of previously inserted biliary stent could affect the treatment strategy. The introduction of covered biliary self-expandable metallic stents (SEMS) has broadened the range of treatment options available due to its removability. Both classifications are important in determining the optimal management strategy for combined biliary and duodenal obstructions.

Combined biliary and duodenal obstruction also occurs in patients with surgically altered anatomy. However, evidence is scarce in this area. One study proposed a new classification for malignant afferent loop obstruction according to the location of the intestinal stricture in relation to the major papilla or bilioenteric anastomosis [13]: type 1, obstruction site located distal to the major papilla or bilioenteric anastomosis; type 2, obstruction site involving the major papilla or bilioenteric anastomosis; and type 3, obstruction site located between bilioenteric and pancreaticoenteric anastomoses. Recently, enteral stenting employing the through-the-scope technique with a short-type balloon-assisted enteroscope and SEMS with a 9-Fr delivery system has become possible [13–16]. Nevertheless, endoscopic biliary stenting remains technically demanding due to difficulties in achieving biliary access. A combination of PTBD or EUS-BD may be required in these situations.

3. Treatment Options for Combined Malignant Biliary and Duodenal Obstruction

3.1. Surgical Approach

Traditionally, double surgical bypass (gastrojejunostomy and hepaticojejunostomy) has been performed for symptomatic treatment of unresectable periampullary cancer [1–3].

However, it has recently been substituted by less invasive endoscopic procedures due to its high morbidity and mortality. A recent systematic review and meta-analysis reported that endoscopic double stenting was associated with higher clinical success (97% vs. 86%) and less adverse events (13% vs. 28%), but with a more frequent need for reintervention (21% vs. 10%) compared with double surgical bypass [17]. Even though endoscopic double stenting has become the standard treatment for combined biliary and duodenal obstruction [18], minimally invasive surgical procedures such as laparoscopic gastrojejunostomy are still favored in patients with a long life expectancy, due to reports suggesting better long-term outcomes [19–21]. On the other hand, data on the efficacy of endoscopic duodenal stenting for patients with long life expectancy are also increasing [22–24]. In addition, EUS-guided gastroenterostomy (EUS-GE) has recently been developed as a novel technique for the management of gastric outlet obstruction, with promising results [25–28]. Further research is needed to determine the optimal management for this population.

3.2. Percutaneous Approach

PTBD including percutaneous transhepatic biliary stenting is a well-established rescue procedure for the palliation of malignant biliary obstruction [29], especially when the endoscopic transpapillary approach is not possible. However, this procedure carries high morbidity. EUS-BD is currently gaining wide acceptance among experienced endosonographers. A multicenter randomized trial reported that procedure-related adverse events were significantly higher in PTBD than in EUS-BD (31.2% vs. 8.8%), with similar efficacy [30]. EUS-BD may be preferable when transpapillary biliary stenting is unsuccessful, if expertise is available.

3.3. Endoscopic Approach

Endoscopic double stenting is the current standard treatment for combined biliary and duodenal obstruction. For malignant biliary obstruction, transpapillary biliary drainage via ERCP and EUS-BD are the two major treatment options. Studies reporting outcomes of endoscopic double stenting including at least 10 subjects are summarized in Table 2. We reclassified biliary drainage procedures that required percutaneous techniques, including PTBD rendezvous technique and percutaneous transhepatic SEMS insertion, as technical failures with respect to endoscopic biliary drainage. In general, the technical success rate was greatly influenced by the biliary drainage method and the proportion of type II obstructions. A systematic review and meta-analysis found that ERCP was associated with similar clinical success and less adverse events (3% vs. 23%) compared to EUS-BD for biliary drainage as part of double stenting [17]. As a result, ERCP remains the preferred treatment option when transpapillary biliary access is possible. While EUS-BD is generally considered a salvage technique for difficult or failed ERCP [31,32], two recent randomized controlled trials reported similar adverse event rates (21.2% vs. 14.7%) in expert hands [33,34].

EUS-BD is especially useful in patients with type II obstruction because transpapillary biliary access is difficult. A retrospective study reported that the technical success rate of EUS-BD was significantly higher than that of transpapillary biliary drainage (95.2% vs. 56.0%) in pancreatic cancer patients with an indwelling duodenal stent [35]. Furthermore, duodenal obstruction has been reported as a risk factor for early transpapillary biliary SEMS dysfunction due to duodenal-biliary reflux [36,37]. Therefore, these two situations are good indications for EUS-BD. The two major EUS-BD techniques are EUS-guided hepatico-gastrostomy (EUS-HGS) and choledocho-duodenostromy (EUS-CDS). A retrospective study comparing the efficacy and safety of EUS-HGS with EUS-CDS suggested that EUS-HGS may be superior to EUS-CDS, with longer stent patency (biliary stent patency: median 133 days vs. 37 days) and fewer adverse events [38]. EUS-CDS was particularly associated with reflux cholangitis, probably due to the closer distance between the duodenal stent and the bilioduodenal fistula relative to EUS-HGS. A recent multicenter randomized controlled study comparing the efficacy and safety of EUS-HGS with EUS-CDS demonstrated that the clinical success, stent patency and adverse events were similar between the two procedures [39]. In summary, disadvantages of EUS-CDS include susceptibility to duodenal-biliary reflux and difficult access in type I obstruction, while those of EUS-HGS include the inability to puncture a non-dilated left intrahepatic bile duct and SEMS occlusion due to bile duct hyperplasia.

Table 2. Results of endoscopic double stenting for combined malignant biliary and duodenal obstruction.

Study	N	Biliary Drainage	Biliary Stent Type	Technical Success (%)		Early Adverse Events
				Biliary Stent	Duodenal Stent	
Kaw et al. [40]	18	ERCP	SEMS	94	94	Bleeding 1
Vanbiervliet et al. [41]	18	ERCP	SEMS	94	Indwelling	None
Maire et al. [42]	23	ERCP	PS, SEMS	91	96	None
Mutignani et al. [5]	64	ERCP	PS, SEMS	97	100	Pancreatitis 1, cholangitis 1, cholecystitis 1, bleeding 1
Kim et al. [4]	24	ERCP	PS, SEMS	54	100	Pancreatitis 3, cholangitis 1
Tonozuka et al. [11]	11	ERCP, EUS-BD	SEMS	100	100	None
Khashab et al. [43]	38	ERCP, EUS-BD	PS, SEMS	66	Indwelling	Cholangitis 1
Yu et al. [44]	17	ERCP	SEMS	100	100	Bleeding 1
Canene et al. [45]	50	ERCP	SEMS	84	100	NA
Hamada et al. [36]	20	ERCP, EUS-BD	PS, SEMS	100	Indwelling	Bleeding 1, pancreatitis 1
Manta et al. [46]	15	ERCP, EUS-BD	SEMS	87	100	None
Ogura et al. [38]	39	EUS-BD	SEMS	100	100	None
Sato et al. [9]	50	ERCP, EUS-BD	SEMS	86	100	NA
Matsumoto et al. [10]	81	ERCP, EUS-BD	PS, SEMS	100	100	NA
Hamada et al. [12]	110	ERCP, EUS-BD	PS, SEMS	100	100	NA
Hori et al. [47]	109	ERCP	SEMS	93	99	Pneumonia 2, pancreatitis 1
Staub et al. [6]	71	ERCP	PS, SEMS	85	Indwelling	Cholangitis 2, perforation 1
Yamao et al. [35]	39	ERCP, EUS-BD	PS, SEMS	87	Indwelling	NA
Debourdeau et al. [48]	31	ERCP, EUS-BD	SEMS	65	100	NA
Mangiavillano et al. [49]	23	EUS-BD, EUS-GBD	SEMS	96	100	None

N, number; ERCP, endoscopic retrograde cholangiopancreatography; EUS-BD, endoscopic ultrasound-guided biliary drainage; EUS-GBD, endoscopic ultrasound-guided gallbladder drainage; PS, plastic stent; SEMS, self-expandable metallic stent; NA, not available.

3.4. Novel Types of Stents

3.4.1. Anti-Reflux Metal Stents

Several types of anti-reflux metal stents (ARMS) have been made to prevent duodenal-biliary reflux [50–56]. Although ARMS was associated with a lower rate of stent occlusion compared to conventional SEMS in several studies on distal malignant biliary obstruction, the results were inconsistent and stent patency rates were low. Recently, two retrospective studies showed that a novel duckbill-type ARMS was more effective in preventing duodenal-biliary reflux than conventional SEMS [57,58]. ARMS may be effective not only for transpapillary biliary stenting, but also for EUS-CDS in patients with combined biliary and duodenal obstruction [59]. Prospective studies are needed to further evaluate the efficacy and safety of AMRS especially in the setting of combined biliary and duodenal obstruction.

3.4.2. Lumen-Apposing Metal Stents

Lumen-apposing metal stents (LAMS), designed for transluminal drainage of nonadherent lumens, were first reported by Binmoeller and Shah in 2011 [60]. Although this stent was initially created for drainage of pancreatic fluid collections, use of LAMS has been reported in gallbladder drainage, biliary drainage (EUS-CDS) and the creation of gastrointestinal fistulae [61]. Recently, a retrospective study reported the technical feasibility of LAMS insertion through the mesh of an indwelling duodenal stent with a technical success rate of 95.6% in 23 patients [49]. Prospective studies with larger sample sizes are needed to further evaluate these LAMS applications.

3.5. EUS-GE

EUS-GE using LAMS has recently received attention as a new alternative for the treatment of gastric outlet obstruction. Several techniques including the direct technique, the device-assisted technique and EUS-guided double balloon-occluded gastrojejunostomy bypass have been reported [62–66]. Each technique involves the LAMS being placed between the stomach and the small intestine distal to the obstructed bowel under EUS and fluoroscopic guidance. Limitations of the traditional approaches (surgical bypass and enteral stent placement) include surgical morbidity and risk of stent occlusion due to tumor ingrowth/overgrowth. Potential advantages of EUS-GE over traditional approaches include less invasiveness (versus surgery) and longer stent patency (versus enteral stent placement). An international, multicenter, retrospective study comparing EUS-GE with laparoscopic GE showed that EUS-GE had similar technical and clinical success rates with reduced time to oral intake, shorter hospital duration and fewer adverse events [67]. A systematic review and meta-analysis comparing EUS-GE and enteral stenting showed that EUS-GE was associated with a significantly lower rate of reintervention despite a comparable technical/clinical success and safety profile [68]. A systematic review and meta-analysis comparing EUS-GE with surgical bypass and enteral stenting demonstrated that EUS-GE was associated with improved outcomes compared to enteral stenting and with shorter hospital stays compared to surgical bypass.

Several case reports have also described the efficacy of EUS-GE in combination with EUS-BD for the management of combined biliary and duodenal obstruction [69–71]. Important advantages of these EUS-guided procedures are the ability to bypass the tumor, reducing the risk of stent occlusion due to tumor ingrowth/overgrowth. Thus, a combination of EUS-BD and EUS-GE may become the optimal procedure for combined biliary and duodenal obstruction in the future. However, several issues remain unresolved. First, EUS-GE is technically challenging, requiring considerable expertise in both EUS and ERCP. Second, development of dedicated accessories and standardization of the procedure are needed for widespread use. Third, EUS-GE may be technically difficult when malignancies invade the fourth part of the duodenum or the jejunum near the ligament of Treitz. Fourth, EUS-GE is contraindicated in patients with significant ascites.

4. Treatment Strategies for Combined Malignant Biliary and Duodenal Obstruction

Based on the above-mentioned evidence, transpapillary stenting and enteral stenting is currently the standard option, whereas to date, EUS-guided procedures are generally reserved for failed or refractory cases to conventional stenting. EUS-GE is especially reserved for selected specialized high-volume centers with extensive experience.

In type I obstruction, transpapillary stenting is possible if the endoscope can pass through the duodenal stricture or an indwelling duodenal stent. Dilation of the duodenal stricture by a balloon or insertion of a duodenal stent prior to ERCP can facilitate scope insertion. When transpapillary stenting fails, EUS-HGS is the next preferred option. Adding EUS-antegrade stenting to EUS-HGS may allow for longer stent patency [72,73].

In type II obstruction, transpapillary stenting is very difficult because the duodenal obstruction involves the major papilla. Although there are several techniques for transpapillary biliary access including RV techniques under PTBD or EUS guidance, success rates are suboptimal. Furthermore, type II obstruction is reported to be susceptible to duodenal-biliary reflux. Double stenting with EUS-HGS or EUS-CDS using ARMS are potential solutions to overcome this issue.

In type III obstruction, transpapillary stenting is not hindered by duodenal obstruction, which is located distal to the major papilla. As with type II obstruction, type III obstruction is reported to present a high risk of duodenal-biliary reflux. Transpapillary stenting using ARMS may be preferable in this context. EUS-HGS or EUS-CDS using ARMS are also possible alternatives in this scenario.

5. Conclusions

Endoscopic double stenting (transpapillary stenting and enteral stenting) is the current standard of care for combined biliary and duodenal obstruction. However, reports on the usefulness of EUS-guided procedures have recently been increasing. An important advantage of EUS-guided procedures is the ability to create a fistula away from the obstructing tumor. With the development of dedicated devices and standardization of the procedure, EUS-guided procedures including EUS-HGS, EUS-CDS and EUS-GE can potentially become the standard of care treatment in the future. The development of new stent types, including ARMS and LAMS, also plays an important role in the management of combined biliary and duodenal obstruction.

Author Contributions: Conceptualization, T.T. and T.S.; writing—original draft preparation, T.T.; writing—review and editing, T.S. and T.O.; supervision, N.S. All authors have read and agreed to the published version of the manuscript.

Funding: This research received no external funding.

Institutional Review Board Statement: Not applicable.

Informed Consent Statement: Not applicable.

Data Availability Statement: Not applicable.

Conflicts of Interest: T.S. has received honoraria from Boston Scientific Japan, Cook Medical, Kawasumi Laboratories, Century Medical, MEDICO'S HIRATA, SUMITOMO BAKELITE, CREATE MEDIC. N.S. has received honararia from Boston Scientific Japan, Cook Medical, Kawasumi Laboratories, Gadelius Medical and consultancies from Gadelius Medical. The other authors declare no conflict of interest.

References

1. Bartlett, E.K.; Wachtel, H.; Fraker, D.L.; Vollmer, C.M.; Drebin, J.A.; Kelz, R.R.; Karakousis, G.C.; Roses, R.E. Surgical palliation for pancreatic malignancy: Practice patterns and predictors of morbidity and mortality. *J. Gastrointest. Surg.* **2014**, *18*, 1292–1298. [CrossRef] [PubMed]
2. Kohan, G.; Ocampo, C.G.; Zandalazini, H.I.; Klappenbach, R.; Yazyi, F.; Ditulio, O.; Coturel, A.; Canullán, C.; Porras, L.T.C.; Rodriguez, J.A. Laparoscopic hepaticojejunostomy and gastrojejunostomy for palliative treatment of pancreatic head cancer in 48 patients. *Surg. Endosc.* **2015**, *29*, 1970–1975. [CrossRef]
3. Lyons, J.M.; Karkar, A.; Correa-Gallego, C.C.; D'Angelica, M.I.; DeMatteo, R.P.; Fong, Y.; Kingham, T.P.; Jarnagin, W.R.; Brennan, M.F.; Allen, P.J. Operative procedures for unresectable pancreatic cancer: Does operative bypass decrease requirements for postoperative procedures and in-hospital days? *HPB* **2012**, *14*, 469–475. [CrossRef] [PubMed]
4. Kim, K.O.; Kim, T.N.; Lee, H.C. Effectiveness of combined biliary and duodenal stenting in patients with malignant biliary and duodenal obstruction. *Scand. J. Gastroenterol.* **2012**, *47*, 962–967. [CrossRef]
5. Mutignani, M.; Tringali, A.; Shah, S.G.; Perri, V.; Familiari, P.; Iacopini, F.; Spada, C.; Costamagna, G. Combined endoscopic stent insertion in malignant biliary and duodenal obstruction. *Endoscopy* **2007**, *39*, 440–447. [CrossRef]
6. Staub, J.; Siddiqui, A.; Taylor, L.J.; Loren, D.; Kowalski, T.; Adler, D.G. ERCP performed through previously placed duodenal stents: A multicenter retrospective study of outcomes and adverse events. *Gastrointest. Endosc.* **2018**, *87*, 1499–1504. [CrossRef] [PubMed]
7. Yao, J.F.; Zhang, L.; Wu, H. Analysis of high risk factors for endoscopic retrograde cholangiopancreatography biliary metallic stenting after malignant duodenal stricture SEMS implantation. *J. Biol. Regul. Homeost. Agents* **2016**, *30*, 743–748.
8. Hamada, T.; Nakai, Y.; Isayama, H.; Sasaki, T.; Kogure, H.; Kawakubo, K.; Sasahira, N.; Yamamoto, N.; Togawa, O.; Mizuno, S.; et al. Duodenal metal stent placement is a risk factor for biliary metal stent dysfunction: An analysis using a time-dependent covariate. *Surg. Endosc.* **2013**, *27*, 1243–1248. [CrossRef]
9. Sato, T.; Hara, K.; Mizuno, N.; Hijioka, S.; Imaoka, H.; Yogi, T.; Tsutsumi, H.; Fujiyoshi, T.; Niwa, Y.; Tajika, M.; et al. Type of Combined Endoscopic Biliary and Gastroduodenal Stenting Is Significant for Biliary Route Maintenance. *Intern. Med.* **2016**, *55*, 2153–2161. [CrossRef]

10. Matsumoto, K.; Kato, H.; Tsutsumi, K.; Mizukawa, S.; Yabe, S.; Seki, H.; Akimoto, Y.; Uchida, D.; Tomoda, T.; Yamamoto, N.; et al. Long-term outcomes and risk factors of biliary stent dysfunction after endoscopic double stenting for malignant biliary and duodenal obstructions. *Dig. Endosc.* **2017**, *29*, 617–625. [CrossRef]
11. Tonozuka, R.; Itoi, T.; Sofuni, A.; Itokawa, F.; Moriyasu, F. Endoscopic double stenting for the treatment of malignant biliary and duodenal obstruction due to pancreatic cancer. *Dig. Endosc.* **2013**, *25* (Suppl. 2), 100–108. [CrossRef]
12. Hamada, T.; Nakai, Y.; Lau, J.Y.; Moon, J.H.; Hayashi, T.; Yasuda, I.; Hu, B.; Seo, D.W.; Kawakami, H.; Kuwatani, M.; et al. International study of endoscopic management of distal malignant biliary obstruction combined with duodenal obstruction. *Scand. J. Gastroenterol.* **2018**, *53*, 46–55. [CrossRef] [PubMed]
13. Sasaki, T.; Yamada, I.; Matsuyama, M.; Sasahira, N. Enteral stent placement for malignant afferent loop obstruction by the through-the-scope technique using a short-type single-balloon enteroscope. *Endosc. Int. Open* **2018**, *6*, E806–E811. [CrossRef] [PubMed]
14. Shimatani, M.; Takaoka, M.; Tokuhara, M.; Kato, K.; Miyoshi, H.; Ikeura, T.; Okazaki, K. Through-the-scope self-expanding metal stent placement using newly developed short double-balloon endoscope for the effective management of malignant afferent-loop obstruction. *Endoscopy* **2016**, *48* (Suppl. 1), E6–E7. [CrossRef]
15. Minaga, K.; Kitano, M.; Takenaka, M. Through-the-scope enteral metal stent placement using a short-type single-balloon enteroscope for malignant surgically reconstructed jejunal stenosis (with video). *Dig. Endosc.* **2016**, *28*, 758. [CrossRef] [PubMed]
16. Tsutsumi, K.; Kato, H.; Okada, H. Impact of a Newly Developed Short Double-Balloon Enteroscope on Stent Placement in Patients with Surgically Altered Anatomies. *Gut Liver* **2017**, *11*, 306–311. [CrossRef]
17. Fábián, A.; Bor, R.; Gede, N.; Bacsur, P.; Pécsi, D.; Hegyi, P.; Tóth, B.; Szakács, Z.; Vincze, Á.; Ruzsics, I.; et al. Double Stenting for Malignant Biliary and Duodenal Obstruction: A Systematic Review and Meta-Analysis. *Clin. Transl. Gastroenterol.* **2020**, *11*, e00161. [CrossRef] [PubMed]
18. Moon, J.H.; Choi, H.J. Endoscopic double-metallic stenting for malignant biliary and duodenal obstructions. *J. Hepatobiliary Pancreat Sci.* **2011**, *18*, 658–663. [CrossRef]
19. Jeurnink, S.M.; Steyerberg, E.W.; van Hooft, J.E.; van Eijck, C.H.; Schwartz, M.P.; Vleggaar, F.P.; Kuipers, E.J.; Siersema, P.D.; Dutch Sustent Study Group. Surgical gastrojejunostomy or endoscopic stent placement for the palliation of malignant gastric outlet obstruction (SUSTENT study): A multicenter randomized trial. *Gastrointest. Endosc.* **2010**, *71*, 490–499. [CrossRef]
20. Manuel-Vázquez, A.; Latorre-Fragua, R.; Ramiro-Pérez, C.; López-Marcano, A.; la Plaza-Llamas, R.; Ramia, J.M. Laparoscopic gastrojejunostomy for gastric outlet obstruction in patients with unresectable hepatopancreatobiliary cancers: A personal series and systematic review of the literature. *World J. Gastroenterol.* **2018**, *24*, 1978–1988. [CrossRef]
21. Min, S.H.; Son, S.Y.; Jung, D.H.; Lee, C.M.; Ahn, S.H.; Park, D.J.; Kim, H.H. Laparoscopic gastrojejunostomy versus duodenal stenting in unresectable gastric cancer with gastric outlet obstruction. *Ann. Surg. Treat. Res.* **2017**, *93*, 130–136. [CrossRef] [PubMed]
22. Kobayashi, S.; Ueno, M.; Nagashima, S.; Sano, Y.; Kawano, K.; Fukushima, T.; Asama, H.; Tezuka, S.; Morimoto, M. Association between time to stent dysfunction and the anti-tumour effect of systemic chemotherapy following stent placement in patients with pancreaticobiliary cancers and malignant gastric outlet obstruction: A retrospective cohort study. *BMC Cancer* **2021**, *21*, 576. [CrossRef] [PubMed]
23. Yoshida, Y.; Fukutomi, A.; Tanaka, M.; Sugiura, T.; Kawata, N.; Kawai, S.; Kito, Y.; Hamauchi, S.; Tsushima, T.; Yokota, T.; et al. Gastrojejunostomy versus duodenal stent placement for gastric outlet obstruction in patients with unresectable pancreatic cancer. *Pancreatology* **2017**, *17*, 983–989. [CrossRef]
24. Matsumoto, K.; Kato, H.; Horiguchi, S.; Tsutsumi, K.; Saragai, Y.; Takada, S.; Mizukawa, S.; Muro, S.; Uchida, D.; Tomoda, T.; et al. Efficacy and safety of chemotherapy after endoscopic double stenting for malignant duodenal and biliary obstructions in patients with advanced pancreatic cancer: A single-institution retrospective analysis. *BMC Gastroenterol.* **2018**, *18*, 157. [CrossRef]
25. Iqbal, U.; Khara, H.S.; Hu, Y.; Kumar, V.; Tufail, K.; Confer, B.; Diehl, D.L. EUS-guided gastroenterostomy for the management of gastric outlet obstruction: A systematic review and meta-analysis. *Endosc. Ultrasound* **2020**, *9*, 16–23. [CrossRef]
26. Chen, Y.I.; Itoi, T.; Baron, T.H.; Nieto, J.; Haito-Chavez, Y.; Grimm, I.S.; Ismail, A.; Ngamruengphong, S.; Bukhari, M.; Hajiyeva, G.; et al. EUS-guided gastroenterostomy is comparable to enteral stenting with fewer re-interventions in malignant gastric outlet obstruction. *Surg. Endosc.* **2017**, *31*, 2946–2952. [CrossRef]
27. Chen, Y.I.; Kunda, R.; Storm, A.C.; Aridi, H.D.; Thompson, C.C.; Nieto, J.; James, T.; Irani, S.; Bukhari, M.; Gutierrez, O.B.; et al. EUS-guided gastroenterostomy: A multicenter study comparing the direct and balloon-assisted techniques. *Gastrointest. Endosc.* **2018**, *87*, 1215–1221. [CrossRef] [PubMed]
28. Ge, P.S.; Young, J.Y.; Dong, W.; Thompson, C.C. EUS-guided gastroenterostomy versus enteral stent placement for palliation of malignant gastric outlet obstruction. *Surg. Endosc.* **2019**, *33*, 3404–3411. [CrossRef]
29. Oikarinen, H.; Leinonen, S.; Karttunen, A.; Tikkakoski, T.; Hetemaa, T.; Mäkelä, J.; Päivänsalo, M. Patency and complications of percutaneously inserted metallic stents in malignant biliary obstruction. *J. Vasc. Interv. Radiol.* **1999**, *10*, 1387–1393. [CrossRef]
30. Lee, T.H.; Choi, J.H.; Park, D.H.; Song, T.J.; Kim, D.U.; Paik, W.H.; Hwangbo, Y.; Lee, S.S.; Seo, D.W.; Lee, S.K.; et al. Similar Efficacies of Endoscopic Ultrasound-guided Transmural and Percutaneous Drainage for Malignant Distal Biliary Obstruction. *Clin. Gastroenterol. Hepatol.* **2016**, *14*, 1011–1019. [CrossRef]
31. Wang, K.; Zhu, J.; Xing, L.; Wang, Y.; Jin, Z.; Li, Z. Assessment of efficacy and safety of EUS-guided biliary drainage: A systematic review. *Gastrointest. Endosc.* **2016**, *83*, 1218–1227. [CrossRef] [PubMed]

32. Khashab, M.A.; Van der Merwe, S.; Kunda, R.; El Zein, M.H.; Teoh, A.Y.; Marson, F.P.; Fabbri, C.; Tarantino, I.; Varadarajulu, S.; Modayil, R.J.; et al. Prospective international multicenter study on endoscopic ultrasound-guided biliary drainage for patients with malignant distal biliary obstruction after failed endoscopic retrograde cholangiopancreatography. *Endosc. Int. Open* **2016**, *4*, E487–E496. [CrossRef]
33. Park, J.K.; Woo, Y.S.; Noh, D.H.; Yang, J.I.; Bae, S.Y.; Yun, H.S.; Lee, J.K.; Lee, K.T.; Lee, K.H. Efficacy of EUS-guided and ERCP-guided biliary drainage for malignant biliary obstruction: Prospective randomized controlled study. *Gastrointest. Endosc.* **2018**, *88*, 277–282. [CrossRef] [PubMed]
34. Bang, J.Y.; Navaneethan, U.; Hasan, M.; Hawes, R.; Varadarajulu, S. Stent placement by EUS or ERCP for primary biliary decompression in pancreatic cancer: A randomized trial (with videos). *Gastrointest. Endosc.* **2018**, *88*, 9–17. [CrossRef] [PubMed]
35. Yamao, K.; Kitano, M.; Takenaka, M.; Minaga, K.; Sakurai, T.; Watanabe, T.; Kayahara, T.; Yoshikawa, T.; Yamashita, Y.; Asada, M.; et al. Outcomes of endoscopic biliary drainage in pancreatic cancer patients with an indwelling gastroduodenal stent: A multicenter cohort study in West Japan. *Gastrointest. Endosc.* **2018**, *88*, 66–75. [CrossRef] [PubMed]
36. Hamada, T.; Isayama, H.; Nakai, Y.; Togawa, O.; Kogure, H.; Kawakubo, K.; Tsujino, T.; Sasahira, N.; Hirano, K.; Yamamoto, N.; et al. Transmural biliary drainage can be an alternative to transpapillary drainage in patients with an indwelling duodenal stent. *Dig. Dis. Sci.* **2014**, *59*, 1931–1938. [CrossRef]
37. Hamada, T.; Isayama, H.; Nakai, Y.; Togawa, O.; Kogure, H.; Kawakubo, K.; Takeshi, T.; Sasahira, N.; Hirano, K.; Yamamoto, N.; et al. Duodenal invasion is a risk factor for the early dysfunction of biliary metal stents in unresectable pancreatic cancer. *Gastrointest. Endosc.* **2011**, *74*, 548–555. [CrossRef]
38. Ogura, T.; Chiba, Y.; Masuda, D.; Kitano, M.; Sano, T.; Saori, O.; Yamamoto, K.; Imaoka, H.; Imoto, A.; Takeuchi, T.; et al. Comparison of the clinical impact of endoscopic ultrasound-guided choledochoduodenostomy and hepaticogastrostomy for bile duct obstruction with duodenal obstruction. *Endoscopy* **2016**, *48*, 156–163. [CrossRef] [PubMed]
39. Minaga, K.; Ogura, T.; Shiomi, H.; Imai, H.; Hoki, N.; Takenaka, M.; Nishikiori, H.; Yamashita, Y.; Hisa, T.; Kato, H.; et al. Comparison of the efficacy and safety of endoscopic ultrasound-guided choledochoduodenostomy and hepaticogastrostomy for malignant distal biliary obstruction: Multicenter, randomized, clinical trial. *Dig. Endosc.* **2019**, *31*, 575–582. [CrossRef]
40. Kaw, M.; Singh, S.; Gagneja, H. Clinical outcome of simultaneous self-expandable metal stents for palliation of malignant biliary and duodenal obstruction. *Surg. Endosc.* **2003**, *17*, 457–461. [CrossRef]
41. Vanbiervliet, G.; Demarquay, J.F.; Dumas, R.; Caroli-Bosc, F.X.; Piche, T.; Tran, A. Endoscopic insertion of biliary stents in 18 patients with metallic duodenal stents who developed secondary malignant obstructive jaundice. *Gastroenterol. Clin. Biol.* **2004**, *28*, 1209–1213. [CrossRef]
42. Maire, F.; Hammel, P.; Ponsot, P.; Aubert, A.; O'toole, D.; Hentic, O.; Levy, P.; Ruszniewski, P. Long-term outcome of biliary and duodenal stents in palliative treatment of patients with unresectable adenocarcinoma of the head of pancreas. *Am. J. Gastroenterol.* **2006**, *101*, 735–742. [CrossRef] [PubMed]
43. Khashab, M.A.; Valeshabad, A.K.; Leung, W.; Camilo, J.; Fukami, N.; Shieh, F.; Diehl, D.; Attam, R.; Vleggaar, F.P.; Saxena, P.; et al. Multicenter experience with performance of ERCP in patients with an indwelling duodenal stent. *Endoscopy* **2014**, *46*, 252–255. [CrossRef] [PubMed]
44. Yu, J.; Hao, J.; Wu, D.; Lang, H. Retrospective evaluation of endoscopic stenting of combined malignant common bile duct and gastric outlet-duodenum obstructions. *Exp. Ther. Med.* **2014**, *8*, 1173–1177. [CrossRef]
45. Canena, J.; Coimbra, J.; Carvalho, D.; Rodrigues, C.; Silva, M.; Costa, M.; Horta, D.; Dias, A.M.; Seves, I.; Ramos, G.; et al. Endoscopic bilio-duodenal bypass: Outcomes of primary and revision efficacy of combined metallic stents in malignant duodenal and biliary obstructions. *Dig. Dis. Sci.* **2014**, *59*, 2779–2789. [CrossRef] [PubMed]
46. Manta, R.; Conigliaro, R.; Mangiafico, S.; Forti, E.; Bertani, H.; Frazzoni, M.; Galloro, G.; Mutignani, M.; Zullo, A. A multimodal, one-session endoscopic approach for management of patients with advanced pancreatic cancer. *Surg. Endosc.* **2016**, *30*, 1863–1868. [CrossRef] [PubMed]
47. Hori, Y.; Naitoh, I.; Hayashi, K.; Kondo, H.; Yoshida, M.; Shimizu, S.; Hirano, A.; Okumura, F.; Ando, T.; Jinno, N.; et al. Covered duodenal self-expandable metal stents prolong biliary stent patency in double stenting: The largest series of bilioduodenal obstruction. *J. Gastroenterol. Hepatol.* **2018**, *33*, 696–703. [CrossRef]
48. Debourdeau, A.; Caillol, F.; Zemmour, C.; Winkler, J.P.; Decoster, C.; Pesenti, C.; Ratone, J.P.; Boher, J.M.; Giovannini, M. Endoscopic management of concomitant biliary and duodenal malignant obstruction: Impact of the timing of drainage for one vs. two procedures and the modalities of biliary drainage. *Endosc. Ultrasound* **2021**, *10*, 124–133. [CrossRef]
49. Mangiavillano, B.; Kunda, R.; Robles-Medranda, C.; Oleas, R.; Anderloni, A.; Sportes, A.; Fabbri, C.; Binda, C.; Auriemma, F.; Eusebi, L.H.; et al. Lumen-apposing metal stent through the meshes of duodenal metal stents for palliation of malignant jaundice. *Endosc. Int. Open* **2021**, *9*, E324–E330. [CrossRef]
50. Boumitri, C.; Gaidhane, M.; Kahaleh, M. Antireflux metallic biliary stents: Where do we stand? *Gastrointest. Endosc.* **2016**, *83*, 413–415. [CrossRef]
51. Dua, K.S.; Reddy, N.D.; Rao, V.G.; Banerjee, R.; Medda, B.; Lang, I. Impact of reducing duodenobiliary reflux on biliary stent patency: An in vitro evaluation and a prospective randomized clinical trial that used a biliary stent with an antireflux valve. *Gastrointest. Endosc.* **2007**, *65*, 819–828. [CrossRef] [PubMed]

2. Lee, K.J.; Chung, M.J.; Park, J.Y.; Lee, D.H.; Jung, S.; Bang, B.W.; Park, S.W.; Chung, J.B.; Song, S.Y.; Bang, S. Clinical advantages of a metal stent with an S-shaped anti-reflux valve in malignant biliary obstruction. *Dig. Endosc.* **2013**, *25*, 308–312. [CrossRef] [PubMed]
3. Hu, B.; Wang, T.T.; Wu, J.; Shi, Z.M.; Gao, D.J.; Pan, Y.M. Antireflux stents to reduce the risk of cholangitis in patients with malignant biliary strictures: A randomized trial. *Endoscopy* **2014**, *46*, 120–126. [CrossRef] [PubMed]
4. Lee, Y.N.; Moon, J.H.; Choi, H.J.; Choi, M.H.; Lee, T.H.; Cha, S.W.; Cho, Y.D.; Choi, S.Y.; Lee, H.K.; Park, S.H. Effectiveness of a newly designed antireflux valve metal stent to reduce duodenobiliary reflux in patients with unresectable distal malignant biliary obstruction: A randomized, controlled pilot study (with videos). *Gastrointest. Endosc.* **2016**, *83*, 404–412. [CrossRef]
5. Hamada, T.; Isayama, H.; Nakai, Y.; Iwashita, T.; Ito, Y.; Mukai, T.; Yagioka, H.; Saito, T.; Togawa, O.; Ryozawa, S.; et al. Antireflux covered metal stent for nonresectable distal malignant biliary obstruction: Multicenter randomized controlled trial. *Dig. Endosc.* **2019**, *31*, 566–574. [CrossRef] [PubMed]
6. Hamada, T.; Nakai, Y.; Isayama, H.; Koike, K. Antireflux metal stent for biliary obstruction: Any benefits? *Dig. Endosc.* **2021**, *33*, 310–320. [CrossRef] [PubMed]
7. Kin, T.; Ishii, K.; Okabe, Y.; Itoi, T.; Katanuma, A. Feasibility of biliary stenting to distal malignant biliary obstruction using a novel designed metal stent with duckbill-shaped anti-reflux valve. *Dig. Endosc.* **2021**, *33*, 648–655. [CrossRef] [PubMed]
8. Yamada, Y.; Sasaki, T.; Takeda, T.; Mie, T.; Furukawa, T.; Kasuga, A.; Matsuyama, M.; Ozaka, M.; Igarashi, Y.; Sasahira, N. A novel laser-cut fully covered metal stent with anti-reflux valve in patients with malignant distal biliary obstruction refractory to conventional covered metal stent. *J. Hepatobiliary Pancreat Sci.* **2021**. [CrossRef]
9. Sasaki, T.; Takeda, T.; Sasahira, N. Double stenting with EUS-CDS using a new anti-reflux metal stent for combined malignant biliary and duodenal obstruction. *J. Hepatobiliary Pancreat Sci.* **2020**, *27*, e15–e16. [CrossRef] [PubMed]
10. Binmoeller, K.F.; Shah, J. A novel lumen-apposing stent for transluminal drainage of nonadherent extraintestinal fluid collections. *Endoscopy* **2011**, *43*, 337–342. [CrossRef]
11. Mussetto, A.; Fugazza, A.; Fuccio, L.; Triossi, O.; Repici, A.; Anderloni, A. Current uses and outcomes of lumen-apposing metal stents. *Ann. Gastroenterol.* **2018**, *31*, 535–540. [CrossRef]
12. Khashab, M.A.; Kumbhari, V.; Grimm, I.S.; Ngamruengphong, S.; Aguila, G.; El Zein, M.; Kalloo, A.N.; Baron, T.H. EUS-guided gastroenterostomy: The first U.S. clinical experience (with video). *Gastrointest. Endosc.* **2015**, *82*, 932–938. [CrossRef] [PubMed]
13. Itoi, T.; Ishii, K.; Ikeuchi, N.; Sofuni, A.; Gotoda, T.; Moriyasu, F.; Dhir, V.; Teoh, A.Y.B.; Binmoeller, K.F. Prospective evaluation of endoscopic ultrasonography-guided double-balloon-occluded gastrojejunostomy bypass (EPASS) for malignant gastric outlet obstruction. *Gut* **2016**, *65*, 193–195. [CrossRef] [PubMed]
14. Irani, S.; Itoi, T.; Baron, T.H.; Khashab, M. EUS-guided gastroenterostomy: Techniques from East to West. *VideoGIE* **2020**, *5*, 48–50. [CrossRef]
15. Itoi, T.; Baron, T.H.; Khashab, M.A.; Tsuchiya, T.; Irani, S.; Dhir, V.; Bun Teoh, A.Y. Technical review of endoscopic ultrasonography-guided gastroenterostomy in 2017. *Dig. Endosc.* **2017**, *29*, 495–502. [CrossRef] [PubMed]
16. Marino, A.; Bessissow, A.; Miller, C.; Valenti, D.; Boucher, L.; Chaudhury, P.; Barkun, J.; Forbes, N.; Khashab, M.A.; Martel, M.; et al. Modified endoscopic ultrasound-guided double-balloon-occluded gastroenterostomy bypass (M-EPASS): A pilot study. *Endoscopy* **2021**. [CrossRef]
17. Bronswijk, M.; Vanella, G.; van Malenstein, H.; Laleman, W.; Jaekers, J.; Topal, B.; Daams, F.; Besselink, M.G.; Arcidiacono, P.G.; Voermans, R.P.; et al. Laparoscopic versus EUS-guided gastroenterostomy for gastric outlet obstruction: An international multicenter propensity score-matched comparison (with video). *Gastrointest. Endosc.* **2021**. [CrossRef] [PubMed]
18. Chandan, S.; Khan, S.R.; Mohan, B.P.; Shah, A.R.; Bilal, M.; Ramai, D.; Bhogal, N.; Dhindsa, B.; Kassab, L.L.; Singh, S.; et al. EUS-guided gastroenterostomy versus enteral stenting for gastric outlet obstruction: Systematic review and meta-analysis. *Endosc. Int. Open* **2021**, *9*, E496–E504. [CrossRef]
19. Kongkam, P.; Luangsukrerk, T.; Harinwan, K.; Vanduangden, K.; Plaidum, S.; Rerknimitr, R.; Kullavanijaya, P. Combination of endoscopic-ultrasound guided choledochoduodenostomy and gastrojejunostomy resolving combined distal biliary and duodenal obstruction. *Endoscopy* **2020**. [CrossRef]
20. Lajin, M. EUS-guided choledocoduodenostomy and gastroenterostomy to palliate simultaneous biliary and duodenal obstruction due to pancreatic cancer. *Endosc. Int. Open* **2020**, *8*, E1681–E1682. [CrossRef]
21. Platt, K.D.; Bhalla, S.; Sondhi, A.R.; Millet, J.D.; Law, R.J. EUS-guided gastrojejunostomy and hepaticogastrostomy for malignant duodenal and biliary obstruction. *VideoGIE* **2021**, *6*, 95–97. [CrossRef] [PubMed]
22. Imai, H.; Takenaka, M.; Omoto, S.; Kamata, K.; Miyata, T.; Minaga, K.; Yamao, K.; Sakurai, T.; Nishida, N.; Watanabe, T.; et al. Utility of Endoscopic Ultrasound-Guided Hepaticogastrostomy with Antegrade Stenting for Malignant Biliary Obstruction after Failed Endoscopic Retrograde Cholangiopancreatography. *Oncology* **2017**, *93* (Suppl. 1), 69–75. [CrossRef] [PubMed]
23. Yamamoto, K.; Itoi, T.; Tsuchiya, T.; Tanaka, R.; Tonozuka, R.; Honjo, M.; Mukai, S.; Fujita, M.; Asai, Y.; Matsunami, Y.; et al. EUS-guided antegrade metal stenting with hepaticoenterostomy using a dedicated plastic stent with a review of the literature (with video). *Endosc. Ultrasound* **2018**, *7*, 404–412. [CrossRef] [PubMed]

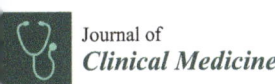

Article

Clinical Outcomes of Early Endoscopic Transpapillary Biliary Drainage for Acute Cholangitis Associated with Disseminated Intravascular Coagulation

Akihiro Sekine [1], Kazunari Nakahara [1,*], Junya Sato [1], Yosuke Michikawa [1], Keigo Suetani [2], Ryo Morita [3], Yosuke Igarashi [1] and Fumio Itoh [1]

1. Department of Gastroenterology and Hepatology, St. Marianna University School of Medicine, Kawasaki 216-8511, Japan; akihiro.sekine@marianna-u.ac.jp (A.S.); j2sato@marianna-u.ac.jp (J.S.); y2michikawa@marianna-u.ac.jp (Y.M.); y2igarashi@marianna-u.ac.jp (Y.I.); fitoh@marianna-u.ac.jp (F.I.)
2. Department of Gastroenterology and Hepatology, Kawasaki Municipal Tama Hospital, Kawasaki 214-8525, Japan; k2suetani@marianna-u.ac.jp
3. Department of Gastroenterology, Morita Hospital, Sagamihara 252-0159, Japan; r2morita@marianna-u.ac.jp
* Correspondence: nakahara@marianna-u.ac.jp; Tel.: +81-44-977-8111

Abstract: Acute cholangitis (AC) is often associated with disseminated intravascular coagulation (DIC), and endoscopic transpapillary biliary drainage (EBD) under endoscopic retrograde cholangiopancreatography (ERCP) is a treatment of choice. However, no evidence exists on the outcomes of EBD for AC associated with DIC. Therefore, we retrospectively evaluated the treatment outcomes of early EBD and compared endoscopic biliary stenting (EBS) and endoscopic nasobiliary drainage (ENBD). We included 62 patients who received early EBD (EBS: 30, ENBD: 32) for AC, associated with DIC. The rates of clinical success for AC and DIC resolution at 7 days after EBD were 90.3% and 88.7%, respectively. Mean hospitalization period was 31.7 days, and in-hospital mortality rate was 4.8%. ERCP-related adverse events developed in 3.2% of patients (bleeding in two patients). Comparison between EBS and ENBD groups showed that the ENBD group included patients with more severe cholangitis, and acute physiology and chronic health evaluation II score, systemic inflammatory response syndrome score, and serum bilirubin level were significantly higher in this group. However, no significant difference was observed in clinical outcomes between the two groups; both EBS and ENBD were effective. In conclusion, early EBD is effective and safe for patients with AC associated with DIC.

Keywords: acute cholangitis; disseminated intravascular coagulation; endoscopic biliary drainage; endoscopic retrograde cholangiopancreatography; clinical outcome

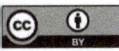

1. Introduction

Acute cholangitis (AC) is often associated with disseminated intravascular coagulation (DIC), which can be fatal without prompt and appropriate treatment intervention. Treatment of the primary disease causing DIC remains the most important factor in the resolution of the pathological conditions underlying DIC, and the prognosis of patients with DIC may be markedly affected by the treatment outcome of the primary disease [1].

Endoscopic transpapillary biliary drainage (EBD) under endoscopic retrograde cholangiopancreatography (ERCP) is the first choice of treatment for AC [2,3]. Endoscopic sphincterotomy (EST) is generally performed before EBD to facilitate insertion of a device into the bile duct or prevention of post-ERCP pancreatitis [4,5]. Moreover, bile outflow can be expected not only through the stent but also through the papilla opened by EST. Nevertheless, when AC is combined with DIC, EBD without EST is generally required because of the high risk for post-EST bleeding. Furthermore, in severe AC associated with DIC, poor drainage or clogging in the stent due to the high viscosity of infected bile and hemobilia associated with contact of the device with the bile duct is a concern in EBD.

EBD methods include endoscopic biliary stenting (EBS) and endoscopic nasobiliary drainage (ENBD). EBS is an internal drainage method with no discomfort and no loss of electrolytes or fluid. In contrast, ENBD is an external drainage method with the advantages of monitoring the bile, performing bile cultures, and washing the catheter. However, patients undergoing ENBD treatment will be uncomfortable because of the transnasal tube and may even pull it out. A few studies compared EBS and ENBD in cases of severe AC. The majority of previous reports demonstrated that no difference existed in the safety and efficacy between EBS and ENBD [6–9], but a report that ENBD demonstrates better drainage than EBS also exists [10]; nonetheless, no sufficient evidence exists. Furthermore, no study exists on the treatment outcomes of EBD for AC associated with DIC.

Therefore, we conducted this study to evaluate the treatment outcomes of early EBD performed within 24 h after the diagnosis of AC associated with DIC and to further compare the outcomes between EBS and ENBD. This is a single-center, retrospective study. To our knowledge, this study is the first to evaluate the role of EBD in AC associated with DIC.

2. Materials and Methods

2.1. Patients

In this retrospective study, we investigated the clinical data of 5637 consecutive patients who received ERCP between April 2006 and March 2019 at St. Marianna University School of Medicine Hospital. The inclusion criteria were (1) EBD performed for AC associated with DIC; (2) initial EBD for naïve papilla; (3) EBD performed within 24 h after the diagnosis of AC associated with DIC; and (4) age ≥ 20 years. The exclusion criteria were (1) past history of choledochojejunostomy; (2) history of EST; (3) placement of biliary stent or nasobiliary drainage catheter; (4) EBD performed at >24 h after the diagnosis of AC, and (5) lack of sufficient data in the medical record.

All patients provided written informed consent for the endoscopic procedures. This study was approved by the institutional review board of St. Marianna University School of Medicine (approval number: 5357).

2.2. Endoscopic Procedures

ERCP was performed using a duodenoscope with patients under moderate/deep sedation. In general, we performed bile duct cannulation by contrast cannulation or wire-guided cannulation. When biliary cannulation was difficult, we attempted the pancreatic guidewire method or the pancreatic stent placement method. In principle, precut, EST, or stone removal was not performed for patients with DIC. However, the decision to perform precut, EST, or stone removal was left to the discretion of the attending physician. We placed a 7-Fr plastic stent for EBS or a 6-Fr nasodrainage catheter for ENBD. All patients received blood tests 3 h after ERCP.

All ERCP procedures were conducted under the supervision of an expert who performed ≥ 1000 ERCP procedures (initials: K.N., Y.M., K.S. and R.M.).

2.3. Measurements

We retrospectively examined the following parameters: patient backgrounds, details of endoscopic procedures, clinical outcomes including the clinical success rate for AC, DIC resolution rate, mortality rate, and ERCP-related adverse events. Then, we and compared these factors between patients who received EBS (EBS group) and those who received ENBD (ENBD group).

2.4. Definitions

The diagnosis and severity of AC were determined according to the Tokyo Guidelines 2018 [11]. The diagnosis of DIC was based on a DIC score of ≥ 4 according to the DIC diagnostic criteria in Japan [12] (Table 1). Early ERCP was defined as ERCP performed within 24 h after the diagnosis of AC associated with DIC. For bile duct cannulation, the conventional method included contrast cannulation and wire-guided cannulation. The duration of procedure time measured from insertion to removal of the scope by reviewing the nursing records. DIC resolution was defined as a decrease in the DIC score to ≤3 within 7 days after EBD. Clinical success of AC was defined as a reduction in serum bilirubin and inflammation parameters and disappearance of signs of cholangitis such as abdominal pain and fever within 7 days after EBD. The diagnosis and severity of adverse events, including pancreatitis, bleeding, and perforation, were determined according to the consensus guidelines provided by Cotton et al. [13]. Hyperamylasemia was defined as an increase in the serum amylase level that was three-fold or higher than the normal limit (>396 IU/L) without associated abdominal pain after ERCP. The hospitalization period included the time required for endoscopic stone removal in additional ERCP sessions.

Table 1. Diagnostic criteria for disseminated intravascular coagulation as defined by the Japanese Association for Acute Medicine.

Diagnostic Criteria for Disseminated Intravascular Coagulation	Points
Systemic inflammatory response syndrome (SIRS) criteria *	
>3	1
0–2	0
Platelet count (PLT), ×103/L	
<80 or >50% decrease within 24 h	3
>80 and <120; or >30% decrease within 24 h	1
>120	0
Prothrombin time international-normalized ratio (PT-INR)	
>1.2	1
<1.2	0
Fibrin/fibrinogen degradation products (FDPs), µg/L	
>25	3
>10 and <25	1
<10	0
Diagnosis of disseminated intravascular coagulation ≥4 points	

* Systemic inflammatory response syndrome (SIRS) criteria
- Fever > 38 °C or < 36 °C
- Heart rate > 90 beats per minute
- Respiratory rate > 20 breaths per minute or a $PaCO_2$ < 32 mmHg
- White blood cell count > 12,000/µL or < 4000/µL or > 10% bands

2.5. Statistical Analysis

Categorical variables were compared using chi-squared test and Fisher's exact test. Continuous parameters were compared using Student's t-test. p values of <0.05 were considered to indicate significance. The statistical analysis was performed using R version 3.4.1 (R Foundation, Vienna, Austria).

3. Results
3.1. Patient Characteristics

Among 5637 patients who received ERCP during the study period, 627 patients received ERCP for AC. Of these 627 patients, 90 (14.4%) presented with AC complicated with DIC. Among these 90 patients, 28 were excluded due to the following conditions: post-pancreatoduodenectomy (one patient), post-EBD (three patients), history of EST (17 patients), bile duct cannulation failure (two patients), no stent/catheter placement (five patients). Finally, 62 patients fulfilled the eligibility criteria and were included in the analysis (Figure 1).

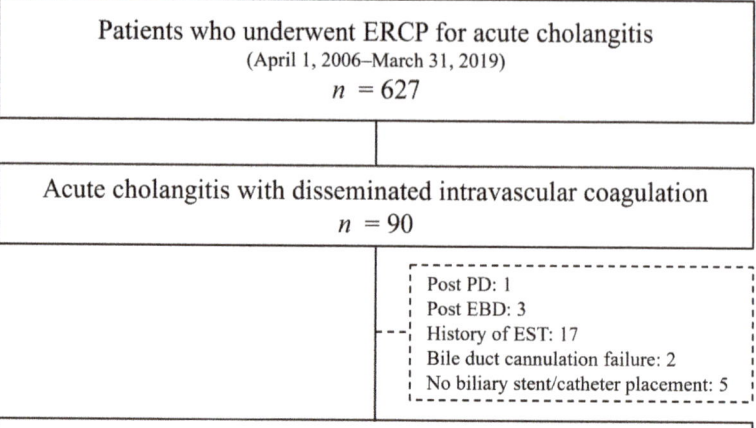

Figure 1. Flowchart of the patient-selection process. ERCP, endoscopic retrograde cholangiopancreatography; PD, pancreatoduodenectomy; EST, endoscopic sphincterotomy; EBD, endoscopic transpapillary drainage.

Table 2 shows the patient's characteristics. Their mean age was 78 years, and 65% were men. The predominant cause of AC was bile duct stone (80.6%). AC was found to be severe in 50 (80.6%), moderate in 10 (16.1%), and mild in 2 (3.2%) patients. The mean acute physiology and chronic health evaluation II (APACHE II) score, DIC score, and systemic inflammatory response syndrome (SIRS) score were 13.8, 5.5, and 2.7, respectively. The most used antibiotic was meropenem (62.9%). As an anticoagulant therapy for DIC, recombinant soluble human thrombomodulin and antithrombin were administered in 45 (72.6%) and 35 (56.5%) patients, respectively (there is some overlapping).

3.2. Endoscopic Procedures

The details of the endoscopic procedures are presented in Table 3. Selective bile duct cannulation was achieved by the conventional method in 50 patients (80.6%). Only one patient (1.6%) received pre-cut and achieved successful bile duct cannulation. Although procedures for the papilla and stone removal were not performed in most cases, EST and stone removal were performed in seven (11.3%) and four (6.5%) patients, respectively. The patients who underwent EST did not meet the diagnostic criteria of DIC before ERCP due to lack of blood test items, but were diagnosed with DIC by a blood test 3 h after ERCP. EBS and ENBD were performed in 30 (48.4%) and 32 (51.6%) patients, respectively. Pancreatic stent for the prevention of post-ERCP pancreatitis was placed in 13 patients (21.0%). The mean procedure duration for ERCP was 31.4 min.

Table 2. Patient backgrounds.

	n = 62
Age (mean ± SD)	77.7 ± 9.4
Sex (Male/Female)	40/22
Etiology of acute cholangitis	
Bile duct stone/Malignant biliary stricture	50/12
Severity of acute cholangitis	
Mild/Moderate/Severe	2/10/50
APACHE II score (mean ± SD)	13.8 ± 6.4
DIC score (mean ± SD)	5.5 ± 1.3
SIRS score (mean ± SD)	2.7 ± 1.1
Serum parameters (mean ± SD)	
WBC ($\times 10^3$/µL)	15.2 ± 8.6
CRP (mg/dL)	13.7 ± 6.4
T-bil (mg/dL)	4.8 ± 3.1
AST (IU/L)	312.2 ± 393.6
ALT (IU/L)	252.4 ± 264.3
Plt ($\times 10^4$/L)	11.1 ± 8.4
FDP (µg/mL)	27.6 ± 20.9
PT-INR	1.47 ± 0.52
Antibiotics	
Carbapenem	46
Sulbactam/Cefoperazone	8
Tazobactam/Piperacillin	3
Others	5
Anticoagulant drugs	
Thrombomodulin	45
Antithrombin	35
Gabexate	39
Gamma globulin	42

SD, standard deviation; APACHE, acute physiology and chronic health evaluation; DIC, disseminated intravascular coagulation; SIRS, systemic inflammatory response syndrome.

Table 3. Endoscopic procedures.

	n = 62
Bile duct cannulation	
Conventional method	50
Pancreatic guidewire method	10
Pancreatic stent placement method	1
Precut	1
Procedure for papilla	
EST	7
Incision range (small/moderate)	3/4
EPBD	2
Biliary drainage	
EBS	30
ENBD	32
Stone removal	4
Use of mechanical lithotripsy	0
Incidental pancreatography	29
Prophylactic pancreatic stenting	13
Procedure time (min, mean ± SD)	31.4 ± 19.8

EST, endoscopic sphincterotomy; EPBD, endoscopic papillary balloon dilation; EBS, endoscopic biliary stenting; ENBD, endoscopic nasobiliary drainage; SD, standard deviation.

3.3. Clinical Outcomes

Table 4 shows the clinical outcomes. The clinical success rate for AC and the DIC resolution rate on day 7 were 90.3% and 88.7%, respectively. Changes in the DIC score and SIRS score, the parameters related to DIC, and the parameters related to AC are shown in

Figures 2–4, respectively. All these parameters showed significant improvement on day 7 compared with those on day 1 of the diagnosis of AC associated with DIC.

The mean hospitalization period was 31.7 days, and the in-hospital mortality rate was 4.8%. Two patients died due to exacerbation of AC and DIC, and another patient died due to ventilator-associated pneumonia. Of the 50 cases with bile duct stone, 47 cases underwent stone removal during the same hospital stay. In the first ERCP session, four patients in the ENBD group underwent stone removal. After improvement of AC and DIC, 23 patients in the EBS group and 20 patients in the ENBD group underwent stone removal. No patient underwent cholecystectomy during the same hospital stay.

Table 4. Clinical outcomes.

	$n = 62$
Clinical success rate for acute cholangitis (% (n))	90.3 (56)
DIC resolution rate (% (n))	88.7 (55)
Number of ERCP sessions (mean ± SD)	2.0 ± 0.6
Hospitalization period (day, mean ± SD)	31.7 ± 21.4
Mortality rate (% (n))	4.8 (3)

DIC, disseminated intravascular coagulation; ERCP, endoscopic retrograde cholangiopancreatography; SD, standard deviation.

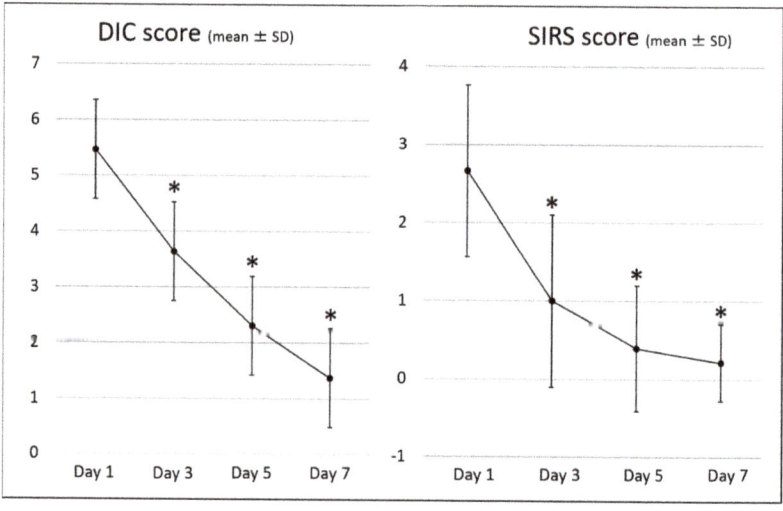

Figure 2. DIC scores and SIRS scores. DIC, disseminated intravascular coagulation; SIRS, systemic inflammatory response syndrome; * $p < 0.05$ vs. baseline.

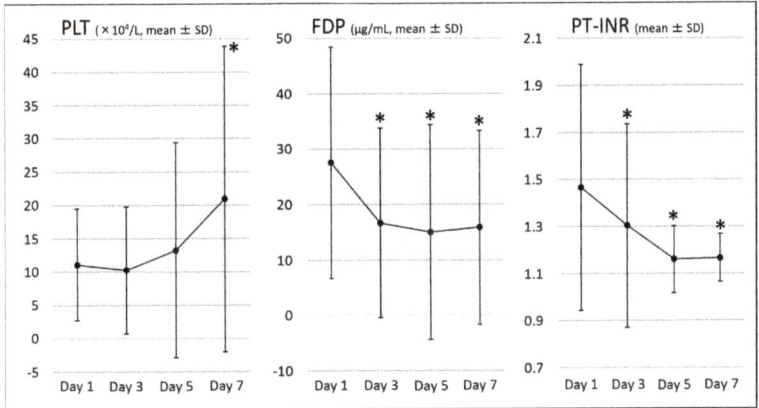

Figure 3. Parameters related to disseminated intravascular coagulation. PLT, platelet; FDP, fibrin degradation product; PT-INR, prothrombin time-international normalized ratio; * $p < 0.05$ vs. baseline.

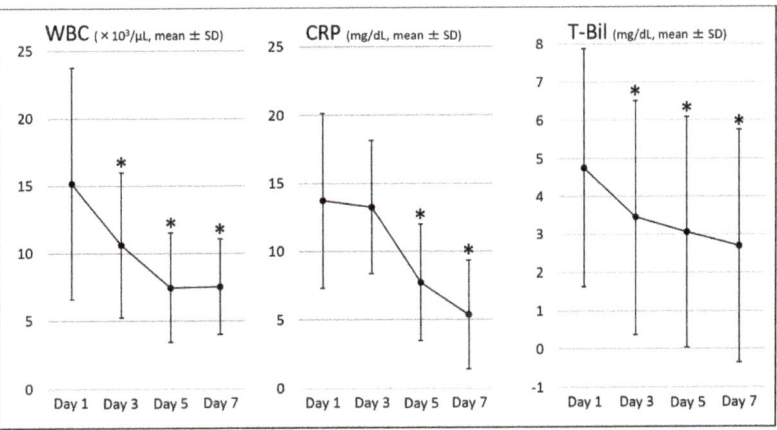

Figure 4. Parameters related to acute cholangitis. WBC, white blood cell; CRP, C-reactive protein; T-Bil, total bilirubin; * $p < 0.05$ vs. baseline.

3.4. Adverse Events

The adverse events are presented in Table 5. The rate of ERCP-related adverse events was 3.2% (2/62). Post-EST bleeding and Mallory–Weiss bleeding occurred in one patient each during endoscopic procedure. Bleeding could be controlled by endoscopic hemostasis by clipping without blood transfusion in both patients. The patient with EST bleeding received anticoagulant therapy with recombinant thrombomodulin, while the patient with Mallory–Weiss did not receive anticoagulant therapy. There was no rebleeding in both cases. Although hyperamylasemia was observed in six patients (6.4%), no patient developed pancreatitis. Two patients pulled out the ENBD catheter, of which one received additional EBS, and the other received stone removal without stent placement.

Table 5. Adverse events.

	n = 62
Total ERCP-related adverse events (% (n))	3.2 (2)
Pancreatitis (% (n))	0 (0)
Bleeding (% (n))	3.2 (2)
Perforation (% (n))	0 (0)
Stent dysfunction (% (n))	3.2 (2)
Hyperamylasemia (% (n))	6.4 (4)

ERCP, endoscopic retrograde cholangiopancreatography.

3.5. Comparison of EBS and ENBD Groups

Comparison between EBS and ENBD groups is presented in Table 6. In the patient backgrounds, the ENBD group contained patients with significantly more severe cholangitis ($p = 0.02$). Moreover, the APACHE II score ($p < 0.01$), the SIRS score ($p = 0.04$), and the total bilirubin level ($p < 0.01$) were significantly higher in the ENBD group. Although no statistically significant difference was found, the DIC score tended to be higher in the ENBD group (5.1 vs. 5.8, $p = 0.09$). These results indicated that ENBD was selected for more critically ill patients with hyperbilirubinemia.

Table 6. Comparison between EBS and ENBD groups.

	EBS Group (n = 30)	ENBD Group (n = 32)	p-Value
Patient backgrounds			
Age (mean ± SD)	79.2 ± 8.7	76.5 ± 9.9	0.27
Etiology of acute cholangitis			
Bile duct stone/Malignant disease	24/6	26/6	1.00
Severity of acute cholangitis			
Mild/Moderate/Severe	2/8/20	0/2/30	0.02
APACHE II score (mean ± SD)	11.4 ± 3.9	16.2 ± 7.4	<0.01
DIC score (mean ± SD)	5.1 ± 0.9	5.8 ± 1.3	0.09
SIRS score (mean ± SD)	2.3 ± 1.0	2.9 ± 1.1	0.04
Serum parameters (mean ± SD)			
WBC ($\times 10^3/\mu L$)	15.0 ± 8.9	15.3 ± 8.6	0.90
CRP (mg/dL)	12.7 ± 6.9	14.7 ± 5.8	0.23
T-bil (mg/dL)	3.4 ± 1.7	6.0 ± 3.6	<0.01
AST (IU/L)	344.0 ± 515.6	290.6 ± 240.5	0.61
ALT (IU/L)	268.3 ± 306.6	243.5 ± 224.8	0.72
Plt ($\times 10^4/L$)	11.2 ± 5.7	11.0 ± 10.4	0.90
FDP (µg/mL)	25.1 ± 15.7	29.9 ± 24.9	0.41
PT-INR	1.50 ± 0.71	1.43 ± 0.26	0.62
Antibiotics			
Carbapenem	22	24	0.89
Sulbactam/Cefoperazone	4	4	0.78
Tazobactam/Piperacillin	2	1	0.95
Others	2	3	0.94
Endoscopic procedures			
Conventional cannulation	24	27	0.33
EST	4	3	1.00
Stone removal	0	4	0.11
Procedure time (min, mean ± SD)	32.5 ± 20.0	30.38 ± 19.89	0.67
Clinical outcomes			
Clinical success for acute cholangitis (% (n))	96.7 (29)	84.4 (27)	0.36
DIC resolution rate (% (n))	93.3 (28)	84.4 (27)	0.67
Number of ERCP sessions (mean ± SD)	2.0 ± 0.61	2.0 ± 0.57	0.83
Hospitalization period (mean ± SD)	27.6 ± 11.8	35.6 ± 26.9	0.15
Mortality rate (% (n))	0 (0)	9.4 (3)	0.24
Adverse events			
Bleeding (% (n))	3.3 (1)	3.1 (1)	1.00
Stent dysfunction (% (n))	0 (0)	6.3 (2)	0.49

EBS, endoscopic biliary stenting; ENBD, endoscopic nasobiliary drainage; SD, standard deviation; APACHE, acute physiology and chronic health evaluation; DIC, disseminated intravascular coagulation; SIRS, systemic inflammatory response syndrome; EST, endoscopic sphincterotomy; ERCP, endoscopic retrograde cholangiopancreatography.

In contrast, although the duration of hospitalization tended to be longer in the ENBD group (27.6 days vs. 35.6 days, $p = 0.15$), no significant difference was found in endoscopic procedures, clinical outcomes, and adverse events between the EBS and ENBD groups.

4. Discussion

DIC is a life-threatening condition that necessitates prompt and appropriate treatment. Because controlling the primary disease that caused DIC is the most essential treatment for DIC [1,14,15], EBD is the most important treatment for AC associated with DIC. However, a concern related to EBD for patients with severe AC associated with DIC is poor drainage or clogging in the stent due to the high viscosity of infected bile and hemobilia associated with contact of the device with the bile duct, and no report exists regarding the treatment outcomes of EBD for AC associated with DIC. Therefore, in the present study, we evaluated the treatment outcomes of early EBD for AC associated with DIC. We found that EBD performed within 24 h after the diagnosis of AC associated with DIC is effective and safe, with a clinical success rate for AC of 90.3%, a DIC resolution rate of 88.7%, and an ERCP-related adverse event rate of 3.3%. The DIC score, the parameters related to DIC, and the parameters related to AC were improved within 7 days after EBD. A previous meta-analysis reported that early EBD performed within 24 h from presentation was associated with reduced mortality in patients with AC [16], and our study results also showed that early EBD performed within 24 h is effective for patients with AC associated with DIC.

For patients with AC associated DIC, EBD without EST is generally required because of the high risk for post-EST bleeding. In the present study, seven patients (11.3%) received EST, and among them, one patient (14.3%) developed post-EST bleeding. A meta-analysis conducted by Sawas et al. [17] reported that EBD with EST carries higher risks for post-ERCP bleeding and EBD with and without EST are equally effective drainage methods for severe AC. Theoretically, the concern about performing EBD without EST is the development of post-ERCP pancreatitis from pancreatic duct orifice blockage. However, no case of post-ERCP pancreatitis was found in this study. Moreover, a meta-analysis showed no significant difference in the incidence of post-ERCP pancreatitis [17]. Therefore, EST may not be feasible during an acute phase of AC associated with DIC.

EBD is performed by either EBS or ENBD. A few studies compared EBS and ENBD in cases of severe AC [6–10]. Most previous reports, including randomized controlled trials (RCTs) [6,7], showed that no difference was found between EBS and ENBD in terms of their safety and efficacy in severe AC. However, an RCT conducted by Zang et al. [10] reported an increased rate of blockage in the EBS group and a greater decrease in liver enzyme levels in the ENBD group; nonetheless, no sufficient evidence exists on this subject. Furthermore, for AC associated with DIC, no report that compared EBS and ENBD exists. Therefore, in the present study, we compared the patient backgrounds, the safety and effectiveness between EBS and ENBD in patients with AC associated with DIC, and our results showed that EBS and ENBD were equally effective and safe for this condition. Nevertheless, ENBD was selected for more critically ill patients, such as those with severe cholangitis, high APACHE II score, and high total bilirubin level. ENBD may be more appropriate for such patients because it is an external drainage procedure with advantages of the ability to monitor, aspirate, and wash the bile through the catheter. However, because of patient discomfort due to the transnasal catheter, the possibility of self-extraction of the catheter in ENBD exists, especially in elderly or confused patients. In the present study, two patients with a confused mental state pulled out the nasobiliary catheter and required re-ERCP. Therefore, for confused or elderly patients who cannot tolerate an ENBD, an EBS may be a better option.

Although treating the primary disease of DIC is the most important point when managing infection-related DIC [1], the efficacy of anticoagulant drugs for DIC, such as recombinant human soluble thrombomodulin and antithrombin, has been reported [18–23]. In this study, treatment outcomes may be affected by anticoagulant therapy. However, only a few reports on anticoagulant therapy for AC-induced DIC exist [14,15,24,25], so very little evidence exists that can form a basis for the selection of anticoagulant agents for this condition.

Several limitations were present in this study. An accurate comparison of the drainage ability between EBS and ENBD was not possible because the patient backgrounds were different between the two groups, i.e., more critically ill patients belonged to the ENBD group. A selection may have caused bias in the endoscopic procedures, such as EST, stone removal, and the method of EBD, because the endoscopic procedures were left to the discretion of the attending endoscopist. Treatment outcomes may be affected by anticoagulant therapy and antibiotics [14,15,24,25]. Furthermore, this study used a retrospective design, and the number of patients was small because of the rare nature of the subject disease, thereby indicating that a large-scale, prospective study is necessary to confirm our findings. However, to our knowledge, this study is the first to evaluate the role of EBD in AC associated with DIC, and we believe that this study contains useful information.

In conclusion, early EBD performed within 24 h after the diagnosis of AC associated with DIC is effective and safe for treating patients with AC associated with DIC.

Author Contributions: K.N. designed the report; A.S., K.N. and J.S. contributed to analysis and interpretation of data; K.N., J.S., Y.M., K.S., R.M. and Y.I. assisted in the preparation of the manuscript; F.I. organized the report; and A.S. wrote the report. All authors have read and agreed to the published version of the manuscript.

Funding: This research received no external funding.

Institutional Review Board Statement: The study was conducted according to the guidelines of the Declaration of Helsinki, and approved by the Institutional Review Board of St. Marianna University School of Medicine (approval number: 5357, approval data: 8 July 2021).

Informed Consent Statement: All patients provided written informed consent for the procedure.

Data Availability Statement: The data presented in this study are available in the article.

Conflicts of Interest: The authors declare no conflict of interest.

References

1. Wada, H.; Asakura, H.; Okamoto, K.; Iba, T.; Uchiyama, T.; Kawasugi, K.; Koga, S.; Mayumi, T.; Koike, K.; Gando, S.; et al. Expert consensus for the treatment of disseminated intravascular coagulation in Japan. *Thromb. Res.* **2010**, *125*, 6–11. [CrossRef]
2. Miura, F.; Okamoto, K.; Takada, T.; Strasberg, S.M.; Asbun, H.J.; Pitt, H.A.; Gomi, H.; Solomkin, J.S.; Schlossberg, D.; Han, H.S.; et al. Tokyo Guidelines 2018: Initial management of acute biliary infection and flowchart for acute cholangitis. *J. Hepatobiliary Pancreat Sci.* **2018**, *25*, 31–40. [CrossRef]
3. Mukai, S.; Itoi, T.; Baron, T.H.; Takada, T.; Strasberg, S.M.; Pitt, H.A.; Ukai, T.; Shikata, S.; Teoh, A.Y.B.; Kim, M.H.; et al. Indications and techniques of biliary drainage for acute cholangitis in updated Tokyo Guidelines 2018. *J. Hepatobiliary Pancreat Sci.* **2017**, *24*, 537–549. [CrossRef]
4. Simmons, D.T.; Petersen, B.T.; Gostout, C.J.; Levy, M.J.; Topazian, M.D.; Baron, T.H. Risk of pancreatitis following endoscopically placed large-bore plastic biliary stents with and without biliary sphincterotomy for management of postoperative bile leaks. *Surg. Endosc.* **2008**, *22*, 1459–1463. [CrossRef]
5. Cui, P.J.; Yao, J.; Zhao, Y.J.; Han, H.Z.; Yang, J. Biliary stenting with or without sphincterotomy for malignant biliary obstruction: A meta-analysis. *World J. Gastroenterol.* **2014**, *20*, 14033–14039. [CrossRef] [PubMed]
6. Lee, D.W.; Chan, A.C.; Lam, Y.H.; Ng, E.K.; Lau, J.Y.; Law, B.K.; Lai, C.W.; Sung, J.J.; Chung, S.C. Biliary decompression by nasobiliary catheter or biliary stent in acute suppurative cholangitis: A prospective randomized trial. *Gastrointest Endosc.* **2002**, *56*, 361–365. [CrossRef]
7. Sharma, B.C.; Kumar, R.; Agarwal, N.; Sarin, S.K. Endoscopic biliary drainage by nasobiliary drain or by stent placement in patients with acute cholangitis. *Endoscopy* **2005**, *37*, 439–443. [CrossRef] [PubMed]
8. Park, S.Y.; Park, C.H.; Cho, S.B.; Yoon, K.W.; Lee, W.S.; Kim, H.S.; Choi, S.K.; Rew, J.S. The safety and effectiveness of endoscopic biliary decompression by plastic stent placement in acute suppurative cholangitis compared with nasobiliary drainage. *Gastrointest Endosc.* **2008**, *68*, 1076–1080. [CrossRef]
9. Kumar, R.; Sharma, B.C.; Singh, J.; Sarin, S.K. Endoscopic biliary drainage for severe acute cholangitis in biliary obstruction as a result of malignant and benign diseases. *J. Gastroenterol. Hepatol.* **2004**, *19*, 994–997. [CrossRef] [PubMed]
10. Zhang, R.L.; Cheng, L.; Cai, X.B.; Zhao, H.; Zhu, F.; Wan, X.J. Comparison of the safety and effectiveness of endoscopic biliary decompression by nasobiliary catheter and plastic stent placement in acute obstructive cholangitis. *Swiss Med. Wkly.* **2013**, *143*, w13823. [CrossRef]

1. Kiriyama, S.; Kozaka, K.; Takada, T.; Strasberg, S.M.; Pitt, H.A.; Gabata, T.; Hata, J.; Liau, K.H.; Miura, F.; Horiguchi, A.; et al. Tokyo Guidelines 2018: Diagnostic criteria and severity grading of acute cholangitis (with videos). *J. Hepatobiliary Pancreat Sci.* **2018**, *25*, 17–30. [CrossRef]
2. Gando, S.; Iba, T.; Eguchi, Y.; Ohtomo, Y.; Okamoto, K.; Koseki, K.; Mayumi, T.; Murata, A.; Ikeda, T.; Ishikura, H.; et al. A multicenter, prospective validation of disseminated intravascular coagulation diagnostic criteria for critically ill patients: Comparing current criteria. *Crit. Care Med.* **2006**, *34*, 625–631. [CrossRef]
3. Cotton, P.B.; Lehman, G.; Vennes, J.; Geenen, J.E.; Russell, R.C.; Meyers, W.C.; Liguory, C.; Nickl, N. Endoscopic sphincterotomy complications and their management: An attempt at consensus. *Gastrointest Endosc.* **1991**, *37*, 383–393. [CrossRef]
4. Nakahara, K.; Okuse, C.; Adachi, S.; Suetani, K.; Kitagawa, S.; Okano, M.; Michikawa, Y.; Takagi, R.; Shigefuku, R.; Itoh, F. Use of antithrombin and thrombomodulin in the management of disseminated intravascular coagulation in patients with acute cholangitis. *Gut Liver* **2013**, *7*, 363–370. [CrossRef]
5. Suetani, K.; Okuse, C.; Nakahara, K.; Michikawa, Y.; Noguchi, Y.; Suzuki, M.; Morita, R.; Sato, N.; Kato, M.; Itoh, F. Thrombomodulin in the management of acute cholangitis-induced disseminated intravascular coagulation. *World J. Gastroenterol.* **2015**, *21*, 533–540. [CrossRef]
6. Du, L.; Cen, M.; Zheng, X.; Luo, L.; Siddiqui, A.; Kim, J.J. Timing of Performing Endoscopic Retrograde Cholangiopancreatography and Inpatient Mortality in Acute Cholangitis: A Systematic Review and Meta-Analysis. *Clin. Transl. Gastroenterol.* **2020**, *11*, e00158. [CrossRef] [PubMed]
7. Sawas, T.; Arwani, N.; Al Halabi, S.; Vargo, J. Sphincterotomy with endoscopic biliary drainage for severe acute cholangitis: A meta-analysis. *Endosc. Int. Open* **2017**, *5*, E103–E109. [CrossRef]
8. Saito, H.; Maruyama, I.; Shimazaki, S.; Yamamoto, Y.; Aikawa, N.; Ohno, R.; Hirayama, A.; Matsuda, T.; Asakura, H.; Nakashima, M.; et al. Efficacy and safety of recombinant human soluble thrombomodulin (ART-123) in disseminated intravascular coagulation: Results of a phase III, randomized, double-blind clinical trial. *J. Thromb. Haemost.* **2007**, *5*, 31–41. [CrossRef] [PubMed]
9. Aikawa, N.; Shimazaki, S.; Yamamoto, Y.; Saito, H.; Maruyama, I.; Ohno, R.; Hirayama, A.; Aoki, Y.; Aoki, N. Thrombomodulin alfa in the treatment of infectious patients complicated by disseminated intravascular coaglation: Subanalysis from the phase 3 trial. *Shock* **2011**, *35*, 349–354. [CrossRef] [PubMed]
10. Vincent, J.L.; Ramesh, M.K.; Ernest, D.; LaRosa, S.P.; Pachl, J.; Aikawa, N.; Hoste, E.; Levy, H.; Hirman, J.; Levi, M.; et al. A randomized, double-blind, placebo-controlled, Phase 2b study to evaluate the safety and efficacy of recombinant human soluble thrombomodulin, ART-123, in patients with sepsis and suspected disseminated intravascular coagulation. *Crit. Care Med.* **2013**, *41*, 2069–2079. [CrossRef] [PubMed]
11. Yamakawa, K.; Aihara, M.; Ogura, H.; Yuhara, H.; Hamasaki, T.; Shimazu, T. Recombinant human soluble thrombomodulin in severe sepsis: A systematic review and meta-analysis. *J. Thromb. Haemost.* **2015**, *13*, 508–519. [CrossRef] [PubMed]
12. Kienast, J.; Juers, M.; Wiedermann, C.J.; Hoffmann, J.N.; Ostermann, H.; Strauss, R.; Keinecke, H.O.; Warren, B.L.; Opal, S.M.; KyberSept Investigators. Treatment effects of high-dose antithrombin without concomitant heparin in patients with severe sepsis with or without disseminated intravascular coagulation. *J. Thromb. Haemost.* **2006**, *4*, 90–97. [CrossRef] [PubMed]
13. Warren, B.L.; Eid, A.; Singer, P.; Pillay, S.S.; Carl, P.; Novak, I.; Chalupa, P.; Atherstone, A.; Pénzes, I.; Kübler, A.; et al. Caring for the critically ill patient. High-dose antithrombin III in severe sepsis: A randomized controlled trial. *JAMA* **2001**, *286*, 1869–1878. [CrossRef]
14. Morita, N.; Nakahara, K.; Morita, R.; Suetani, K.; Michikawa, Y.; Sato, J.; Tsuji, K.; Ikeda, H.; Matsunaga, K.; Watanabe, T.; et al. Efficacy of Combined Thrombomodulin and Antithrombin in Anticoagulant Therapy for Acute Cholangitis-induced Disseminated Intravascular Coagulation. *Intern. Med.* **2019**, *58*, 907–914. [CrossRef] [PubMed]
15. Ogura, T.; Eguchi, T.; Nakahara, K.; Kanno, Y.; Omoto, S.; Itonaga, M.; Kuroda, T.; Hakoda, A.; Ikeoka, S.; Takagi, M.; et al. Clinical impact of recombinant thrombomodulin administration on disseminated intravascular coagulation due to severe acute cholangitis (Recover-AC study). *J. Hepatobiliary Pancreat Sci.* **2021**. [CrossRef]

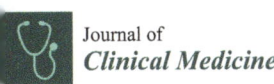

Article

Outcomes of Endoscopic Ultrasound-Guided Biliary Drainage in a General Hospital for Patients with Endoscopic Retrograde Cholangiopancreatography-Difficult Transpapillary Biliary Drainage

Naosuke Kuraoka [1,*], Satoru Hashimoto [1], Shigeru Matsui [1] and Shuji Terai [2]

1 Department of Gastroenterology, Saiseikai Kawaguchi General Hospital, 5-11-5 Nishikawaguchi, Kawaguchi 332-8558, Saitama, Japan; shashim@saiseikai.gr.jp (S.H.); mshigerum@saiseikai.gr.jp (S.M.)
2 Department of Gastroenterology and Hepatology, Graduate School of Medical and Dental Sciences, Niigata University, 1-757 Asahimachidori, Niigata 951-8510, Japan; terais@med.niigata-u.ac.jp
* Correspondence: kuraoka0926@gmail.com; Tel.: +81-(48)-253-1551

Abstract: Endoscopic ultrasound-guided biliary drainage (EUS-BD) has been developed as an alternative treatment for percutaneous transhepatic biliary drainage for patients with bile duct stenosis. At specialized hospitals, the high success rate and effectiveness of EUS-BD as primary drainage has been reported. However, the procedure is highly technical and difficult, and it has not been generally performed. In this study, we retrospectively examined the effectiveness of EUS-BD in ERCP-difficult patients with distal bile duct stenosis. We retrospectively examined 24 consecutive cases in which EUS-BD was performed at our hospital for distal bile duct stenosis from October 2018 to December 2020. EUS-guided choledochoduodenostomy (EUS-CDS) was selected for cases that could be approached from the duodenal bulb, and EUS-HGS was selected for other cases. In the EUS-CDS and EUS-HGS groups, the technical success rates were 83.3% (10/12) and 91.7% (11/12), respectively. An adverse event occurred in one case in the EUS-CDS group, which developed severe biliary peritonitis. The stent patency period was 91 and 101 days in the EUS-CDS and EUS-HGS groups, respectively. EUS-BD for ERCP-difficult patients with distal bile duct stenosis is considered to be an effective alternative for biliary drainage that can be performed not only in specialized hospitals but also in general hospitals.

Keywords: EUS-BD; EUS-CDS; EUS-HGS; biliary stenosis; ERCP

1. Introduction

Endoscopic ultrasound-guided biliary drainage (EUS-BD) has been developed as an alternative treatment to percutaneous transhepatic biliary drainage (PTBD) for patients with difficult or unsuccessful transpapillary biliary drainage using endoscopic retrograde cholangiopancreatography (ERCP) [1,2]. EUS-BD, which is performed in many specialized hospitals, is generally classified into EUS-guided choledochoduodenostomy (EUS-CDS) and EUS-guided hepaticogastrostomy (EUS-HGS). At these hospitals, it has been reported that performing EUS-BD as the primary drainage is effective and had a high success rate. However, at present, the procedure is still highly technical and difficult, and it has not been widely used in other medical facilities [3–6]. Therefore, the success rate and safety of EUS-BD in general hospitals are currently unknown. In this study, we retrospectively examined the effectiveness of EUS-BD for patients with distal bile duct stenosis at our institution in whom performing an ERCP was difficult.

2. Materials and Methods

We retrospectively examined 24 consecutive cases in which EUS-BD was performed at our hospital for distal bile duct stenosis from October 2018 to December 2020. All cases

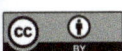

underwent EUS-BD instead of ERCP due to the difficult procedure of the latter. EUS-CDS was performed for cases that could be approached from the duodenal bulb, whereas EUS-HGS was selected for other cases. The endoscopic procedures were performed by a skilled endoscopist who had more than 1000 cases of ERCP experience, more than 1000 cases of observation EUS experiences and more than 200 cases of EUS-guided fine needle aspiration.

This study was approved by the Institutional Review Board of the Saiseikai Kawaguchi General Hospital. The primary endpoint of this study was the technical success rate of EUS-BD, and the secondary endpoints were the rate of adverse events, stent patency period, and re-intervention.

For the EUS-CDS procedure, the extrahepatic bile duct was visualized from the duodenal bulb using a linear endoscopic ultrasound (GF-UCT260; Olympus Medical Japan, Tokyo, Japan). The extrahepatic bile duct was punctured using a 19-G puncture needle, and a guidewire was placed in the bile duct. The fistula was then dilated using a dilation device, and a plastic stent (PS) or a self-expandable metal stent (SEMS) was deployed (Figure 1).

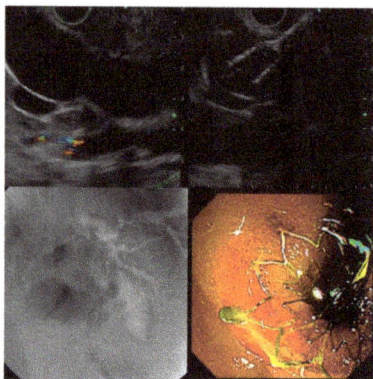

Figure 1. Procedure of endoscopic ultrasound-guided choledochoduodenostomy.

For the EUS-HGS procedure, the intrahepatic bile ducts (B2 or B3) were visualized from the stomach using linear endoscopic ultrasound (GF-UCT260; Olympus Medical Ja-pan, Tokyo, Japan). The intrahepatic bile duct was punctured with a 19-G or 22-G puncture needle, and a guidewire was placed. After cholangiography, fistula dilation was performed using a dilation device, and the PS or SEMS was deployed. Alternatively, the PS or SEMS was placed without dilating the fistula (Figure 2).

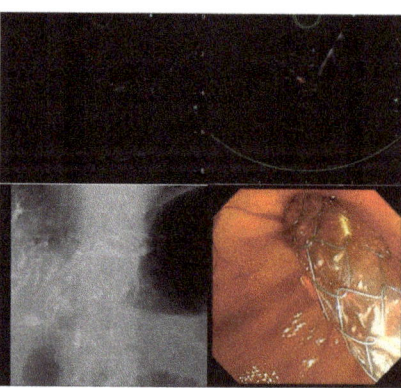

Figure 2. Procedure of endoscopic ultrasound-guided hepaticogastrostomy.

Technical success was defined as a case in which PS or SEMS could be placed during EUS-BD. Clinical success was defined as a case in which cholangitis was alleviated or the total bilirubin level improved. Adverse events were defined as all complications that occurred after procedure (e.g., bleeding, stent migration, peritonitis, stent dysfunction, and so on). Early and late complications were defined as adverse events that occurred <30 days and >30 days after treatment, respectively. Re-intervention was defined as performing another endoscopic or percutaneous treatment due to recurrence of cholangitis or obstructive jaundice. The stent patency period was defined as the period before the recurrence of cholangitis and jaundice. Patients who died due to the current illness were treated as censored. The performance status refers to the Eastern Cooperative Oncology Group performance status [7]. The adverse events were graded using the American Society for Gastrointestinal Endoscopy lexicon severity grading system [8].

A specialized hospital was defined as a university hospital, a cancer center, and a tertiary medical institution. On the other hand, a general hospital was defined as a medical institution other than university hospitals, cancer centers, and tertiary medical institutions. Saiseikai Kawaguchi General Hospital was defined as a general hospital.

The results are presented as numerical values (%), while continuous variables are presented as median values (range). This study performed an intention-to-treat analysis, and the median of the stent patency periods was calculated using the Kaplan–Meier method. All statistical analyses were performed using the Statistical Product and Service Solutions (SPSS, IBM, Tokyo, Japan).

3. Results

Among the cases in which ERCP was performed for distal bile duct stenosis from October 2018 to December 2020, 24 consecutive ERCP-difficult cases in which EUS-BD was instead performed were retrospectively examined.

3.1. Patient Characteristics

The EUS-CDS and EUS-HGS groups had 12 patients each. Pancreatic cancer was the most common background disease in both groups (EUS-CDS: 9/12, 66.7%; EUS-HGS: 7/12, 58.3%). The mean total bilirubin level before treatment was 9.49 mg/dL in the EUS-CDS group and 6.72 mg/dL in the EUS-HGS group. In the EUS-CDS group, an extrahepatic bile duct was punctured, and the average bile duct diameter was 14.9 mm. The average diameter of the intrahepatic bile duct in the EUS-HGS group was 5.1 mm. In most cases, 19-G needles were used as puncture needles in both the EUS-CDS and EUS-HGS groups; 22-G needles were used in two cases in the EUS-HGS group (Table 1).

3.2. Outcomes

The technical success rates in the EUS-CDS and EUS-HGS groups were 10/12 (83.3%) and 11/12 (91.7%), respectively. Both groups were effective in stent-placeable cases, and the clinical success rates were similar. SEMS was deployed in 9 of the 10 cases in the EUS-CDS group in which the stent could be inserted. In the EUS-HGS group, SEMS was deployed in four cases whereas PS was deployed in the rest. Regarding fistula dilation, electrocautery dilation was performed in the EUS-CDS group, while non-electrocautery dilation was performed in the EUS-HGS group. In addition, non-dilation of the fistula was also performed in two cases in the EUS-HGS group (Table 2). An adverse event occurred in only one case in the EUS-CDS group, which developed severe biliary peritonitis (Table 3). The median stent patency period was 91 days and 101 days in the EUS-CDS and EUS-HGS groups, respectively, showing no significant difference (Figure 3). After stent insertion, resection and chemotherapy was performed in two and five patients (41.7%), respectively, in the EUS-HGS group. Meanwhile, chemotherapy was administered to five patients in the EUS-CDS group. Re-intervention was performed in five patients in the EUS-CDS group, and the technical success rate was 100%. In the EUS-CDS group, re-intervention was performed by replacing the stent or changing the position of the stent. In the EUS-HGS group, re-intervention was performed in six patients, and the technical success rate was also 100%. However, a new EUS-HGS route was required in one patient (Table 4).

Table 1. Patient characteristics.

	EUS-CDS (n = 12)	EUS-HGS (n = 12)
Median age (range)	76.5 (57–75)	76.5 (60–85)
Sex, male, n (%)	4 (33.3)	7 (58.3)
Diagnosis, n (%)		
Pancreatic cancer	9 (66.7)	7 (58.3)
Cholangiocarcinoma	0	1 (8.3)
Dissemination of cancer	3 (33.3)	2 (16.7)
Bile duct stones	0	2 (16.7)
Pre-total Bilirubin, mean, mg/dL (range)	9.49 (3.29–16.06)	6.72 (0.48–13.65)
Performance status (PS)		
Performance status < 2, n (%)	7 (58.3)	8 (66.7)
Performance status > 3, n (%)	5 (41.7)	4 (33.3)
Diameter of bile duct		
Extrahepatic bile duct, mean, mm (range)	14.9 (11–20)	N/A
Intrahepatic bile duct, mean, mm (range)	N/A	5.1 (2.6–7)
Size of needle		
19G, n (%)	12 (100)	10 (83.3)
22G, n (%)	0	2 (16.7)

EUS-CDS: endoscopic ultrasound-guided choledochoduodenostomy; EUS-HGS: endoscopic ultrasound-guided hepaticogastrostomy; PS: plastic stent.

Table 2. Outcomes of EUS-CDS and EUS-HGS.

	EUS-CDS (n = 12)	EUS-HGS (n = 12)
Technical success, n (%)	10/12 (83.3)	11/12 (91.7)
Clinical success, n (%)	10/12 (83.3)	11/12 (91.7)
Deployment of SEMS, n (%)	9 (75)	4 (33.3)
Deployment of PS	1 (8.3)	7 (58.3)
Dilatation		
Electrocautery dilation, n (%)	10 (83.3)	0
Non-electrocautery dilation, n (%)	1 (8.3)	8 (66.7)
Non-dilation, n (%)	0	3 (25)
Stent patency, median days	91	101

EUS-CDS: endoscopic ultrasound-guided choledochoduodenostomy, EUS-HGS: endoscopic ultrasound-guided hepaticogastrostomy. SEMS: self-expandable metal stent.

Table 3. Adverse events.

	EUS-CDS (n = 12)	EUS-HGS (n = 12)
Overall adverse events, n (%)	1/12 (8.3)	0/12 (0)
Type of adverse events, grade	bile peritonitis, severe	
Early adverse events, n (%)	1/12 (8.3)	0/12 (0)
Late adverse events, n (%)	0/12 (0)	0/12 (0)

EUS-CDS: endoscopic ultrasound-guided choledochoduodenostomy, EUS-HGS: endoscopic ultrasound-guided hepaticogastrostomy.

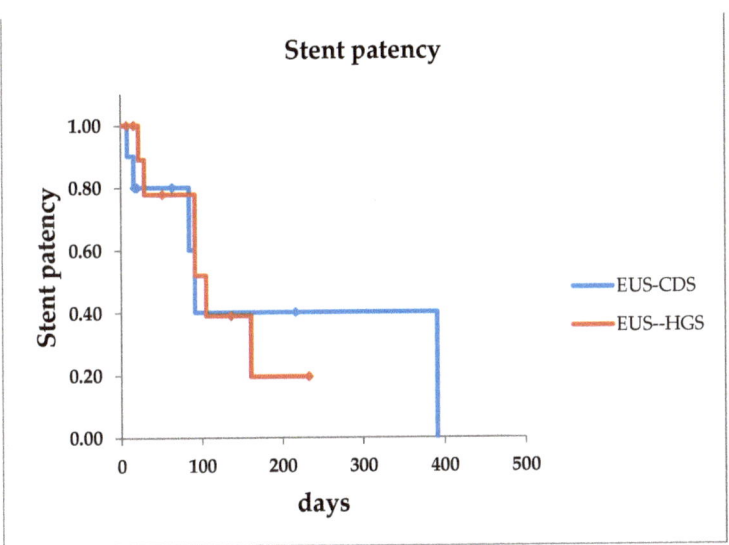

Figure 3. Stent patency of EUS-CDS and EUS-HGS. The stent patency period is 91 days in the EUS-CDS group and 101 days in the EUS-HGS group. EUS-CDS: endoscopic ultrasound-guided choledochoduodenostomy, EUS-HGS: endoscopic ultrasound-guided hepaticogastrostomy.

Table 4. Treatment after the procedures and re-intervention.

	EUS-CDS (n = 12)	EUS-HGS (n = 12)
Treatment		
Resection, n (%)	0	2/12 (16.7)
Chemotherapy	5/12 (41.7)	5/12 (41.7)
Re-intervention, n (%)	5 (41.7)	6 (50)
Technical success	5/5 (80)	6/6 (100)
Re-intervention, n (%)		
Stent exchange	3/5 (60)	5/6 (83.3)
Stent direction change	2/5 (40)	0
Another EUS-BD	0	1/6 (16.7)

EUS-BD: endoscopic ultrasound-guided biliary drainage. EUS-CDS: endoscopic ultrasound-guided choledochoduodenostomy, EUS-HGS: endoscopic ultrasound-guided hepaticogastrostomy.

4. Discussion

EUS-BD has been developed as an alternative treatment for ERCP-difficult cases. After Wiersema et al. reported cholangiography as an endosonography-guided cholangiopancreatography in 1999, Giovannini et al. first reported biliary drainage as EUS-guided bilioduodenal anastomosis in 2001 [9,10]. Since then, numerous EUS-BDs have been performed at specialized facilities, with some EUS-BDs being reported as the primary drainage as well as an alternative treatment for ERCP-difficult patients [3–6]. However, in many facilities, the EUS-BD has not been introduced, which hinders the widespread and generalized use of the procedure.

This study examined the initial results after the introduction of EUS-BD. Most of the target patients had malignant biliary stenosis. In addition, many of them were elderly with a decreased performance status, and there were many cases in which chemotherapy could not be initiated. The technical success rates of EUS-CDS and EUS-HGS was reported to be 90.9–100% [3–6] and over 90% [11–14]. In our study, the technical success rates for EUS-CDS and EUS-HGS were 83.3 and 91.7%, respectively, which is considered to be equivalent to previous studies. During the introduction of EUS-HGS, biliary drainage was performed by using a PS, but the placement of SEMS increased with the advent of small-diameter stents. In addition, many EUS-CDS detentions were performed using SEMS. In our study, EUS-CDS showed severe bile leakage in one case. Although the incidence of adverse events was 8.3% in EUS-CDS, only one case of adverse events was severe bile leakage. On the other hand, in EUS-HGS, no adverse events were observed.

Regarding the stent patency period, the median patency periods were 91 and 101 days in the EUS-CDS and EUS-HGS groups, respectively. The reason for the short patency period of the EUS-CDS group was considered to be due to the stent direction being changed early after the procedure. As mentioned above, the introduction of EUS-BD has been highly successful in many specialized hospitals, but the current situation is that the procedure has not been generally applied. The results at our hospital, which is a general hospital, are the initial results of the introduction of EUS-BD, which can be an index for facilities considering the introduction of EUS-BD. The technical success, which is the primary endpoint, was as high as previously reported. The rate of adverse events was low enough, and re-intervention was possible in this study. Although this study was a small number of case studies, no adverse events were observed in EUS-HGS. EUS-HGS is possibly more secure in initial introduction of EUS-BD than EUS-CDS.

In addition, EUS-BD cannot be performed by a skilled endoscopist alone, and an assistant who is familiar with both the procedure and biliary tract treatment tools and equipment is required. The advent of EUS-BD-dedicated devices may alleviate these difficulties. Recently, EUS-CDS using lumen-apposing metal stents that has a high technical success rate and low rate of adverse events has been reported [15–17].

This study had several limitations. This was a retrospective single-center study in which an endoscopic procedure was performed by a skilled endoscopist. Moreover, there were a small number of case studies. In the future, in order to generalize our results and the application of EUS-BD, it is necessary to carry out prospective multicenter research.

5. Conclusions

In conclusion, EUS-BD in ERCP-difficult patients with distal bile duct stenosis is considered to be an effective alternative for biliary drainage that might be possibly performed not only in specialized hospitals but also in general hospitals. However, adverse events have been observed, and the development of EUS-BD dedicated devices is desirable for the general application of this procedure.

Author Contributions: N.K. performed the endoscopic examinations and drafted the manuscript; S.H. revised the manuscript; S.M. revised the manuscript and approved the final draft; S.T. revised the manuscript and approved the final draft. All authors have read and agreed to the published version of the manuscript.

Funding: This research received no external funding.

Institutional Review Board Statement: The study was conducted according to the guidelines of the Declaration of Helsinki and approved by the Institutional Review Board of Saiseikai Kawa-guchi General Hospital (protocol code 2021-21, 28 July 2021).

Informed Consent Statement: Informed consent was obtained from all subjects involved in the study.

Data Availability Statement: The data presented in this study are available on request from the corresponding author. The data are not publicly available due to ethical and privacy restrictions.

Conflicts of Interest: The authors declare no conflict of interest.

References

1. Mallery, S.; Matlock, J.; Freeman, M.L. EUS-Guided Rendezvous Drainage of Obstructed Biliary and Pancreatic Ducts: Report of 6 Cases. *Gastrointest. Endosc.* **2004**, *59*, 100–107. [CrossRef]
2. Kawakubo, K.; Isayama, H.; Kato, H.; Itoi, T.; Kawakami, H.; Hanada, K.; Ishiwatari, H.; Yasuda, I.; Kawamoto, H.; Itokawa, F.; et al. Multicenter Retrospective Study of Endoscopic Ultrasound-Guided Biliary Drainage for Malignant Biliary Obstruction in Japan. *J. Hepato-Biliary-Pancreat. Sci.* **2014**, *21*, 328–334. [CrossRef] [PubMed]

5. Kuraoka, N.; Hara, K.; Okuno, N.; Kuwahara, T.; Mizuno, N.; Shimizu, Y.; Niwa, Y.; Terai, S. Outcomes of EUS-Guided Choledochoduodenostomy as Primary Drainage for Distal Biliary Obstruction With Covered Self-Expandable Metallic Stents. *Endosc. Int. Open* **2020**, *8*, E861–E868. [CrossRef] [PubMed]
6. Nakai, Y.; Isayama, H.; Kawakami, H.; Ishiwatari, H.; Kitano, M.; Ito, Y.; Yasuda, I.; Kato, H.; Matsubara, S.; Irisawa, A.; et al. Prospective Multicenter Study of Primary EUS-Guided Choledochoduodenostomy Using a Covered Metal Stent. *Endosc. Ultrasound* **2019**, *8*, 111–117. [PubMed]
7. Bang, J.Y.; Navaneethan, U.; Hasan, M.; Hawes, R.; Varadarajulu, S. Stent Placement by EUS or ERCP for Primary Biliary Decompression in Pancreatic Cancer: A Randomized Trial (With Videos). *Gastrointest. Endosc.* **2018**, *88*, 9–17. [CrossRef] [PubMed]
8. Paik, W.H.; Lee, T.H.; Park, D.H.; Choi, J.H.; Kim, S.O.; Jang, S.; Kim, D.U.; Shim, J.H.; Song, T.J.; Lee, S.S.; et al. EUS-Guided Biliary Drainage Versus ERCP for the Primary Palliation of Malignant Biliary Obstruction: A Multicenter Randomized Clinical Trial. *Am. J. Gastroenterol.* **2018**, *113*, 987–997. [CrossRef] [PubMed]
9. Oken, M.M.; Creech, R.H.; Tormey, D.C.; Horton, J.; Davis, T.E.; McFadden, E.T.; Carbone, P.P. Toxicity and Response Criteria of the Eastern Cooperative Oncology Group. *Am. J. Clin. Oncol.* **1982**, *5*, 649–655. [CrossRef] [PubMed]
10. Cotton, P.B.; Eisen, G.M.; Aabakken, L.; Baron, T.H.; Hutter, M.M.; Jacobson, B.C.; Mergener, K.; Nemcek, A.; Petersen, B.T.; Petrini, J.L.; et al. A Lexicon for Endoscopic Adverse Events: Report of an ASGE Workshop. *Gastrointest. Endosc.* **2010**, *71*, 446–454. [CrossRef] [PubMed]
11. Wiersema, M.J.; Sandusky, D.; Carr, R.; Wiersema, L.M.; Erdel, W.C.; Frederick, P.K. Endosonography-Guided Cholangiopancreatography. *Gastrointest. Endosc.* **1996**, *43 Pt 1*, 102–106. [CrossRef]
12. Giovannini, M.; Moutardier, V.; Pesenti, C.; Bories, E.; Lelong, B.; Delpero, J.R. Endoscopic Ultrasound-Guided Bilioduodenal Anastomosis: A New Technique for Biliary Drainage. *Endoscopy* **2001**, *33*, 898–900. [CrossRef] [PubMed]
13. Paik, W.H.; Park, D.H.; Choi, J.H.; Choi, J.H.; Lee, S.S.; Seo, D.W.; Lee, S.K.; Kim, M.H.; Lee, J.B. Simplified Fistula Dilation Technique and Modified Stent Deployment Maneuver for EUS-Guided Hepaticogastrostomy. *World J. Gastroenterol.* **2014**, *20*, 5051–5059. [CrossRef] [PubMed]
14. Artifon, E.L.A.; Marson, F.P.; Gaidhane, M.; Kahaleh, M.; Otoch, J.P. Hepaticogastrostomy or Choledochoduodenostomy for Distal Malignant Biliary Obstruction after Failed ERCP: Is There Any Difference? *Gastrointest. Endosc.* **2015**, *81*, 950–959. [CrossRef] [PubMed]
15. Nakai, Y.; Isayama, H.; Yamamoto, N.; Matsubara, S.; Ito, Y.; Sasahira, N.; Hakuta, R.; Umefune, G.; Takahara, N.; Hamada, T.; et al. Safety and Effectiveness of a Long, Partially Covered Metal Stent for Endoscopic Ultrasound-Guided Hepaticogastrostomy in Patients With Malignant Biliary Obstruction. *Endoscopy* **2016**, *48*, 1125–1128. [CrossRef] [PubMed]
16. Ogura, T.; Chiba, Y.; Masuda, D.; Kitano, M.; Sano, T.; Saori, O.; Yamamoto, K.; Imaoka, H.; Imoto, A.; Takeuchi, T.; et al. Comparison of the Clinical Impact of Endoscopic Ultrasound-Guided Choledochoduodenostomy and Hepaticogastrostomy for Bile Duct Obstruction With Duodenal Obstruction. *Endoscopy* **2016**, *48*, 156–163. [PubMed]
17. Anderloni, A.; Fugazza, A.; Troncone, E.; Auriemma, F.; Carrara, S.; Semeraro, R.; Maselli, R.; Di Leo, M.; D'Amico, F.; Sethi, A.; et al. Single-Stage EUS-Guided Choledochoduodenostomy Using a Lumen-Apposing Metal Stent for Malignant Distal Biliary Obstruction. *Gastrointest. Endosc.* **2019**, *89*, 69–76. [CrossRef] [PubMed]
18. Tsuchiya, T.; Teoh, A.Y.B.; Itoi, T.; Yamao, K.; Hara, K.; Nakai, Y.; Isayama, H.; Kitano, M. Long-Term Outcomes of EUS-Guided Choledochoduodenostomy Using a Lumen-Apposing Metal Stent for Malignant Distal Biliary Obstruction: A Prospective Multicenter Study. *Gastrointest. Endosc.* **2018**, *87*, 1138–1146. [CrossRef] [PubMed]
19. El Chafic, A.H.; Shah, J.N.; Hamerski, C.; Binmoeller, K.F.; Irani, S.; James, T.W.; Baron, T.H.; Nieto, J.; Romero, R.V.; Evans, J.A.; et al. EUS-Guided Choledochoduodenostomy for Distal Malignant Biliary Obstruction Using Electrocautery-Enhanced Lumen-Apposing Metal Stents: First US, Multicenter Experience. *Dig. Dis. Sci.* **2019**, *64*, 3321–3327. [CrossRef] [PubMed]

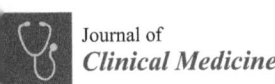

Article

Impact of the Coronavirus Disease-2019 Pandemic on Pancreaticobiliary Disease Detection and Treatment

Muneo Ikemura, Ko Tomishima, Mako Ushio, Sho Takahashi, Wataru Yamagata, Yusuke Takasaki, Akinori Suzuki, Koichi Ito, Kazushige Ochiai, Shigeto Ishii, Hiroaki Saito, Toshio Fujisawa, Akihito Nagahara and Hiroyuki Isayama *

Department of Gastroenterology, Graduate School of Medicine, Juntendo University, 2-1-1 Hongo, Bunkyo-ku, Tokyo 113-8421, Japan; m-ikemura@juntendo.ac.jp (M.I.); tomishim@juntendo.ac.jp (K.T.); m-ushio@juntendo.ac.jp (M.U.); sho-takahashi@juntendo.ac.jp (S.T.); w.yamagata.mx@juntendo.ac.jp (W.Y.); ytakasa@juntendo.ac.jp (Y.T.); suzukia@juntendo.ac.jp (A.S.); kitoh@juntendo.ac.jp (K.I.); k.ochiai.qd@juntendo.ac.jp (K.O.); sishii@juntendo.ac.jp (S.I.); hiloaki@juntendo.ac.jp (H.S.); t-fujisawa@juntendo.ac.jp (T.F.); nagahara@juntendo.ac.jp (A.N.)
* Correspondence: h-isayama@juntendo.ac.jp; Tel.: +81-33-813-3111; Fax: +81-33-813-8862

Abstract: The emergency declaration (ED) associated with the coronavirus disease-2019 (COVID-19) pandemic in Japan had a major effect on the management of gastrointestinal endoscopy. We retrospectively compared the number of pancreaticobiliary endoscopies and newly diagnosed pancreaticobiliary cancers before (1 April 2018 to 6 April 2020), during (7 April 2020 to 25 May), and after the ED (26 May to 31 July). Multiple comparisons of the three groups were performed with respect to the presence or absence of symptoms and clinical disease stage. There were no significant differences among the three groups (Before/During/After the ED) in the mean number of diagnoses of pancreatic cancer and biliary cancer per month in each period (8.0/7.5/7.5 cases, $p = 0.5$, and 4.0/3.5/3.0 cases, $p = 0.9$, respectively). There were no significant differences among the three groups in the number of pancreaticobiliary endoscopies (EUS: endoscopic ultrasonography/ERCP: endoscopic retrograde cholangiopancreatography) per month (67.8/62.5/69.0 cases, $p = 0.7$ and 89.8/51.5/86.0 cases, $p = 0.06$, respectively), whereas the number of EUS cases decreased by 42.7% between before and during the ED. There were no significant differences among the three groups in the presence or absence of symptoms at diagnosis or clinical disease stage. There was no significant reduction in the newly diagnosed pancreaticobiliary cancer, even during the ED. The number of ERCP cases was not significantly reduced as a result of urgent procedures, but the number of EUS cases was significantly reduced.

Keywords: COVID-19; ERCP; EUS; pancreaticobiliary disease; pandemic; SARS-CoV-2

1. Introduction

COVID-19 is an infectious disease that can lead to serious respiratory disorders caused by severe acute respiratory syndrome coronavirus-2 (SARS-CoV-2) and which spread worldwide from China (Wuhan) around November 2019, causing a pandemic. SARS-CoV-2 is transmitted through droplet infection and contact infection, but airborne transmission via aerosolized SARS-CoV-2 is also a concern [1,2]. In Japan, infection spread from around January 2020, and an emergency declaration (ED) was issued for the period between 7 April 2020 and 25 May 2020. To prevent the spread of infection, the following was requested: refraining from going outside, closing of schools, and restrictions on the use of facilities where many people gather, such as department stores and movie theaters.

During gastroenterological endoscopy, an aerosol generated by coughing during endoscope insertion is a risk because of the proximity of medical workers and patients. SARS-CoV-2 can survive for several hours in the air and may be transmitted by prolonged exposure to high concentrations of contaminated aerosols in enclosed spaces, such as the endoscope room [3]. Additionally, there is potential for fecal virus shedding [4,5], which is a potential risk of infection in colonoscopy. Therefore, the number of endoscopies for gastrointestinal screening has decreased, possibly delaying detection of gastrointestinal cancer [6]. Emergency endoscopic procedures should be performed under strict infection control. Especially in the field of pancreaticobiliary disease, such as severe cholangitis, delay is dangerous, and it is necessary to commence diagnosis and treatment promptly, considering the poor prognosis of pancreaticobiliary cancer. Pancreaticobiliary cancer is often at an advanced stage at diagnosis, which contributes to the poor prognosis. Because endoscopic treatment for pancreaticobiliary cancer is usually in a symptomatic context, it is important to examine the changes in endoscopic examination of the bile and pancreas under COVID-19 to evaluate the usefulness of screening for asymptomatic pancreaticobiliary cancer.

We compared the number of cases of pancreaticobiliary endoscopy before and after the ED and the number of newly diagnosed pancreaticobiliary cancers, and examined the period-by-period correlation between the presence of symptoms and tumor progression.

2. Methods

2.1. Study Design

This was a single-center retrospective study and was approved by our institutional review board (ethical code 20-232). We reviewed the chart and database of endoscopy and radiological procedures. All authors had access to the study data and approved the final manuscript.

We examined the number of endoscopic treatments for pancreaticobiliary disease (EUS: endoscopic ultrasonography/ERCP: endoscopic retrograde cholangiopancreatography) and newly diagnosed pancreaticobiliary cancer (BTC: biliary tract cancer/PC: pancreatic cancer) in our hospital. We analyzed BTC including intrahepatic bile duct cancer, hilar bile duct cancer, distal bile duct cancer, gallbladder cancer, and papilla of vater cancer. We surveyed three periods: before (1 April 2018 to 6 April 2020), during (7 April to 25 May 2020), and after the ED (26 May to 31 July). We retrospectively compared the age, sex, clinical stage, and symptoms of patients with pancreaticobiliary cancer diagnosed during each period. Symptoms were defined as jaundice, fever, abdominal pain, and weight loss.

2.2. Infection Protection Measures of Endoscopic for Coronavirus in Our Hospital

During the COVID-19 period, patients were required to wear masks with face-shields (or goggles and masks), gloves, caps, and gowns (long sleeves) when undergoing endoscopy. After the examination and treatment were completed, the fingers and elbows were cleaned thoroughly and disinfected with alcohol. All procedures were performed with medical staff wearing N95 masks and surgical masks. For high-risk patients (positive PCR or antigen test; persistent fever and/or dyspnea; computed tomography (CT) findings of pneumonia, dysgeusia, and/or dysosmia; and close contact with COVID-19 patients within 2 weeks), endoscopic treatment was performed in a continuous negative pressure room with double-layer gloves, covering on the whole body, and ventilation as recommended by the Ministry of Health, Labor, and Welfare (30 m^3 per person per hour) [7,8]. The minimum number of endoscopists, assistants, and nurses were used for the procedure.

2.3. Statistical Analysis

The number of endoscopic procedures (ERCP/EUS) and the number of diagnoses of pancreaticobiliary cancer (PC, BTC) and the presence or absence of symptoms, and the proportion of stage III/IV at diagnosis, were compared via Kruskal–Wallis test and the Steel–Dwass method during the three periods. The Mann–Whitney U-test was used for two-group comparisons. The α-level was defined as 0.05, and probability values less than the α-level were considered to be statistically significant.

3. Results

3.1. Details of Newly Diagnosed Pancreaticobiliary Cancer at Each Period

The mean number of diagnoses per month before, during, and after the ED was 8.0, 7.5, and 7.5 cases, respectively, with no significant difference among the three groups ($p = 0.5$). The mean age at the time of pancreatic cancer diagnosis was 69.6, 69.7, and 71.6 years, and the proportion of males was 51.5%, 53.3%, and 55.6%, with no significant difference among the three groups. The presence of symptoms at diagnosis and the clinical stage of cancer (rate of stage III and IV) were more in evidence and more advanced during the ED, but there was no significant difference among the three groups (77.5%/93.3%/80.0%, $p = 0.3$ and 72.5%/80.0%/60.0%, $p = 0.9$, respectively) (Table 1).

Table 1. Details of pancreaticobiliary Cancer at Each Period.

	Before the ED	During the ED	After the ED	p Value
Duration	1 April 2018– 6 April 2020	7 April 2020– 25 May 2020	26 May 2020– 31 July 2020	
PC cases, total	96	15	15	
PC cases, average/m	8.0	7.5	7.5	0.5
Age average	69.6	69.7	71.6	0.3
Sex (Male), %	51.5	53.3	55.6	0.4
Symptomatic case, %	77.5	93.3	80	0.3
Stage III/IV, %	72.5	80	60	0.9
BTC cases, total	48	7	6	
BTC cases, average/m	4.0	3.5	3.0	0.9
Age average	71.8	71.4	71.8	0.3
Sex (Male), %	67.3	71.4	66.7	0.3
Symptomatic case, %	82.5	57.1	100	0.4
Stage III/IV, %	62	83	88	0.5

ED: emergency declaration, BTC: biliary tract cancer, PC: pancreatic cancer.

The mean number of diagnoses of biliary tract cancer per month was 4.0, 3.5, and 3.0, and there was no significant difference among the three groups ($p = 0.9$). The mean age at the time of diagnosis of biliary tract cancer was 71.8, 71.4, and 71.8, and the rate of males was 67.3%, 71.4%, and 66.7%, showing no significant difference among the three groups. The rate of symptoms was 82.5%, 57.1%, and 100%, which tended to be slightly but non-significantly lower during the ED, but there was no significant difference ($p = 0.4$). There was no significant difference in stage III and IV disease (62.0%/83.0%/88.0%) ($p = 0.5$) (Table 1).

3.2. The Average Number of Biliary and Pancreatic Endoscopes at Each Period (Monthly Average)

The number of biliary and pancreatic endoscopies decreased. There was no significant difference in the number of pancreaticobiliary endoscopies performed per month among the three groups (67.8/62.5/69.0 cases), whereas the number of EUSs was 89.8, 51.5, and 86.0, a 42.7% decrease between before and during the ED. Multiple comparisons showed a significant reduction between before and during the ED ($p = 0.04$, Figure 1). The number of EUS-guided fine needle aspiration (EUS-FNA) cases also tended to be lower (17.8, 11.5, and 18.5 cases) during the ED, but the difference was not significant ($p = 0.7$) (Table 2).

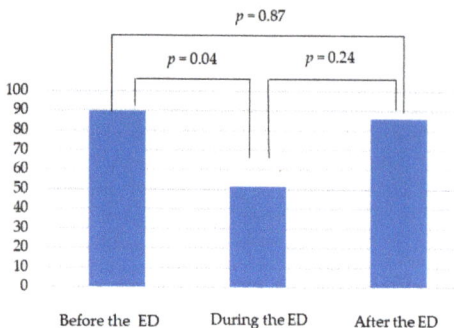

Figure 1. There were no significant differences among the three groups in the number of EUS per month (89.8/51.5/86.0 cases). Multiple comparisons showed a significant reduction between before and during the ED ($p = 0.04$).

Table 2. The number of biliary and pancreatic endoscopes at each period (monthly average).

	Before the ED	During the ED	After the ED	p Value
Duration	1 April 2018– 6 April 2020	7 April 2020– 25 May 2020	26 May 2020– 31 July 2020	
EUS	89.8	51.5	86.0	0.06
EUS-FNA	15.0	11.5	18.5	0.3
ERCP	67.8	62.5	69.0	0.7

EUS: endoscopic ultrasounds, EUS-FNA: EUS-guided fine needle aspiration, ERCP: endoscopic retrograde cholangiopancreatography.

3.3. The Breakdown of ERCP during and Post Emergency Declaration (Monthly Average)

The ERCP breakdown between during and after the ED showed no change in the treatment of malignant tumor, benign biliary tract workup, or stone. Regarding cholecystitis, one patient was treated percutaneously during the ED. Endoscopic transpapillary gallbladder drainage (ETGBD) was enforced for four cases of cholecystitis after the ED (Table 3).

Table 3. The breakdown of ERCP during and post emergency declaration (monthly average).

	During the ED	After the ED	p Value
Duration	7 April 2020– 25 May 2020	26 May 2020– 31 July 2020	
Malignant stricture			
Diagnosis	15.0	15.0	0.2
Exchange stent	10.0	9.0	0.6
Benign stricture			
Diagnosis	1.0	5.0	0.3
Exchange stent	19.0	16.5	1.0
CBDS	11.5	15.0	0.2
ETGBD	0.5	2.0	0.6

CBDS: common bile duct stones, ETGBD: endoscopic transpapillary gallbladder drainage.

4. Discussion

All upper gastrointestinal endoscopies (including ERCP/EUS) have a risk of aerosol generation. To prevent aerosols caused by the cough reflex, sedation is recommended. For pancreaticobiliary endoscopic procedures such as EUS and ERCP, the procedure duration is longer than other upper endoscopic procedures. Caution is also needed with regards to aerosols when placing and removing a number of devices in and from the working channel.

In these aspects, pancreaticobiliary endoscopic procedures may be associated with a higher risk than upper gastrointestinal endoscopies. At the time of the emergency declaration, it was recommended that the decision for examination and treatment of each case should take into account the extent of COVID-19 infection, the triage and risk of infection by case, and the circumstances of the hospital setting [9].

In this study, we investigated the impact of coronavirus epidemics on the diagnosis of malignancy using the number of endoscopic examinations and the number of newly diagnosed pancreaticobiliary cancer our hospital. The results showed no significant difference in the number of diagnoses of pancreatic cancer and biliary tract cancer before, during, and after the ED. The functioning of the hospital and the maintenance of a similar diagnosis rate for pancreaticobiliary cancer to that of before the ED, without a cluster, were considered to be due to adequate triage and protection against infection. However, more than 60% of the cases were stage III or higher at diagnosis. This underscores the importance of screening for pancreaticobiliary cancer, given that early diagnosis before symptom onset was not possible. Gastrointestinal cancer can be detected early by screening endoscopy; therefore, a reduction in the rate of screening endoscopy will reduce that of gastrointestinal cancer detection. The number of pancreaticobiliary endoscopies decreased. The rate of EUS was significantly reduced, by 42.7%, and that of EUS-FNA by 23.3% between during and before the ED (Figure 2). This may be due to a shift from EUS to magnetic resonance cholangiopancreatography (MRCP) follow-up, especially in intraductal papillary mucinous neoplasm (IPMN) without high-risk symptoms and asymptomatic choledocholithiasis [10]. Priority was given to symptomatic patients, patients with masses on CT or MRI/MRCP, and those at high suspicion of malignancy [8,11]. Pancreatic cancer should be diagnosed and treated aggressively because of its rapid progression and limited resectability. The European Society of Medical Oncology (ESMO) recommends aggressive workup of pancreatic cancer in patients with suspected cancer on imaging, jaundice, or gastrointestinal obstruction [12]. Although it did not influence the diagnosis rate or stage of malignancy, further studies are needed to determine the magnitude of the delay in the diagnosis of cancer caused by a reduced rate of pancreaticobiliary EUS screening. Regarding the ERCP breakdown, there were no differences between during and after the ED in stent occlusion (benign/malignancy) or symptomatic bile duct stones. Endoscopic drainage (ETGBD) is the first-line modality for cholecystitis, but during the ED, patients were switched to percutaneous transhepatic gallbladder drainage (PTGBD) based on the risk of aerosol generation during endoscopy. There were no clinical problems with switching to PTGBD.

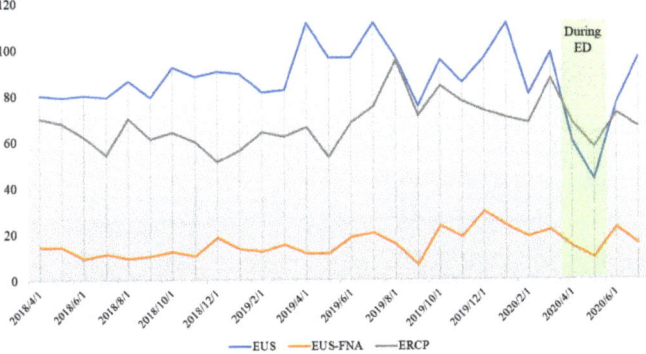

Figure 2. The number of pancreaticobiliary endoscopies decreased. The rate of EUS was significantly reduced by 42.7%, and that of EUS-FNA was reduced by 23.3% between during and before the ED.

Emergency cases in gastroenterology include gastrointestinal bleeding, obstructive jaundice, biliary tract infection, acute pancreatitis, appendicitis, strangulating ileus, and acute large bowel obstruction. If the patient has a fever, we should be sufficiently cautious about delaying treatment of emergency cases. However, if consultations with a specialist are delayed until after a negative COVID-19 test result, it may be too late for theses emergency cases. In our hospital, EUS-hepaticogastrostomy (EUS-HGS) stenting was performed to prevent recurrence of bile duct cancer after surgery, and if the patient visited our hospital because of cholangitis. Because pneumonia was recognized by CT, a patient was put under 1-day observation and an antibiotic agent prescribed until a negative PCR result ensued. However, on day 2, the delayed treatment led to multiple organ failure. Thus, it is important not to miss the window for treatment of these emergency diseases. Especially, patients with malignancies have less spare ability than healthy individuals and are more likely to have severe infections such as cholangitis. In such situations, ERCP, including elective stent replacement procedures, should be performed without delay [13]. Hepatic disorders have been noted in about 20% of patients with COVID-19 symptoms, and differentiation from cholangitis may be difficult in patients with fever and hepatic dysfunction [14,15]. Elevated pancreatic enzymes were reported in 17% of patients [12]. High amylase without abdominal pain is common, and attention must be paid to pancreatic enzymes such as amylase and lipase when examining patients with COVID-19. CT of the abdomen is necessary to rule out pancreatitis. Thus, with regards to pancreaticobiliary disease and COVID-19, it is important to determine whether the disease is aggravated or a side effect of COVID-19, and to perform necessary treatment without delay [12–15].

Limitation

Simple comparisons are difficult because of the different lengths and timing of the three periods compared. It is a limitation that the number of cases was small in the examination of a single department.

5. Conclusions

The diagnosis of pancreaticobiliary cancer should be made with adequate protection against infection in COVID-19. In addition, treatment with symptoms such as cholangitis was appropriately performed during the ED. On the other hand, the number of asymptomatic screening procedures has decreased, and the impact on the early diagnosis of pancreaticobiliary cancer needs further investigation.

Author Contributions: Conceptualization, K.T. and H.I.; methodology, M.U.; software, S.T.; validation, W.Y.; formal analysis, Y.T.; investigation, A.S.; resources, K.I.; data curation, K.O., S.I.; writing—original draft preparation, M.I.; writing—review and editing, K.T.; visualization, H.S., T.F.; supervision, A.N.; project administration, H.I. All authors have read and agreed to the published version of the manuscript.

Funding: This research received no external funding.

Institutional Review Board Statement: This was a single-center retrospective study and was approved by our institutional review board (ethical code 20-232). We reviewed the chart and database of endoscopy and radiological procedures. All authors had access to the study data and approved the final manuscript.

Informed Consent Statement: Informed consent was obtained from all subjects involved in the study.

Conflicts of Interest: The authors declare no conflict of interest.

References

1. Yu, I.T.; Li, Y.; Wong, T.W.; Tam, W.; Chan, A.; Lee, J.H.; Leung, D.Y.; Ho, T. Evidence of Airborne Transmission of the Severe Acute Respiratory Syndrome Virus. *N. Engl. J. Med.* **2004**, *350*, 1731–1739. [CrossRef] [PubMed]
2. Wang, J.; Du, G. COVID-19 may transmit through aerosol. *Ir. J. Med. Sci.* **2020**, *189*, 1143–1144. [CrossRef] [PubMed]
3. Van Doremalen, N.; Bushmaker, T.; Morris, D.H.; Holbrook, M.G.; Gamble, A.; Williamson, B.N. Aerosol and Surface Stability of SARS-CoV-2 as Compared with SARS-CoV-1. *N. Engl. J. Med.* **2020**, *382*, 1564–1567. [CrossRef] [PubMed]
4. Gu, J.; Han, B.; Wang, J. COVID-19: Gastrointestinal Manifestations and Potential Fecal–Oral Transmission. *Gastroenterology* **2020**, *158*, 1518–1519. [CrossRef] [PubMed]

5. Wong, S.H.; Lui, R.N.; Sung, J.J. Covid-19 and the digestive system. *J. Gastroenterol. Hepatol.* **2020**, *35*, 744–748. [CrossRef] [PubMed]
6. Lui, T.K.L.; Leung, K.; Guo, C.G.; Tsui, V.W.M.; Wu, J.T.; Leung, W.K. Impacts of the Coronavirus 2019 Pandemic on Gastrointestinal Endoscopy Volume and Diagnosis of Gastric and Colorectal Cancers: A Population-Based Study. *Gastroenterology* **2020**, *159*, 1164–1166.e1163. [CrossRef] [PubMed]
7. Soetikno, R.; Teoh, A.Y.; Kaltenbach, T.; Lau, J.Y.; Asokkumar, R.; Cabral-Prodigalidad, P.; Shergill, A. Considerations in performing endoscopy during the COVID-19 pandemic. *Gastrointest. Endosc.* **2020**, *92*, 176–183. [CrossRef] [PubMed]
8. Repici, A.; Maselli, R.; Colombo, M.; Gabbiadini, R.; Spadaccini, M.; Anderloni, A.; Carrara, S.; Fugazza, A.; Di Leo, M.; Galtieri, P.A.; et al. Coronavirus (COVID-19) outbreak: What the department of endoscopy should know. *Gastrointest. Endosc.* **2020**, *92*, 192–197. [CrossRef]
9. Prachand, V.N.; Milner, R.; Angelos, P.; Posner, M.C.; Fung, J.J.; Agrawal, N.; Jeevanandam, V.; Matthews, J.B. Medically Necessary, Time-Sensitive Procedures: Scoring System to Ethically and Efficiently Manage Resource Scarcity and Provider Risk During the COVID-19 Pandemic. *J. Am. Coll. Surg.* **2020**, *231*, 281–288. [CrossRef] [PubMed]
10. Buxbaum, J.L.; Abbas Fehmi, S.M.; Sultan, S.; Fishman, D.S.; Qumseya, B.J.; Cortessis, V.K. ASGE guideline on the role of endoscopy in the evaluation and manage-ment of choledocholithiasis. *Gastrointest. Endosc.* **2019**, *89*, 1075–1105.e1015. [CrossRef] [PubMed]
11. Ang, T.L.; Li, J.W.; Vu CK, F.; Ho, G.H.; Chang, J.P.E.; Chong, C.H. Chapter of Gastroenterologists professional guidance on risk mitigation for gastrointes-tinal endoscopy during COVID-19 pandemic in Singapore. *Singap. Med. J.* **2020**, *61*, 345–349. [CrossRef] [PubMed]
12. Catanese, S.; Pentheroudakis, G.; Douillard, J.-Y.; Lordick, F. ESMO Management and treatment adapted recommendations in the COVID-19 era: Pancreatic Cancer. *ESMO Open* **2020**, *5* (Suppl. 3), e000804. [CrossRef] [PubMed]
13. Khamaysi, I.; Michlin, S. Increased mortality in patients waiting for biliary stent replacement during the COVID-19 pan-demic. *Endoscopy* **2020**, *52*, 708. [PubMed]
14. Sultan, S.; Altayar, O.; Siddique, S.M.; Davitkov, P.; Feuerstein, J.D.; Lim, J.K.; Falck-Ytter, Y.; El-Serag, H.B. AGA Institute Rapid Review of the Gastrointestinal and Liver Manifestations of COVID-19, Meta-Analysis of International Data, and Recommendations for the Consultative Management of Patients with COVID-19. *Gastroenterology* **2020**, *159*, 320–334.e27. [CrossRef] [PubMed]
15. Mao, R.; Qiu, Y.; He, J.-S.; Tan, J.-Y.; Li, X.-H.; Liang, J.; Shen, J.; Zhu, L.-R.; Chen, Y.; Iacucci, M.; et al. Manifestations and prognosis of gastrointestinal and liver involvement in patients with COVID-19: A systematic review and meta-analysis. *Lancet Gastroenterol. Hepatol.* **2020**, *5*, 667–678. [CrossRef]

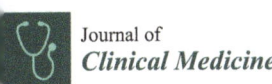

Review

Role of lncRNAs in the Development of an Aggressive Phenotype in Gallbladder Cancer

Pablo Pérez-Moreno [1,†], Ismael Riquelme [2,†], Priscilla Brebi [3] and Juan Carlos Roa [1,*]

1. Department of Pathology, School of Medicine, Pontificia Universidad Católica de Chile, Santiago 8380000, Chile; pablo.perezm@uc.cl
2. Institute of Biomedical Sciences, Faculty of Health Sciences, Universidad Autónoma de Chile, Temuco 4810101, Chile; ismael.riquelme@uautonoma.cl
3. Laboratory of Integrative Biology (LiBi), Centro de Excelencia en Medicina Translacional (CEMT), Scientific and Technological Bioresource Nucleus (BIOREN), Universidad de la Frontera, Temuco 4810296, Chile; priscilla.brebi@ufrontera.cl
* Correspondence: jcroa@med.puc.cl; Tel.: +56-22354-1061
† These authors contributed equally to this work.

Abstract: Long non-coding RNAs are sequences longer than 200 nucleotides that are involved in different normal and abnormal biological processes exerting their effect on proliferation and differentiation, among other cell features. Functionally, lncRNAs can regulate gene expression within the cells by acting at transcriptional, post-transcriptional, translational, or post-translational levels. However, in pathological conditions such as cancer, the expression of these molecules is deregulated, becoming elements that can help in the acquisition of tumoral characteristics in the cells that trigger carcinogenesis and cancer progression. Specifically, in gallbladder cancer (GBC), recent publications have shown that lncRNAs participate in the acquisition of an aggressive phenotype in cancer cells, allowing them to acquire increased malignant capacities such as chemotherapy resistance or metastasis, inducing a worse survival in these patients. Furthermore, lncRNAs are useful as prognostic and diagnostic biomarkers since they have been shown to be differentially expressed in tumor tissues and serum of individuals with GBC. Therefore, this review will address different lncRNAs that could be promoting malignant phenotypic characteristics in GBC cells and lncRNAs that may be useful as markers due to their capability to predict a poor prognosis in GBC patients.

Keywords: long non-coding RNAs; lncRNA; prognosis; gallbladder cancer

1. Introduction

In the last decades, the study of aggressive malignant characteristics in cancer has involved mainly protein-coding RNAs (mRNA encoded from genes), which have been associated with different mechanisms that promote an aggressive phenotype in cancer cells [1]. However, in recent years a new group of molecules named non-coding RNAs (ncRNAs) has been described to play an important role in the development of cancer due to its implication in several malignant cellular processes [2]. These ncRNAs include microRNAs (miRNAs), small-nuclear RNAs (snRNA), small-nucleolar RNAs (snoRNAs), ribosomal RNAs (rRNAs), small-interfering RNAs (siRNAs), PIWI-interacting RNAs (piRNAs), and long non-coding RNAs (lncRNAs), all with different action mechanisms able to regulate gene expression within the cells in both homeostatic and pathological conditions [3].

LncRNAs are defined as RNA sequences of more than 200 nucleotides that typically do not possess functional open reading frames (ORFs) and most are transcribed by RNA polymerase II [4]. These transcripts act by epigenetically regulating the gene expression at post-transcriptional, transcriptional, translational and post-translational levels by forming structures of RNA:RNA, RNA:DNA, and RNA:Protein that allow them to participate in different cellular processes [5,6]. The expression of lncRNAs has been associated with different types of cancers by inducing the acquisition of more aggressive characteristics, such as higher tumorigenic capacity, higher metastatic capacity, induction of epithelial-mesenchymal-transition (EMT) features, drug resistance, and stem-like phenotype, all of them directly related to poor prognosis in cancer patients [7–10]. These characteristics are frequently observed in different cancers such as breast, lung, colorectal, and gallbladder cancer [3,11]. Specifically, in gallbladder cancer (GBC), it has been shown that the expression of certain lncRNAs can promote the development of malignant features in cancer cells, correlating with a worsening of clinicopathological characteristics. Examples of this are the ROR and UCA1 lncRNAs, which have been shown to promote greater proliferative and invasive capacity, correlating with a worse prognosis in GBC patients [12,13]. For this reason, this review will address different malignant phenotypic characteristics that may be induced by lncRNAs in GBC cells and that may be useful to predict a more aggressive tumor phenotype in patients.

2. Search and Selection of Literature

A comprehensive search of the literature was performed by authors using online databases including PubMed and Web of Science. The search terms were as follows: (lncRNA OR long noncoding RNA) AND (gallbladder cancer OR gallbladder neoplasia OR gallbladder carcinoma) AND (poor prognosis OR aggressive phenotype OR metastasis OR drug resistance OR stem OR tumorigenesis OR invasion OR Migration OR proliferation).

Selection criteria for lncRNAs in GBC were as follows: (1) lncRNA expression detected in tissues or serum from GBC patients; (2) lncRNAs related to aggressive phenotypic features in GBC (e.g., proliferation, invasion, epithelial-mesenchymal transition, tumorigenicity, migration, stemness, drug resistance and metastasis); and (3) lncRNAs related to some clinicopathological features (e.g., overall survival, TNM stage, tumor size, histological grade, distant metastasis, and lymphatic invasion). Those studies about lncRNAs not related directly to GBC were excluded from this article. The search diagram used in this article is shown in Figure 1.

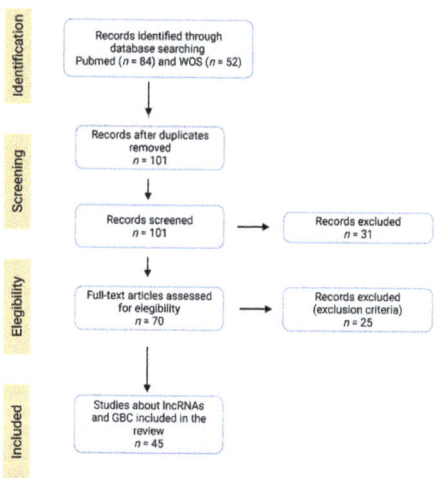

Figure 1. Search diagram used in the systematic review.

3. Long Non-Coding RNAs: Mechanisms of Action

LncRNAs are divided into five broad categories according to the location relative to nearby protein-coding genes: intergenic, intronic, bidirectional, antisense and sense [14–16]. LncRNAs can exert their functions within the cells in both the nucleus and the cytoplasm. In the nucleus, lncRNAs actively participate interacting with *cis* or *trans* binding sites that induce the transcription or silencing of specific genes. In this regard, many lncRNAs can interact with the nuclear epigenetic machinery as the polycomb repressive complex 2 (PRC2) resulting in the control of gene expression [17–19]. For example, HOTAIR mediates the transcriptional silencing of HOXD locus via recruitment of the PRC2, promoting the subsequent invasion and metastasis in breast cancer [20]. Meanwhile, in the cytoplasm, these transcripts participate in the stabilization of mRNAs and the regulation of translation, for instance, by interacting with RNA binding proteins (RBPs) that lead to several alterations in the mRNA stability, splicing, protein stability and subcellular localization [21–23].

As mentioned above, lncRNAs are capable of physically interacting with different molecules, including DNA, RNA and proteins, generating complexes that allow the regulation of the function and expression of these macromolecules. Based on this, five main mechanisms in which this type of non-coding RNAs participates have been described [24]. First, lncRNAs can be signal molecules. This implies that they can increase or decrease against different stimuli determining a specific cellular context, for example, as indicators of transcriptional activity. In addition, this type of lncRNA can interact with DNA sites allowing the binding of different proteins, such as specific transcription factors, which allow regulation in the transcription of downstream genes. Second, lncRNAs can act as guides by binding to effector proteins that allow directing the target to a specific site. As an example, lncRNAs often interact with transcription factors that guide them to their target site to regulate gene expression. Third, lncRNAs can function as decoys since they can bind and sequester different target proteins preventing their normal function. Fourth, lncRNAs can function as scaffolds, because they can bind to proteins and mediate the formation of protein complexes regulating gene expression. Finally, lncRNAs can function as a competitive endogenous RNA network (ceRNA) since it has been shown that they can sponge miRNAs and prevent their binding to their mRNA target, causing an increase in the stability of the mRNA [25,26]. To improve understanding of these processes the mechanisms described above are summarized in Figure 2.

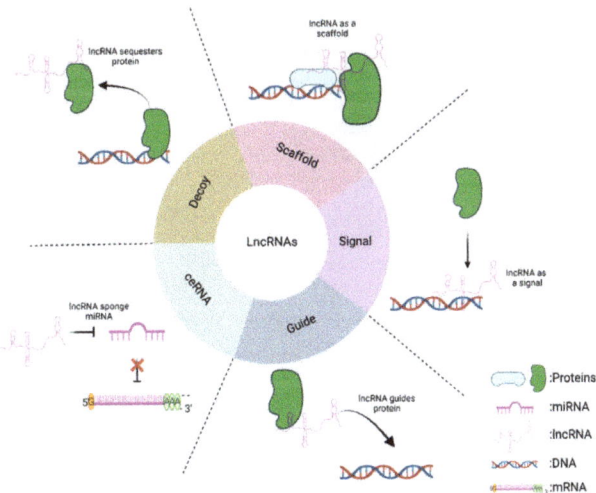

Figure 2. Scheme of the mechanisms of action of lncRNAs. This diagram shows the different forms in which lncRNAs can regulate different molecular processes. Decoy: lncRNA can sequester a protein of interest, interfering with its normal function. Scaffold: lncRNA can interact with different proteins allowing the formation of protein complexes. Signal: lncRNA acts as a tag for the recruitment of a protein to a specific site. Guide: lncRNA drives a protein of interest to its specific site of action. ceRNA: lncRNA acts as a competitive molecule that binds a miRNA sequence preventing the binding of this miRNA to its target (mRNA), allowing that the mRNA increases its stability and expression.

4. LncRNAs in Gallbladder Cancer

Gallbladder cancer has a mortality of 85,000 deaths worldwide and an incidence rate of 0.9 cases per 100,000 individuals [27]. The incidence of GBC varies among the different geographical areas of the world, showing a higher incidence among descendants of North and South American natives, and in several Asian countries [28]. The highest GBC incidence rate is found in Chile between individuals who descend from the Mapuche people, with 12.3 cases per 100,000 in men and 27.3 cases per 100,000 in women [28,29].

Unfortunately, as symptomatology is unspecific and routine biochemical assays are not accurate, GBC is usually diagnosed late, sometimes as an accidental finding in patients with cholelithiasis. Due to this late diagnosis, GBC is generally found in an advanced stage, which causes that these patients have a poor prognosis and short life expectancy [28]. For instance, the 5-year survival rate of GBC in advanced stages (T3 and T4 stages) is less than 5%, while if this cancer were detected in the initial stages (T1 stage) there would be an increase up to 75% in this 5-year survival rate [28].

The research about lncRNAs and their participation in the acquisition of a malignant tumor phenotype has evidenced a dramatic increase because a large number of them have been demonstrated to actively participate in several mechanisms that contribute to the progression of cancer [11]. Regarding this, the development of metastatic and tumorigenic characteristics is closely related to a more aggressive phenotype in cancer because these features provide cancer cells the capacity of expanding to other tissues and form new tumors, indicating a worse prognosis in cancer patients [1].

Due to the reasons previously stated, the search for new biomarkers that can help in the diagnosis and prognosis of the GBC cases is urgently necessary. In this search for more suitable biomarkers in the follow-up of GBC, lncRNAs seem to be molecules that are worth exploring in greater depth.

Next, we will classify each lncRNA described according to its expression in GBC tissues

4.1. Upregulated lncRNAs in GBC

Since the discovery of the first lncRNA in 1990 [30], many other lncRNAs have been described to date, using the latest technologies in molecular biology and due to large databases that have been able to provide a large amount of information on their molecular characteristics and biological functions in cancer [31]. Regarding the GBC, AFAP1-AS1, is a lncRNA that is overexpressed in GBC tissues and its expression levels are significantly associated with tumor size. The long-rank Kaplan—Meier analysis suggests that higher expression of AFAP1-AS1 is a poor prognosis factor in these patients. Functionally, the knockdown of AFAP1-AS1 may inhibit proliferation and invasion, and decrease Twist1 and Vimentin expression in GBC cell lines, indicating that AFAP1-AS1 may participate in cancer progression [32]. Similarly, ANRIL has been found upregulated in GBC tissues compared to adjacent normal tissues and has been also shown to increase proliferation and tumor size in a murine model, which is consistent with the correlation of its expression with overall survival in these patients [33].

CCAT1 has been described in different cancers, including gastric and colorectal cancer [34]. This lncRNA has been shown to be upregulated in GBC tissues compared with adjacent normal tissues. Furthermore, CCAT1 is more highly expressed in tumors in advanced stages than (T3 + T4) early stages (T1 + T2), and more highly expressed in tumors spread to lymph nodes (N1/2) compared with tumors localized only in the gallbladder (N0). CCAT1 expression is significantly correlated with tumor status, lymph node invasion and advanced tumor node metastasis (TNM) stage, suggesting that CCAT1 expression is related to poor prognosis in GBC. In addition, in vitro experiments show that the knockdown of CCAT1 decreases S-phase, invasion and tumor growth in vivo. Mechanistically, the authors propose that CCAT1 increases the expression of Bmi1 through competitively sponging miRNA-218-5p [35].

Along with this, current evidence has shown that those tumor tissues with a higher expression of cancer stem cell (CSCs) markers are prone to developing a greater tumorigenic and metastatic capacity and are directly associated with a worse life expectancy of patients [36–40]. Only one overexpressed lncRNA has been described in GBC patient tissues that promote the expression of markers associated with the stem-like cell population. DILC is overexpressed in gallbladder CSCs and GBC tissues and its knockdown decreased stem-like CD44$^+$/CD133$^+$ cell population and diminished sphere-forming capacity in GBC cells. Consistently, the expression of stemness-associated transcription factors and CSC markers (ABCG2, MDR-1, Oct4 and CD34) were also inhibited by DILC knockdown in GBC spheroids. Moreover, DILC knockdown decreased proliferation, migration and invasion in vitro, as well as tumor growth and CSC number in NOD/SCID xenograft model. In addition, the knockdown of DILC reduced metastasis capacity in vivo by activating Wnt/β-catenin pathway. This suggests that DILC promotes stem-like properties in GBC and can subsequently induce a pro-metastatic and pro-tumorigenic phenotype in this neoplasm [41].

Another lncRNA implicated in the development of aggressive features in cancer is DGCR5 [42–46]. This lncRNA is upregulated in GBC tissues and cell lines and has been associated with proliferation migration, invasion, colony formation, and tumor growth in vivo in GBC. Mechanistically, when DGCR5 is upregulated, a lower expression of ZO-1 and E-cadherin can be induced, whereas the expression levels of N-cadherin, vimentin, MMP-2, and MMP-9 are upregulated. Moreover, the MEK/ERK1/2 and JNK/p38 MAPK pathways may also be involved in the function performed by DGCR5 to induce invasion and EMT processes [47].

FOXD2-AS1 is another lncRNA that has been shown to induce proliferation, tumor growth, migration and invasion due to its effect on recruiting DNMT1, a methyltransferase that subsequently produces promoter methylation in the MLH1 gene, and consequently the inhibition of MLH1 transcription [48]. A study by Cai et al. identified around 457 overexpressed and 266 downregulated lncRNAs in doxorubicin (DOX)-resistant GBC cells. Among the overexpressed lncRNAs, GBCDRlnc1 seemed to be interesting because it was also found highly expressed in GBC tissues compared to adjacent noncancerous tissues. Kaplan—Meier analysis demonstrated that patients with GBCDRlnc1 overexpression have a significantly shorter overall survival than those with lower expression of this lncRNA, which was also correlated with histological grade and TNM stage [49]. In DOX-resistant GBC cell lines, the GBCDRlnc1 overexpression showed to be involved in an increased autophagy activity within the cells by enhancing the conversion from LC3-I into LC3-II and by inhibiting the ubiquitination of phosphoglycerate kinase 1 (PGK1). High GBCDRlnc1 levels were found in DOX-resistant GBC cells inducing a significantly greater resistance to doxorubicin, gemcitabine, and 5-fluorouracil in these cells. Therefore, this study suggests that chemoresistance observed in GBC cells may be related to the increased autophagic activity induced by GBCDRlnc1 [49].

Regarding GALM, this has been observed to be increased in tumor tissues from GBC patients and positively correlated with poorly differentiated cells, lymph node metastases, and TNM staging. Kaplan-Meier analysis revealed that elevated GALM expression is associated with reduced overall survival, suggesting that GALM expression is related to a worse prognosis in GBC. To observe the functional effect of GALM, the authors overexpressed this lncRNA in GBC cell lines, observing a greater migratory and invasive capacity in vitro. It is observed that the overexpression of GALM increased the levels of ZEB1, ZEB2, Vimentin and N-cadherin, suppressing the levels of E-cadherin. Accordingly, in vivo experiments demonstrated an increase in liver metastatic capacity, suggesting that GALM may promote EMT and metastatic ability in GBC. Notably, those cells that overexpressed GALM had a greater extravasation capacity, detected 48 h after intrasplenic injection of these cells in a mice model, suggesting that GALM promotes EMT and metastatic ability in GBC. Mechanistically, the authors showed that GALM functioned as sponges by competitively binding to members of the miR-200 family and binding to IL-1β mRNA, stabilizing it [50]. Similarly, HGBC has been involved in cell proliferation and the promotion of EMT and metastasis in GBC [24]. HGBC knockdown has shown a significantly decreased cell proliferation (over a 5-day culture), and a reduction in the colony formation ability in GBC cell lines. Similar effects have been observed when HGBC-knockdown GBC cell lines were injected subcutaneously into nude mice. The results showed that tumor volume and weight in mice injected with HGBC-knockdown cells were significantly decreased up to 30% compared to control. These data suggest HGBC has a potential role in the promotion of proliferation and tumor growth in GBC [24]. In addition, it has been shown that knockdown of HGBC reduces cell migration, expression of vimentin and N-cadherin, and decreased metastatic liver nodules after injection of cancer cells in the spleen in mice. This effect can be mediated by the binding among HGBC and an RNA-binding protein called Hu Antigen R (HuR). In addition, HGBC expression can be used as a progression and poor prognosis marker in GBC, particularly because the upregulation of HGBC has been positively associated with TNM stage and lymph node metastasis and has been significantly correlated with reduced overall survival [24].

HEGBC is another lncRNA that shares similar characteristics in GBC. HEGBC has been shown to increase their expression significantly in GBC cell lines and tissues compared to controls. Correlation analyses between the expression of HEGBC and clinicopathologic characteristics of GBC patients indicate that high HEGBC expression is positively correlated with lymph node metastasis and TNM stages. A Kaplan—Meier survival analysis has been shown that GBC patients with high HEGBC expression have worse survival than those with low HEGBC expression, suggesting that HEGBC expression is related to poor prognosis. In vitro, ectopic expression of HEGBC increased proliferation and migration, decreasing apoptotic capacity. In vivo experiments have shown that HEGBC overexpression in GBC cell lines significantly increased tumor growth in nude mice. The proliferation marker Ki-67 was higher in tumors that had HEGBC overexpression. Furthermore, GBC cells that stably overexpress HEGBC increased metastatic foci in the liver in nude mice. Mechanistically, it shows that HEGBC binds to the IL-11 promoter, increasing IL-11 transcription promoting an autocrine IL-11 signal, and activating the STAT3 signaling pathway. Furthermore, it has been demonstrated that STAT3 is also bound to the HEGBC promoter and activated HEGBC expression, suggesting that the effects induced by HEGBC are through a HEGBC/IL-11/STAT3 positive regulatory loop in GBC [51].

It has been shown that HOXA-AS2 is actively involved in human cancers [52]. About this, it has been shown a higher expression in GBC tumors and cell lines of HOXA-AS2. In addition, the overexpression of this lncRNA promotes proliferation, colony formation, apoptosis evading, migration, and invasion. Notably, the ectopic expression of HOXA-AS2 induces N-cadherin and Vimentin expression with the consequent decrease of E-cadherin, which suggests that HOXA-AS2 induces aggressiveness and EMT characteristics in GBC [53].

Another lncRNA is HOTAIR, which has been shown to be overexpressed in different cancers and to promote malignant tumor characteristics [54]. HOTAIR is overexpressed in gallbladder cancer tissues compared with adjacent non-tumoral tissues, indicating that HOTAIR is frequently upregulated on GBC. In addition, HOTAIR is more expressed in gallbladder tumors (T3 + T4) compared with tumors (T1 + T2). HOTAIR expression is more expressed in tumors spread to regional lymph nodes (N1) compared to primary tumors, suggesting that HOTAIR expression may be a progression and prognosis marker in GBC patients. Functionally, HOTAIR promotes proliferation and migration in GBC cell lines, correlating positively with the expression of c-Myc and negatively with miRNA-130a, which suggests that this mechanism may participate in cancer progression in GBC patients [54].

H19 is a lncRNA that has been expressed in different cancers in which it has been shown to participate in the acquisition of different oncogenic characteristics [55]. In GBC, H19 expression has been shown to be overexpressed in tumor tissue than in adjacent non-tumor tissue. Its expression is correlated with tumor size, lymphatic metastasis, and a worse prognosis in patients with GBC. Furthermore, H19 knockdown has been shown to decrease proliferation, tumorigenesis, migration, invasion, and EMT, by reducing

Twist expression. Mechanistically, it was observed that overexpression of H19 in GBC cells downregulated miR-194-5p and markedly increased AKT2 expression, as well as enhanced the expression of miR-342-3p targeting FOXM1 through competitively sponging miR-342-3p, which suggests that the oncogenic function of H19 will be through both H19/miR-194-5p/AKT2 and H19/miR-342-3p/FOXM1 axes [56–58].

LINC01694 levels were also found remarkably elevated in GBC tissues, cell lines, and sera of patients with GBC. Patients with high LINC01694 values were more likely to develop stage III + IV and poorly differentiated GBC. Moreover, patients with higher LINC01694 levels had shorter total survival rates, being this transcript subsequently considered an independent factor in the prognosis of GBC patients. In vitro experiments evidenced that the LINC01694 knockdown effectively decreased proliferation and invasion compared to controls. In vivo analyses showed that the overexpression of LINC01694 significantly increased tumor growth in nude mice. Mechanistically, the higher expression of LINC01694 induced a reduction of miR-340-5p expression and, in consequence, a higher expression of SOX4. This result was confirmed in GBC tissues, which showed a positive correlation between LINC01694 y SOX4 expression but an inverse correlation with miR-340-5p expression. These data suggest that the aggressiveness induced by LINC01694 is via the LINC01694/miR-340-5p/SOX4 axis [59]. In a similar way, Loc344887 was found overexpressed in GBC tissues and cell lines compared to controls, and higher levels of Loc344887 were associated with larger tumor size. The Loc344887 knockdown was able to reduce the proliferative, migratory, and invasive features of GBC cells by decreasing the levels of Vimentin, N-Cadherin and Twist, and increasing the levels of E-cadherin, which suggests that Loc344887 promotes EMT and tumor progression in GBC [60].

LINC00152 has been widely described as an inductor of a tumorigenic phenotype in cells of several cancer types [61,62]. LINC00152 levels were found significantly higher in GBC tissues and in four human GBC cell lines compared to controls. The high LINC00152 levels were significantly associated with increased Ki-67-positive staining, a cell proliferation marker in tumors. In addition, the expression of LINC00152 was significantly higher in T3 + T4 compared to T1 + T2 tumors. Overexpression of LINC00152 significantly enhanced cell proliferation and the number of cancer cells in the S-phase in in vitro assays. This feature was confirmed in animal models where the high LINC00152 levels produced a greater tumor growth rate. Regarding the metastatic phenotype, LINC00152 expression levels were higher in metastatic lymph nodes than in primary tumors correlating positively with tumor status progression, lymph node invasion, TNM stage advancement and overall survival [63,64]. Moreover, the ectopic expression of LINC0052 promoted higher migration and invasion in vitro, as well as an increment in the number of peritoneal metastatic nodes in a murine model, accompanied by increased levels of Vimentin protein and decreased levels of E-cadherin protein. Mechanistically, LINC00152 can activate the PI3K pathway in GBC cells and can also act as a molecular sponge for miR-138, which directly suppresses the expression of hypoxia-inducible factor-1a (HIF-1a), suggesting that both the LINC00152/miR-138/HIF-1a axis and the activation of PI3K pathway by LINC00152 might be inducing GBC progression [63,64].

MALAT1 is one of the most studied lncRNAs in cancer [65–67] and has several oncogenic functions as modulates multiple signaling pathways involved in the enhancement of cell proliferation, metastasis, and invasion that commonly results in poor prognosis in cancer patients [68–74]. MALAT1 was found overexpressed in GBC tissue samples versus controls and its upregulation correlated positively with tumor size and lymph node metastasis, while also correlating negatively with overall survival [66,75–78]. The tumorigenic features developed by MALAT1 expression were evidenced by lower proliferation rate, lower colony formation and decreased tumor growth in in vivo models once GBC cells were treated with siRNAs against MALAT1 (siMALAT1) [66]. The metastatic features produced by MALAT1 are demonstrated in the fact that siMALAT1 significantly reduced the migration and invasion in GBC cell lines and produced a diminished expression of matrix metalloproteinase 9 (MMP-9), an enzyme involved in invasion by digesting the extracellular matrix. The confirmation of these results was performed in mice injected with siMALAT1 NOZ cells, which exhibited few metastatic peritoneal nodules at 8 weeks after inoculation, as well as a significant reduction in the levels of phosphorylated MEK1/2, ERK 1/2, MAPK, and JNK 1/2/3. These results suggest that the ERK/MAPK pathway participates in the MALAT1-induced metastasis of GBC cells [66]. Another probable mechanism by which MALAT1 may promote aggressive characteristics in GBC is regulating MCL-1 expression as a competing endogenous RNA for miR-363-3p [78].

MINCR expression is significantly elevated in GBC tissues, being associated with larger tumor size, lymph node metastasis, and shorter overall survival time, which suggests that MINCR is related to poor prognosis in GBC patients. Functionally, the knockdown of MINCR can reduce cell proliferation, migration, invasion, and EMT in vitro. As expected, tumor volume in vivo also significantly decreased in mice injected subcutaneously with GBC si-MINCR cells. This result can be explained because MINCR may be interacting with miRNA ribonucleoprotein complexes (miRNP) that also contain Ago2, and this interplay may modify the ability of miR-26a-5p to bind to EZH2, influencing its expression [79]. Similarly, NEAT1 is another lncRNA that has been found highly expressed in GBC tissues compared to controls. In addition, its knockdown decreases colony formation, migration, invasion in vitro, and tumor growth in vivo. The NEAT1 action mechanism probably involves serving as a sponge of miR-335 to subsequently provoke the increase of Survivin expression [80].

Recently, OIP5-AS1 has been described as a new lncRNA that participates in the acquisition of malignant characteristics in cancer [81–83]. In GBC cells lines (GBC-SD, NOZ, SGC996) this lncRNA has been shown to be significantly overexpressed. Furthermore, this OIP5-AS1 overexpression has been closely related to proliferation, migration, and invasion in GBC cell lines via reduction of miR-143-3p expression [84]. Another lncRNA significantly upregulated in GBC tissues is PVT1 in which expression was associated with advanced TNM stage and distant metastasis as well as correlated with a worse overall survival rate. Univariate and multivariate analyses showed that PVT1 was a potent independent prognostic indicator for GBC patients, suggesting that PVT1 expression is associated with poor prognosis in GBC patients. Additionally, PVT1 knockdown significantly inhibited cell proliferation, colony formation assay, migration, and invasion, inhibiting the expression of two matrix metalloproteinases, MMP-2, and MMP-9, suggesting that PVT1 can regulate EMT and cancer progression. Furthermore, the results demonstrated that these effects may be due to the up-regulation of HK2 by PVT1 through its competitive activity of endogenous RNA (ceRNA) on miR-143. However, other studies have been shown that these effects may be induced by other miRNAs, as miR-18b-5p and miR-30d-5p [85–87]. Another example is PAGBC, which is overexpressed in GBC tissues and is related with poor survival and advanced TNM stage, being considered as an independent prognostic factor for the overall survival of patients. This lncRNA promotes proliferation, colony formation, migration, invasion, and spleen metastasis in a mice model in GBC. This lncRNA can bind competitively to the tumor-suppressor microRNAs miR-133b and miR-511 activating the PI3K/mTOR pathway in GBC cells [88].

Another lncRNA is ROR, which has been involved in the acquisition of a more aggressive phenotype in GBC cases. ROR is upregulated in GBC tissues compared to matched normal tissues. The high expression of ROR has been found significantly associated with tumor size, lymph node metastasis and poorer overall survival time in GBC patients [13]. Also, ROR has been demonstrated to play an important role in cell proliferation, migration, and invasion in GBC cell lines. Silencing of ROR due to a siRNA against this lncRNA (siROR) induced a significant reduction in the number of cells in the S-phase and a decrease in the migration and invasion capacity of GBC cells [13]. To determine whether these aggressive characteristics are related to an EMT process, an siRNA against ROR was perform. The results showed that the mRNA expression of E-cadherin was significantly increased but Twist1 and Vimentin were markedly decreased in GBC cell lines, suggesting that ROR induces EMT in GBC cells [13].

SPRY4-IT1 is another non-coding RNA that is overexpressed in GBC cell lines and tissues versus controls. Its overexpression in GBC cell lines increases migration, proliferation, colony formation and invasion [89]. In a similar way, SNHG6 has been shown to be upregulated in serum from GBC patients and GBC cell lines compared to controls. This transcript has been closely related to poor prognosis because GBC has a correlation with grade of differentiation, TNM stage, tumor invasion, and location. The knockdown of SNHG6 may also decrease proliferation and invasion abilities in vitro, and reduced tumor growth in nude mice. Furthermore, these assays showed a significantly lower expression of N-cadherin, Vimentin and Snail while E-cadherin was significantly upregulated after transfection with siSNHG6, also indicating that SNHG6 can play a role in the development of EMT in GBC cells. This EMT process in GBC tumors may be triggered by SNHG6 via its downregulating effect on miR-26b-5p and the subsequent activation of the Hedgehog signaling pathway [90]. Another lncRNA is SSTR5-AS1 that has been involved in chemoresistance. SSTR5-AS1 has been found highly expressed in gemcitabine-resistant GBC cell lines. Results showed that upregulation of SSTR5-AS1 produced a decrease in apoptosis, specifically because the NONO/SSTR5-AS1 interaction prevents the degradation of NONO by the proteasome, thus suggesting that the apoptosis inhibition caused by SSTR5-AS1 is a signal of the development of drug resistance in GBC cell lines [91]. Moreover, SSTR5-AS1 was also found significantly upregulated in GBC tissues and cell lines compared to adjacent non-tumoral tissues, being associated with a worse overall survival rate in this cohort. Therefore, SSTR5-AS1 may be useful as a marker of prognosis marker in GBC patients [91]. Similarly, TUG1 has been found significantly overexpressed in GBC tissues and cell lines. Functionally, knockdown of TUG1 was able to significantly reduce proliferation and invasion in vitro, as well as inhibiting the Vimentin expression and upregulating the E-cadherin levels through a decrease in the miR-300 expression [92].

Another lncRNA involved in GBC progression is UCA1, whose upregulation has been observed in GBC tissues and GBC cell lines compared to controls. The UCA1 upregulation has been directly and significantly associated with certain clinicopathological characteristics of GBC patients including tumor size, lymph node metastasis, TNM stage, and poor overall survival time compared to patients with lower levels of UCA1 [12]. In tumor tissue injected subcutaneously in mice, the UCA1 overexpression also correlated with immunohistochemical expression of Ki-67, indicating that UCA1 may participate actively in proliferation and tumor growth processes [12]. In addition, UCA1 overexpression significantly promoted the cell migration and invasion of GBC cell lines by inducing the reduced expression of E-cadherin, and the increased Vimentin expression by Western blot. UCA1 expression was observed to be significantly upregulated after GBC cell lines were treated with TGF-β1, an activator o EMT process, which prompts that UCA1 can promote EMT in GBC through the recruitment of enhancer of zeste homolog 2 (EZH2) that subsequently induces the repression of p21 and E-cadherin in this malignancy [12].

TTN-AS and FENDRR are also found highly expressed in GBC tissues compared to controls. The knockdown of TTN-AS1 induced a decrease in migration and invasion capabilities by acting as a sponge to miR-107 and provoking the subsequent upregulation of HMGA1 [93,94]. Finally, CRNDE is a lncRNA that has not been described if its expression increases or decreases in patients with GBC. However, it has been observed that when a DMBT1 knockdown (CRNDE target as scaffold) is performed, the CRNDE expression increases. Furthermore, it has been observed that the expression of DMBT1 decreases in GBC tissues. Thus, these data suggest that CRNDE expression may be increased in GBC patients. Mechanistically, CRNDE acts as a scaffold for DMBT1, promoting migration and invasion through increased activity of the PI3K/AKT pathway [95].

For a better understanding, Table 1 resumes those lncRNAs that induce the acquisition of an aggressive phenotype in GBC.

Table 1. Resume of lncRNAs related to an aggressive phenotype on gallbladder cancer.

Expression	LncRNA	Aggressive Phenotype	Mechanism	Ref.
Up-regulated	AFAP1-AS1	P, I, E	ND	[34]
	ANRIL	P, T	ND	[33]
	CCAT1	I, P	Increases BMI-1 expression through the sponging of miR-218-5p	[35]
	DILC	S, P, I, M, T, ME	Promotes Wnt/β-catenin pathway	[41]
	DGCR5	P, T, I, M, E	Decreases ZO-1 expression and increases MEK/ERK1/2 and JNK/p38 MAPK pathways	[47]
	FENDRR	ND	ND	[94]
	FOXD2-AS1	P, M, T, I	Promotes MLH1 methylation by recruiting DNMT1	[48]
	GBCDRlnc1	D	Increases autophagy activity by enhancing the conversion from LC3-I into LC3-II and by inhibiting the ubiquitination of phosphoglycerate kinase 1(PGK1)	[49]
	GALM	I, M, ME, E	Acts as a sponge by competitively binding to miR-200 family and binding to IL-1β mRNA	[50]
	HGBC	P, T, M, E, ME	Acts through the interaction among HGBC and HuR	[24]
	HEGBC	P, M, T, ME	Acts through a HEGBC/IL-11/STAT3 positive regulatory loop	[51]
	HOXA-AS2	P, M, I, E	ND	[53]
	HOTAIR	M, P	Increases c-Myc expression through the sponging of miR-130a	[54]
	H19	P, T, M, I, E	Acts through both H19/miR-194-5p/AKT2 and H19/miR-342-3p/FOXM1 axes	[56–58]
	LINC01694	P, T, I	Acts via LIN01694/miR-340-5p/SOX4 axis	[59]
	LOC344887	P, M, I, E	ND	[60]
	LINC00152	P, T, E, M, I, ME	Acts through LINC00152/miR-138/HIF-1a axis activating PI3K pathway	[63,64]
	MALAT1	P, T, M, I, ME	MALAT1 regulates MCL-1 expression as a competing endogenous RNA for miR-363-3p	[66,75,76,78]
	MINCR	P, M, T, I, E	Modulates the ability of miR-26a-5p to bind to EZH2	[79]
	NEAT1	P, M, I, T	Increases surviving expression and acts as a sponge of miR-335	[80]
	OIP5-AS1	P, M, I	Reduces miR-143-3p expression	[84]
	PVT1	P, M, I, E	Upregulates HK2 through its competitive endogenous activity on miR-143 as well as miR-18b-5p and miR-30d-5p	[85–87]
	PAGBC	P, M, I, ME	Binds competitively miR-133b and miR-511 activating PI3K/mTOR pathway	[88]
	ROR	P, M, I, E	ND	[13]
	SPRY4-IT1	P, I, M	ND	[89]
	SNHG6	P, I, T, E	Decreases miR-26b-5p expression and regulates Hedgehog signaling pathway	[90]
	SSTR5-AS1	D	NONO/SSTR5_AS1 interaction prevents the degradation of NONO	[91]
	TUG1	P, I, E	Decreases miR-300 expression	[92]

Table 1. Cont.

Expression	LncRNA	Aggressive Phenotype	Mechanism	Ref.
Down-regulated	UCA1	M, T, I, E	Recruits EZH2 and induces p21 repression	[12,77]
	TTN-AS1	M, I	Acts as a sponge to miR-107 and upregulates HMGA1 expression	[93]
	GATA6-AS	P, I	Decreases mir-421 expression through TMP-2	[96]
	GCASPC	P, T	Inhibition of pyruvate carboxylase by GCASPC and miR-17-3p	[97]
	LET	P, I, T	ND	[98]
	MEG3	P, T, E, I	Promotes EZH2 degradation regulating LATS2 and NF-κb pathway	[33,99,100]

ND: not described; P: proliferation; I: invasion; E: epithelial-mesenchymal transition; T: tumorigenicity; M: migration; S: stemness; D: drug resistance; ME: metastasis.

4.2. Downregulated lncRNAs in GBC

As shown above, most of the lncRNAs described in GBC are overexpressed in these patients. However, there are lncRNAs that are also downregulated. An example of this is LET and GATA6-AS, which have been found downregulated in GBC tissues compared to non-tumor tissues. The low LET expression was correlated with less differentiated histology, greater invasion of lymph nodes, and advanced tumor stages. Moreover, multivariate analysis showed that LET expression was an independent prognostic indicator for metastasis and death, suggesting that the low levels of LET can serve as a prognostic indicator. Functionally, LET knockdown was able to increase the invasiveness and proliferative capacities under hypoxic conditions in GBC cells. On the contrary, LET overexpression increased apoptosis and suppressed proliferation and tumor growth in vivo. These results suggest that the lower expression of LET can participate in the progression of GBC [98]. Conversely, GATA6-AS expression was shown to progressively decrease as the gallbladder tumors proceeded to advanced stages, suggesting that GATA6-AS can serve as a marker of tumor progression. Furthermore, the overexpression of GATA6-AS was shown to significantly decrease the proliferative and invasive features in GBC cell lines. This effect can be explained by a decrease in the expression of miR-421 through TMP-2 [96].

Another lncRNA is MEG3 that it has been demonstrated that its expression is downregulated in GBC tissues compared with adjacent non-tumoral tissue. The low expression is related to poor prognosis, lymph node metastasis, and histological grade, suggesting that the low expression of MEG3 is related to poor prognosis in GBC patients. In vitro experiments showed that MEG3 overexpression significantly attenuated cell proliferation, colony formation and induce apoptosis in GBC cell lines. These results are reproduced in vivo since MEG3 overexpression decreases tumorigenesis and Ki-67 marker in the Balb/c nude mice model. In addition, MEG3 overexpression inhibited the invasion of NOZ cells with a significant upregulation of E-cadherin, accompanied by downregulation of N-cadherin and Vimentin. These data indicated that MEG3 inhibited cell invasion and EMT progression in GBC. Mechanistically, MEG3 promotes EZH2 degradation through its ubiquitination, regulating large tumor suppressor 2 (LATS2) as well as NF-κb pathway [33,99,100]. Similarly, GCASPC is a non-coding RNA that is downregulated in GBC tissues, being correlated with tumor size, advanced stage of disease, reduced overall survival (OS) and disease-free survival (DFS) rates. The ectopic expression of GCASPC decreased proliferation and induced significant G1-S arrest in GBC cell lines, while cell lines overexpressing GCASPC developed smaller tumors in nude mice, indicating that high expression of GCASPC reduces tumorigenesis in GBC. The authors mention that the probable mechanism will be via the inhibition of pyruvate carboxylase by the GCASP/miR-17-3p interaction proposing a new mechanism for the acquisition of a malignant phenotype in GBC [97].

In this review, the molecular and clinicopathological findings of lncRNAs described to date in GBC are summarized. Most of the lncRNAs studied in GBC have been selected due to being found overexpressed in GBC tissues and associated with malignant features that explain a worsening survival in GBC patients. Regarding this, a meta-analysis by Zhong et al., [62] describes similar findings to those reviewed in this work. The authors showed that overexpression of certain lncRNAs (e.g., MALAT1, MINCR, ROR, LINC00152, and AFAP1-AS1) can be used as potential predictors of worse survival or can be involved in the regulation of tumor size (e.g., AFAP1-AS1, MALAT1 and ROR). In addition, the overexpression of certain lncRNAs (e.g., LINC00152, HEGBC, MALAT1, and ROR and HEGBC) were found to be positively correlated with lymph node metastases, meanwhile, other lncRNAs such as PVT1 were correlated with a higher TNM stage. In contrast, Zhong et al. also described that the expression of LET and MEG3 was associated with a lower histological grade, lower TNM stage and absence of lymph node metastases, which is consistent with what has been described about the tumor suppressor role of these lncRNAs in other cancers [101,102]. Therefore, the inferences concluded in Zhong et al., corroborate the features described in this review.

For a better understanding of the clinical correlation of these lncRNAs, Table 2 resumes the correlation between lncRNAs and clinicopathological features in GBC.

Table 2. Resume of lncRNAs expression related with clinicopathological features on Gallbladder cancer.

LncRNA	Overall Survival	Tumor Size	TNM Stage	Histological Grade	Distant Metastasis	Lymphatic Invasion	Ref.
AFAP1-AS1	Decrease	Increase	NS	NS	ND	Negative	[34]
ANRIL	Decrease	NS	NS	NS	ND	Negative	[33]
CCAT1	ND	Increase	Advanced	ND	ND	Positive	[35]
GBCDRlnc1	Decrease	NS	Advanced	Poorer	ND	Negative	[49]
GCASPC	Decrease	Increase	Advanced	ND	NS	Positive	[97]
GALM	Decrease	NS	Advanced	Poorer	ND	Positive	[50]
HGBC	Decrease	ND	Advanced	NS	ND	Positive	[24]
HEGBC	Decrease	Increase	Advanced	NS	ND	Positive	[51]
HOTAIR	ND	ND	Advanced	ND	ND	Positive	[54]
H19	Decrease	Increase	NS	NS	ND	Positive	[56–58]
LINC01694	Decrease	NS	Advanced	Poorer	ND	ND	[59]
LET	Decrease	Increase	Advanced	Poorer	ND	Positive	[98]
LINC00152	Decrease	Increase	Advanced	NS	ND	Positive	[63,64]
MALAT1	Decrease	Increase	NS	NS	ND	Positive	[66,75,76,78,103]
MEG3	Decrease	NS	Advanced	Poorer	ND	Positive	[33,99,100]
MINCR	Decrease	Increase	ND	ND	ND	Positive	[79]
PAGBC	Decrease	ND	Advanced	ND	ND	ND	[88]
PVT1	Decrease	NS	Advanced	NS	Increase	ND	[85–87]
ROR	Decrease	Increase	NS	NS	ND	Positive	[13]
SNHG6	ND	Increase	Advanced	Poorer	Increase	Positive	[90]
SSTR5-AS1	Decrease	ND	ND	ND	ND	ND	[91]
UCA1	Decrease	Increase	Advanced	NS	ND	Positive	[12,77]

NS: not significant; ND: not described; Advanced: stage ≥ pT2. The results: decrease, increase, advanced, poorer and positive are expressions statistically significant.

Finally, Figure 3 summarizes all the features associated with an aggressive phenotype and its relationship with the different lncRNAs described to date in GBC.

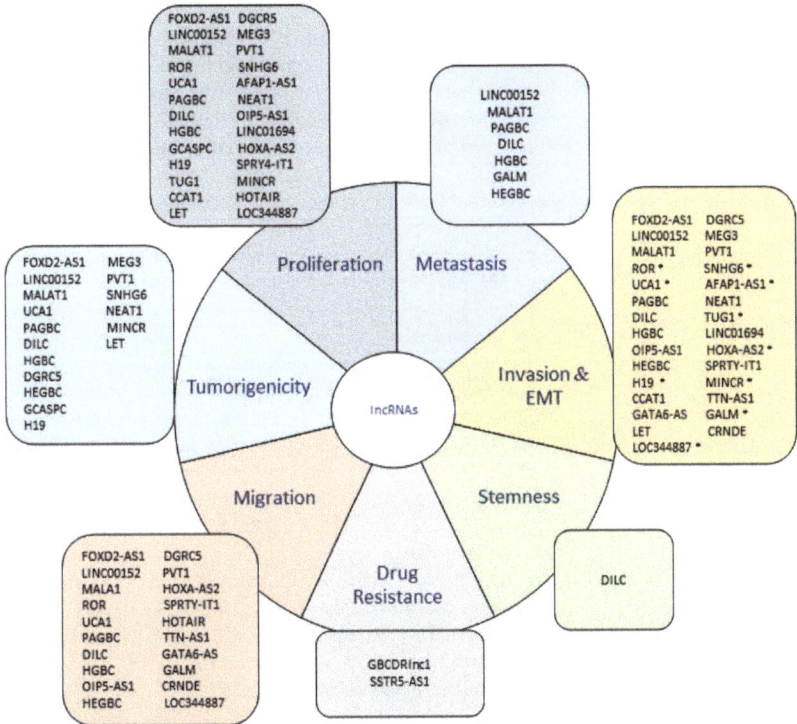

Figure 3. Role of lncRNAs in the aggressive phenotype in gallbladder cancer. LncRNAs associated with aggressive characteristics described in GBC. *: involved in invasion and EMT. lncRNAs without * are involved only in invasion.

5. Conclusions

The discovery of new cancer-related lncRNAs has been accelerated due to the development of high-throughput technologies. In addition, new cellular and molecular biology techniques along with new bioinformatic tools have been useful to describe the functional mechanisms of these lncRNAs in the acquisition of malignant phenotypic characteristics in cancer, such as GBC.

In this review, 30 lncRNAs were described as overexpressed in GBC patients (e.g., MALAT1, MINCR, ROR, AFAP1-AS1, PAGBC, LINC00152, UCA1, HEGBC, and PVT19) and were associated with worse clinical outcomes. Additionally, four lncRNAs were described as downregulated (e.g., LET, GCASPC, and MEG3), also acting as agents whose low expression promotes malignant tumor characteristics in these patients, worsening the overall survival (OS) in these patients. This suggests that lncRNAs can act as tumor suppressor or oncogenic transcripts, which account for complexity and the diversity of cellular processes in which they participate. Another finding is that one of the most relevant mechanisms of action of lncRNAs observed in this review are through ceRNAs (e.g., MALAT-1, PAGBC, LINC00152, MINCR, PAGBC, and PVT1), which is consistent with the mechanisms that can be described for lncRNAs that are upregulated in GBC, suggesting that lncRNAs act mainly as "sponging" against miRNAs, maintaining stability of oncogenic mRNAs and mainly inducing the activation of relevant signaling pathways widely described in cancer, such as PI3K/Akt, Wnt-β-catenin and MAPK.

It is known that the acquisition of a stem-like phenotype in cancer cells leads to the acquisition of an increasingly aggressive phenotype, which has been correlated with a worse prognosis in cancer patients. In this review, DILC was the only lncRNA described as a promoter of a stem-like phenotype in GBC cancer, which was related to increased tumorigenic and metastatic capacity. This data suggests that at least in GBC, there is still a need for more research on the role of lncRNAs in the acquisition of a stem-like phenotype, considering the clinical importance that this involves.

Clinically, the deregulation of these lncRNAs has been associated to poor prognosis evidenced by worsening of clinicopathological features. This correlation is consistent with the cellular phenotypic characteristics found in in vitro and in vivo models since it has been shown that the worsening of the patient's clinical state is due to a greater aggressiveness acquired by cancer cells, in this case, attributed to the role of lncRNAs in cancer. Regarding this, it has been observed that tumor size has been correlated with greater tumorigenic capacity and metastasis (lymphatic or distant) with EMT and invasive capacity. Therefore, the need to use lncRNAs as prognostic or diagnostic biomarkers is becoming an urgent aspect to address.

One of the diagnostic methods that has been growing in recent years is liquid biopsy, which through different studies has demonstrated to be potentially useful for a great variety of clinical analyses, being used mainly for the detection of diagnostic or prognostic biomarkers in cancer patients due to its much easier sample collection. Regarding this, only two lncRNAs (SNHG6 and LINC01694) described in this review were detected in serum samples, which implies that more studies are still needed to determine the helpfulness of these methods as a routinary methodology clinically viable for the detection of lncRNAs in individuals with cancer.

In summary, many lncRNAs are aberrantly expressed in samples from GBC patients and are involved in different oncogenic processes in GBC. However, it is necessary to study the molecular mechanisms in which lncRNAs are involved and the potential utility of these transcripts as clinical biomarkers in GBC cases, more than simply establishing the differential expressions in this cancer.

Author Contributions: Conceptualization, P.P.-M.; writing—original draft preparation, P.P.-M.; writing—review and editing, I.R.; supervision, J.C.R. and P.B.; funding acquisition, J.C.R. All authors have read and agreed to the published version of the manuscript.

Funding: This research has received funding from the European Research Council (ERC) under the European Union's Horizon 2020 research and innovation programme (grant agreement N° 825510), Fondecyt N° 1210440 and Postdoctoral Scholarship ANID N° 3210237.

Conflicts of Interest: The authors declare no conflict of interest.

References

1. Hanahan, D.; Weinberg, R.A. Hallmarks of cancer: The next generation. *Cell* **2011**, *144*, 646–674. [CrossRef] [PubMed]
2. Slack, F.J.; Chinnaiyan, A.M. The Role of Non-coding RNAs in Oncology. *Cell* **2019**, *179*, 1033–1055. [CrossRef] [PubMed]
3. Fang, Y.; Fullwood, M.J. Roles, Functions, and Mechanisms of Long Non-coding RNAs in Cancer. *Genom. Proteom. Bioinform.* **2016**, *14*, 42–54. [CrossRef] [PubMed]
4. Guttman, M.; Amit, I.; Garber, M.; French, C.; Lin, M.F.; Feldser, D.; Huarte, M.; Zuk, O.; Carey, B.W.; Cassady, J.P.; et al. Chromatin signature reveals over a thousand highly conserved large non-coding RNAs in mammals. *Nature* **2009**, *458*, 223–227. [CrossRef] [PubMed]
5. Vance, K.W.; Ponting, C.P. Transcriptional regulatory functions of nuclear long noncoding RNAs. *Trends Genet.* **2014**, *30*, 348–355. [CrossRef]
6. Dykes, I.M.; Emanueli, C. Transcriptional and Post-transcriptional Gene Regulation by Long Non-coding RNA. *Genom. Proteom. Bioinform.* **2017**, *15*, 177–186. [CrossRef] [PubMed]
7. Cheng, Y.; Geng, L.; Wang, K.; Sun, J.; Xu, W.; Gong, S.; Zhu, Y. Long Noncoding RNA Expression Signatures of Colon Cancer Based on the ceRNA Network and Their Prognostic Value. *Dis. Markers* **2019**, *2019*, 7636757. [CrossRef]
8. Li, Y.; Song, Y.; Wang, Z.; Zhang, Z.; Lu, M.; Wang, Y. Long Non-coding RNA LINC01787 Drives Breast Cancer Progression via Disrupting miR-125b Generation. *Front. Oncol.* **2019**, *9*, 1140. [CrossRef]
9. Huarte, M. The emerging role of lncRNAs in cancer. *Nat. Med.* **2015**, *21*, 1253–1261. [CrossRef]

10. Bekric, D.; Neureiter, D.; Ritter, M.; Jakab, M.; Gaisberger, M.; Pichler, M.; Kiesslich, T.; Mayr, C. Long Non-Coding RNAs in Biliary Tract Cancer-An Up-to-Date Review. *J. Clin. Med.* **2020**, *9*, 1200. [CrossRef]
11. Chi, Y.; Wang, D.; Wang, J.; Yu, W.; Yang, J. Long Non-Coding RNA in the Pathogenesis of Cancers. *Cells* **2019**, *8*, 1015. [CrossRef]
12. Cai, Q.; Jin, L.; Wang, S.; Zhou, D.; Wang, J.; Tang, Z.; Quan, Z. Long non-coding RNA UCA1 promotes gallbladder cancer progression by epigenetically repressing p21 and E-cadherin expression. *Oncotarget* **2017**, *8*, 47957–47968. [CrossRef] [PubMed]
13. Wang, S.H.; Zhang, M.D.; Wu, X.C.; Weng, M.Z.; Zhou, D.; Quan, Z.W. Overexpression of LncRNA-ROR predicts a poor outcome in gallbladder cancer patients and promotes the tumor cells proliferation, migration, and invasion. *Tumor Biol.* **2016**, *37*, 12867–12875. [CrossRef]
14. Ponting, C.P.; Oliver, P.L.; Reik, W. Evolution and functions of long noncoding RNAs. *Cell* **2009**, *136*, 629–641. [CrossRef] [PubMed]
15. Rinn, J.L.; Chang, H.Y. Genome regulation by long noncoding RNAs. *Ann. Rev. Biochem.* **2012**, *81*, 145–166. [CrossRef]
16. Yan, B.; Wang, Z. Long noncoding RNA: Its physiological and pathological roles. *DNA Cell Biol.* **2012**, *31* (Suppl. 1), S34–S41. [CrossRef] [PubMed]
17. Marchese, F.P.; Huarte, M. Long non-coding RNAs and chromatin modifiers: Their place in the epigenetic code. *Epigenetics* **2014**, *9*, 21–26. [CrossRef]
18. Guttman, M.; Rinn, J.L. Modular regulatory principles of large non-coding RNAs. *Nature* **2012**, *482*, 339–346. [CrossRef]
19. Khalil, A.M.; Guttman, M.; Huarte, M.; Garber, M.; Raj, A.; Rivea Morales, D.; Thomas, K.; Presser, A.; Bernstein, B.E.; van Oudenaarden, A.; et al. Many human large intergenic noncoding RNAs associate with chromatin-modifying complexes and affect gene expression. *Proc. Natl. Acad. Sci. USA* **2009**, *106*, 11667–11672. [CrossRef]
20. Gupta, R.A.; Shah, N.; Wang, K.C.; Kim, J.; Horlings, H.M.; Wong, D.J.; Tsai, M.C.; Hung, T.; Argani, P.; Rinn, J.L.; et al. Long non-coding RNA HOTAIR reprograms chromatin state to promote cancer metastasis. *Nature* **2010**, *464*, 1071–1076. [CrossRef]
21. Cao, J. The functional role of long non-coding RNAs and epigenetics. *Biol. Proced. Online* **2014**, *16*, 11. [CrossRef]
22. Chen, L.L. Linking Long Noncoding RNA Localization and Function. *Trends Biochem Sci* **2016**, *41*, 761–772. [CrossRef]
23. He, R.Z.; Luo, D.X.; Mo, Y.Y. Emerging roles of lncRNAs in the post-transcriptional regulation in cancer. *Genes Dis.* **2019**, *6*, 6–15. [CrossRef] [PubMed]
24. Hu, Y.P.; Jin, Y.P.; Wu, X.S.; Yang, Y.; Li, Y.S.; Li, H.F.; Xiang, S.S.; Song, X.L.; Jiang, L.; Zhang, Y.J.; et al. LncRNA-HGBC stabilized by HuR promotes gallbladder cancer progression by regulating miR-502-3p/SET/AKT axis. *Mol. Cancer* **2019**, *18*, 167. [CrossRef]
25. Wang, K.C.; Chang, H.Y. Molecular mechanisms of long noncoding RNAs. *Mol. Cell* **2011**, *43*, 904–914. [CrossRef] [PubMed]
26. Gao, N.; Li, Y.; Li, J.; Gao, Z.; Yang, Z.; Liu, H.; Fan, T. Long Non-Coding RNAs: The Regulatory Mechanisms, Research Strategies, and Future Directions in Cancers. *Front. Oncol.* **2020**, *10*, 598817. [CrossRef] [PubMed]
27. Sung, H.; Ferlay, J.; Siegel, R.L.; Laversanne, M.; Soerjomataram, I.; Jemal, A.; Bray, F. Global Cancer Statistics 2020: GLOBOCAN Estimates of Incidence and Mortality Worldwide for 36 Cancers in 185 Countries. *CA Cancer J. Clin.* **2021**, *71*, 209–249. [CrossRef] [PubMed]
28. Hundal, R.; Shaffer, E.A. Gallbladder cancer: Epidemiology and outcome. *Clin. Epidemiol.* **2014**, *6*, 99–109. [CrossRef]
29. Bertran, E.; Heise, K.; Andia, M.E.; Ferreccio, C. Gallbladder cancer: Incidence and survival in a high-risk area of Chile. *Int. J. Cancer* **2010**, *127*, 2446–2454. [CrossRef] [PubMed]
30. Brannan, C.I.; Dees, E.C.; Ingram, R.S.; Tilghman, S.M. The product of the H19 gene may function as an RNA. *Mol. Cell Biol.* **1990**, *10*, 28–36. [CrossRef]
31. Isin, M.; Dalay, N. LncRNAs and neoplasia. *Clin. Chim. Acta* **2015**, *444*, 280–288. [CrossRef] [PubMed]
32. Ma, F.; Wang, S.H.; Cai, Q.; Zhang, M.D.; Yang, Y.; Ding, J. Overexpression of LncRNA AFAP1-AS1 predicts poor prognosis and promotes cells proliferation and invasion in gallbladder cancer. *Biomed. Pharm.* **2016**, *84*, 1249–1255. [CrossRef] [PubMed]
33. Liu, B.; Shen, E.D.; Liao, M.M.; Hu, Y.B.; Wu, K.; Yang, P.; Zhou, L.; Chen, W.D. Expression and mechanisms of long non-coding RNA genes MEG3 and ANRIL in gallbladder cancer. *Tumor Biol.* **2016**, *37*, 9875–9886. [CrossRef]
34. Liu, Z.; Chen, Q.; Hann, S.S. The functions and oncogenic roles of CCAT1 in human cancer. *Biomed. Pharm.* **2019**, *115*, 108943. [CrossRef]
35. Ma, M.Z.; Chu, B.F.; Zhang, Y.; Weng, M.Z.; Qin, Y.Y.; Gong, W.; Quan, Z.W. Long non-coding RNA CCAT1 promotes gallbladder cancer development via negative modulation of miRNA-218-5p. *Cell Death Dis.* **2015**, *6*, e1583. [CrossRef]
36. Ma, Y.C.; Yang, J.Y.; Yan, L.N. Relevant markers of cancer stem cells indicate a poor prognosis in hepatocellular carcinoma patients: A meta-analysis. *Eur. J. Gastroenterol. Hepatol.* **2013**, *25*, 1007–1016. [CrossRef] [PubMed]
37. Joseph, C.; Arshad, M.; Kurozomi, S.; Althobiti, M.; Miligy, I.M.; Al-Izzi, S.; Toss, M.S.; Goh, F.Q.; Johnston, S.J.; Martin, S.G.; et al. Overexpression of the cancer stem cell marker CD133 confers a poor prognosis in invasive breast cancer. *Breast Cancer Res. Treat.* **2019**, *174*, 387–399. [CrossRef]
38. Han, Y.; Xue, X.; Jiang, M.; Guo, X.; Li, P.; Liu, F.; Yuan, B.; Shen, Y.; Zhi, Q.; Zhao, H. LGR5, a relevant marker of cancer stem cells, indicates a poor prognosis in colorectal cancer patients: A meta-analysis. *Clin. Res. Hepatol. Gastroenterol.* **2015**, *39*, 267–273. [CrossRef]
39. Liu, B.; Zhang, Y.; Liao, M.; Deng, Z.; Gong, L.; Jiang, J.; Lynn, L.; Wu, K.; Miao, X. Clinicopathologic and prognostic significance of CD24 in gallbladder carcinoma. *Pathol. Oncol. Res.* **2011**, *17*, 45–50. [CrossRef]
40. Nguyen, L.V.; Vanner, R.; Dirks, P.; Eaves, C.J. Cancer stem cells: An evolving concept. *Nat. Rev. Cancer* **2012**, *12*, 133–143. [CrossRef] [PubMed]

41. Liang, C.; Yang, P.; Han, T.; Wang, R.Y.; Xing, X.L.; Si, A.F.; Ma, Q.Y.; Chen, Z.; Li, H.Y.; Zhang, B. Long non-coding RNA DILC promotes the progression of gallbladder carcinoma. *Gene* **2019**, *694*, 102–110. [CrossRef] [PubMed]
42. Xue, C.; Chen, C.; Gu, X.; Li, L. Progress and assessment of lncRNA DGCR5 in malignant phenotype and immune infiltration of human cancers. *Am. J. Cancer Res.* **2021**, *11*, 1–13.
43. Wang, R.; Dong, H.X.; Zeng, J.; Pan, J.; Jin, X.Y. LncRNA DGCR5 contributes to CSC-like properties via modulating miR-330-5p/CD44 in NSCLC. *J. Cell Physiol.* **2018**, *233*, 7447–7456. [CrossRef] [PubMed]
44. Dong, H.X.; Wang, R.; Jin, X.Y.; Zeng, J.; Pan, J. LncRNA DGCR5 promotes lung adenocarcinoma (LUAD) progression via inhibiting hsa-mir-22-3p. *J. Cell Physiol.* **2018**, *233*, 4126–4136. [CrossRef] [PubMed]
45. Wang, X.L.; Shi, M.; Xiang, T.; Bu, Y.Z. Long noncoding RNA DGCR5 represses hepatocellular carcinoma progression by inactivating Wnt signaling pathway. *J. Cell Biochem.* **2019**, *120*, 275–282. [CrossRef] [PubMed]
46. Jiang, D.; Wang, C.; He, J. Long non-coding RNA DGCR5 incudes tumorigenesis of triple-negative breast cancer by affecting Wnt/β-catenin signaling pathway. *J. BUON* **2020**, *25*, 702–708. [PubMed]
47. Liu, S.; Chu, B.; Cai, C.; Wu, X.; Yao, W.; Wu, Z.; Yang, Z.; Li, F.; Liu, Y.; Dong, P.; et al. DGCR5 Promotes Gallbladder Cancer by Sponging MiR-3619-5p via MEK/ERK1/2 and JNK/p38 MAPK Pathways. *J. Cancer* **2020**, *11*, 5466–5477. [CrossRef] [PubMed]
48. Gao, J.; Dai, C.; Yu, C.; Yin, X.B.; Liao, W.-y.; Huang, Y.; Zhou, F. Silencing of long non-coding RNA FOXD2-AS1 inhibits the progression of gallbladder cancer by mediating methylation of MLH1. *Gene Ther.* **2020**, *28*, 306–318. [CrossRef]
49. Cai, Q.; Wang, S.; Jin, L.; Weng, M.; Zhou, D.; Wang, J.; Tang, Z.; Quan, Z. Long non-coding RNA GBCDRlnc1 induces chemoresistance of gallbladder cancer cells by activating autophagy. *Mol. Cancer* **2019**, *18*, 82. [CrossRef]
50. Li, H.; Hu, Y.; Jin, Y.; Zhu, Y.; Hao, Y.; Liu, F.; Yang, Y.; Li, G.; Song, X.; Ye, Y.; et al. Long noncoding RNA lncGALM increases risk of liver metastasis in gallbladder cancer through facilitating N-cadherin and IL-1β-dependent liver arrest and tumor extravasation. *Clin. Transl. Med.* **2020**, *10*, e201. [CrossRef] [PubMed]
51. Yang, L.; Gao, Q.; Wu, X.; Feng, F.; Xu, K. Long noncoding RNA HEGBC promotes tumorigenesis and metastasis of gallbladder cancer via forming a positive feedback loop with IL-11/STAT3 signaling pathway. *J. Exp. Clin. Cancer Res.* **2018**, *37*, 186. [CrossRef] [PubMed]
52. Wang, J.; Su, Z.; Lu, S.; Fu, W.; Liu, Z.; Jiang, X.; Tai, S. LncRNA HOXA-AS2 and its molecular mechanisms in human cancer. *Clin. Chim. Acta* **2018**, *485*, 229–233. [CrossRef] [PubMed]
53. Zhang, P.; Cao, P.; Zhu, X.; Pan, M.; Zhong, K.; He, R.; Li, Y.; Jiao, X.; Gao, Y. Upregulation of long non-coding RNA HOXA-AS2 promotes proliferation and induces epithelial-mesenchymal transition in gallbladder carcinoma. *Oncotarget* **2017**, *8*, 33137–33143. [CrossRef]
54. Ma, M.Z.; Li, C.X.; Zhang, Y.; Weng, M.Z.; Zhang, M.D.; Qin, Y.Y.; Gong, W.; Quan, Z.W. Long non-coding RNA HOTAIR, a c-Myc activated driver of malignancy, negatively regulates miRNA-130a in gallbladder cancer. *Mol. Cancer* **2014**, *13*, 156. [CrossRef]
55. Ghafouri-Fard, S.; Esmaeili, M.; Taheri, M. H19 lncRNA: Roles in tumorigenesis. *Biomed. Pharm.* **2020**, *123*, 109774. [CrossRef] [PubMed]
56. Wang, S.H.; Wu, X.C.; Zhang, M.D.; Weng, M.Z.; Zhou, D.; Quan, Z.W. Long noncoding RNA H19 contributes to gallbladder cancer cell proliferation by modulated miR-194-5p targeting AKT2. *Tumor Biol.* **2016**, *37*, 9721–9730. [CrossRef]
57. Wang, S.H.; Ma, F.; Tang, Z.H.; Wu, X.C.; Cai, Q.; Zhang, M.D.; Weng, M.Z.; Zhou, D.; Wang, J.D.; Quan, Z.W. Long non-coding RNA H19 regulates FOXM1 expression by competitively binding endogenous miR-342-3p in gallbladder cancer. *J. Exp. Clin. Cancer Res.* **2016**, *35*, 160. [CrossRef]
58. Wang, S.H.; Wu, X.C.; Zhang, M.D.; Weng, M.Z.; Zhou, D.; Quan, Z.W. Upregulation of H19 indicates a poor prognosis in gallbladder carcinoma and promotes epithelial-mesenchymal transition. *Am. J. Cancer Res.* **2016**, *6*, 15–26.
59. Liu, L.; Yan, Y.; Zhang, G.; Chen, C.; Shen, W.; Xing, P. Knockdown of LINC01694 inhibits growth of gallbladder cancer cells via miR-340-5p/Sox4. *Biosci. Rep.* **2020**, *40*. [CrossRef]
60. Wu, X.C.; Wang, S.H.; Ou, H.H.; Zhu, B.; Zhu, Y.; Zhang, Q.; Yang, Y.; Li, H. The NmrA-like family domain containing 1 pseudogene Loc344887 is amplified in gallbladder cancer and promotes epithelial-mesenchymal transition. *Chem. Biol. Drug Des.* **2017**, *90*, 456–463. [CrossRef] [PubMed]
61. Seo, D.; Kim, D.; Kim, W. Long non-coding RNA linc00152 acting as a promising oncogene in cancer progression. *Genom. Inf.* **2019**, *17*, e36. [CrossRef]
62. Zhong, Y.; Wu, X.; Li, Q.; Ge, X.; Wang, F.; Wu, P.; Deng, X.; Miao, L. Long noncoding RNAs as potential biomarkers and therapeutic targets in gallbladder cancer: A systematic review and meta-analysis. *Cancer Cell Int.* **2019**, *19*, 169. [CrossRef]
63. Cai, Q.; Wang, Z.Q.; Wang, S.H.; Li, C.; Zhu, Z.G.; Quan, Z.W.; Zhang, W.J. Upregulation of long non-coding RNA LINC00152 by SP1 contributes to gallbladder cancer cell growth and tumor metastasis via PI3K/AKT pathway. *Am. J. Transl. Res.* **2016**, *8*, 4068–4081.
64. Cai, Q.; Wang, Z.; Wang, S.; Weng, M.; Zhou, D.; Li, C.; Wang, J.; Chen, E.; Quan, Z. Long non-coding RNA LINC00152 promotes gallbladder cancer metastasis and epithelial-mesenchymal transition by regulating HIF-1α via miR-138. *Open Biol.* **2017**, *7*. [CrossRef]
65. Li, Z.X.; Zhu, Q.N.; Zhang, H.B.; Hu, Y.; Wang, G.; Zhu, Y.S. MALAT1: A potential biomarker in cancer. *Cancer Manag. Res.* **2018**, *10*, 6757–6768. [CrossRef] [PubMed]

66. Wu, X.S.; Wang, X.A.; Wu, W.G.; Hu, Y.P.; Li, M.L.; Ding, Q.; Weng, H.; Shu, Y.J.; Liu, T.Y.; Jiang, L.; et al. MALAT1 promotes the proliferation and metastasis of gallbladder cancer cells by activating the ERK/MAPK pathway. *Cancer Biol. Ther.* **2014**, *15*, 806–814. [CrossRef] [PubMed]
67. Sun, Y.; Ma, L. New Insights into Long Non-Coding RNA MALAT1 in Cancer and Metastasis. *Cancers* **2019**, *11*, 216. [CrossRef] [PubMed]
68. Huo, Y.; Li, Q.; Wang, X.; Jiao, X.; Zheng, J.; Li, Z.; Pan, X. MALAT1 predicts poor survival in osteosarcoma patients and promotes cell metastasis through associating with EZH2. *Oncotarget* **2017**, *8*, 46993–47006. [CrossRef]
69. Chen, Q.; Su, Y.; He, X.; Zhao, W.; Wu, C.; Zhang, W.; Si, X.; Dong, B.; Zhao, L.; Gao, Y.; et al. Plasma long non-coding RNA MALAT1 is associated with distant metastasis in patients with epithelial ovarian cancer. *Oncol. Lett.* **2016**, *12*, 1361–1366. [CrossRef]
70. Luan, C.; Li, Y.; Liu, Z.; Zhao, C. Long Noncoding RNA MALAT1 Promotes the Development of Colon Cancer by Regulating. *OncoTargets Ther.* **2020**, *13*, 3653–3665. [CrossRef]
71. Jen, J.; Tang, Y.A.; Lu, Y.H.; Lin, C.C.; Lai, W.W.; Wang, Y.C. Oct4 transcriptionally regulates the expression of long non-coding RNAs NEAT1 and MALAT1 to promote lung cancer progression. *Mol. Cancer* **2017**, *16*, 104. [CrossRef]
72. Schmidt, L.H.; Spieker, T.; Koschmieder, S.; Schäffers, S.; Humberg, J.; Jungen, D.; Bulk, E.; Hascher, A.; Wittmer, D.; Marra, A.; et al. The long noncoding MALAT-1 RNA indicates a poor prognosis in non-small cell lung cancer and induces migration and tumor growth. *J. Thorac. Oncol.* **2011**, *6*, 1984–1992. [CrossRef] [PubMed]
73. Jadaliha, M.; Zong, X.; Malakar, P.; Ray, T.; Singh, D.K.; Freier, S.M.; Jensen, T.; Prasanth, S.G.; Karni, R.; Ray, P.S.; et al. Functional and prognostic significance of long non-coding RNA MALAT1 as a metastasis driver in ER negative lymph node negative breast cancer. *Oncotarget* **2016**, *7*, 40418–40436. [CrossRef] [PubMed]
74. Huang, N.S.; Chi, Y.Y.; Xue, J.Y.; Liu, M.Y.; Huang, S.; Mo, M.; Zhou, S.L.; Wu, J. Long non-coding RNA metastasis associated in lung adenocarcinoma transcript 1 (MALAT1) interacts with estrogen receptor and predicted poor survival in breast cancer. *Oncotarget* **2016**, *7*, 37957–37965. [CrossRef] [PubMed]
75. Lin, N.; Yao, Z.; Xu, M.; Chen, J.; Lu, Y.; Yuan, L.; Zhou, S.; Zou, X.; Xu, R. Long noncoding RNA MALAT1 potentiates growth and inhibits senescence by antagonizing ABI3BP in gallbladder cancer cells. *J. Exp. Clin. Cancer Res.* **2019**, *38*, 244. [CrossRef] [PubMed]
76. Wang, S.H.; Zhang, W.J.; Wu, X.C.; Zhang, M.D.; Weng, M.Z.; Zhou, D.; Wang, J.D.; Quan, Z.W. Long non-coding RNA Malat1 promotes gallbladder cancer development by acting as a molecular sponge to regulate miR-206. *Oncotarget* **2016**, *7*, 37857–37867. [CrossRef]
77. Zhang, T.; Chen, L.; Xu, X.; Shen, C. Knockdown of Long Noncoding RNA. *Cancer Biother. Radiopharm.* **2020**. [CrossRef]
78. Wang, S.H.; Zhang, W.J.; Wu, X.C.; Weng, M.Z.; Zhang, M.D.; Cai, Q.; Zhou, D.; Wang, J.D.; Quan, Z.W. The lncRNA MALAT1 functions as a competing endogenous RNA to regulate MCL-1 expression by sponging miR-363-3p in gallbladder cancer. *J. Cell Mol. Med.* **2016**, *20*, 2299–2308. [CrossRef]
79. Wang, S.H.; Yang, Y.; Wu, X.C.; Zhang, M.D.; Weng, M.Z.; Zhou, D.; Wang, J.D.; Quan, Z.W. Long non-coding RNA MINCR promotes gallbladder cancer progression through stimulating EZH2 expression. *Cancer Lett.* **2016**, *380*, 122–133. [CrossRef]
80. Yang, F.; Tang, Z.; Duan, A.; Yi, B.; Shen, N.; Bo, Z.; Yin, L.; Zhu, B.; Qiu, Y.; Li, J. Long Non-coding RNA. *OncoTargets Ther.* **2020**, *13*, 2357–2367. [CrossRef]
81. Meng, X.; Ma, J.; Wang, B.; Wu, X.; Liu, Z. Long non-coding RNA OIP5-AS1 promotes pancreatic cancer cell growth through sponging miR-342-3p via AKT/ERK signaling pathway. *J. Physiol. Biochem.* **2020**, *76*, 301–315. [CrossRef] [PubMed]
82. Ma, Y.S.; Chu, K.J.; Ling, C.C.; Wu, T.M.; Zhu, X.C.; Liu, J.B.; Yu, F.; Li, Z.Z.; Wang, J.H.; Gao, Q.X.; et al. Long Noncoding RNA OIP5-AS1 Promotes the Progression of Liver Hepatocellular Carcinoma via Regulating the hsa-miR26a-3p/EPHA2 Axis. *Mol. Ther. Nucleic Acids* **2020**, *21*, 229–241. [CrossRef] [PubMed]
83. Wang, Y.; Dou, L.; Qin, Y.; Yang, H.; Yan, P. OIP5-AS1 contributes to tumorigenesis in hepatocellular carcinoma by miR-300/YY1-activated WNT pathway. *Cancer Cell Int.* **2020**, *20*, 440. [CrossRef] [PubMed]
84. Li, J.; Zhang, H.; Luo, H. Long Non-Coding RNA OIP5-AS1 Contributes to Gallbladder Cancer Cell Invasion and Migration by miR-143-3p Suppression. *Cancer Manag. Res.* **2020**, *12*, 12983–12992. [CrossRef]
85. Chen, J.; Yu, Y.; Li, H.; Hu, Q.; Chen, X.; He, Y.; Xue, C.; Ren, F.; Ren, Z.; Li, J.; et al. Long non-coding RNA PVT1 promotes tumor progression by regulating the miR-143/HK2 axis in gallbladder cancer. *Mol. Cancer* **2019**, *18*, 33. [CrossRef] [PubMed]
86. Liu, K.; Xu, Q. LncRNA PVT1 regulates gallbladder cancer progression through miR-30d-5p. *J. Biol. Regul. Homeost. Agents* **2020**, *34*, 875–883. [CrossRef] [PubMed]
87. Jin, L.; Cai, Q.; Wang, S.; Wang, J.; Quan, Z. Long noncoding RNA PVT1 promoted gallbladder cancer proliferation by epigenetically suppressing miR-18b-5p via DNA methylation. *Cell Death Dis.* **2020**, *11*, 871. [CrossRef]
88. Wu, X.S.; Wang, F.; Li, H.F.; Hu, Y.P.; Jiang, L.; Zhang, F.; Li, M.L.; Wang, X.A.; Jin, Y.P.; Zhang, Y.J.; et al. LncRNA-PAGBC acts as a microRNA sponge and promotes gallbladder tumorigenesis. *EMBO Rep.* **2017**, *18*, 1837–1853. [CrossRef]
89. Yang, L.; Cheng, X.; Ge, N.; Guo, W.; Feng, F.; Wan, F. Long non-coding RNA SPRY4-IT1 promotes gallbladder carcinoma progression. *Oncotarget* **2017**, *8*, 3104–3110. [CrossRef]
90. Liu, X.F.; Wang, K.; Du, H.C. LncRNA SNHG6 regulating Hedgehog signaling pathway and affecting the biological function of gallbladder carcinoma cells through targeting miR-26b-5p. *Eur. Rev. Med. Pharm. Sci.* **2020**, *24*, 7598–7611. [CrossRef]

91. Xue, Z.; Yang, B.; Xu, Q.; Zhu, X.; Qin, G. Long non-coding RNA SSTR5-AS1 facilitates gemcitabine resistance via stabilizing NONO in gallbladder carcinoma. *Biochem. Biophys. Res. Commun.* **2020**, *522*, 952–959. [CrossRef]
92. Ma, F.; Wang, S.H.; Cai, Q.; Jin, L.Y.; Zhou, D.; Ding, J.; Quan, Z.W. Long non-coding RNA TUG1 promotes cell proliferation and metastasis by negatively regulating miR-300 in gallbladder carcinoma. *Biomed. Pharm.* **2017**, *88*, 863–869. [CrossRef] [PubMed]
93. Lin, Z.; Li, Y.; Shao, R.; Hu, Y.; Gao, H. LncRNA TTN-AS1 acts as a tumor promoter in gallbladder carcinoma by regulating miR-107/HMGA1 axis. *World J. Surg. Oncol.* **2021**, *19*, 163. [CrossRef]
94. Zhang, L.; Geng, Z.; Meng, X.; Meng, F.; Wang, L. Screening for key lncRNAs in the progression of gallbladder cancer using bioinformatics analyses. *Mol. Med. Rep.* **2018**, *17*, 6449–6455. [CrossRef] [PubMed]
95. Shen, S.; Liu, H.; Wang, Y.; Wang, J.; Ni, X.; Ai, Z.; Pan, H.; Shao, Y. Long non-coding RNA CRNDE promotes gallbladder carcinoma carcinogenesis and as a scaffold of DMBT1 and C-IAP1 complexes to activating PI3K-AKT pathway. *Oncotarget* **2016**, *7*, 72833–72844. [CrossRef] [PubMed]
96. Li, K.; Tang, J.; Hou, Y. LncRNA GATA6-AS inhibits cancer cell migration and invasion in gallbladder cancer by downregulating miR-421. *OncoTargets Ther.* **2019**, *12*, 8047–8053. [CrossRef] [PubMed]
97. Ma, M.Z.; Zhang, Y.; Weng, M.Z.; Wang, S.H.; Hu, Y.; Hou, Z.Y.; Qin, Y.Y.; Gong, W.; Zhang, Y.J.; Kong, X.; et al. Long Noncoding RNA GCASPC, a Target of miR-17-3p, Negatively Regulates Pyruvate Carboxylase-Dependent Cell Proliferation in Gallbladder Cancer. *Cancer Res.* **2016**, *76*, 5361–5371. [CrossRef]
98. Ma, M.Z.; Kong, X.; Weng, M.Z.; Zhang, M.D.; Qin, Y.Y.; Gong, W.; Zhang, W.J.; Quan, Z.W. Long non-coding RNA-LET is a positive prognostic factor and exhibits tumor-suppressive activity in gallbladder cancer. *Mol. Carcinog.* **2015**, *54*, 1397–1406. [CrossRef]
99. Bao, D.; Yuan, R.X.; Zhang, Y. Effects of lncRNA MEG3 on proliferation and apoptosis of gallbladder cancer cells through regulating NF-κB signaling pathway. *Eur. Rev. Med. Pharm. Sci.* **2020**, *24*, 6632–6638. [CrossRef]
100. Jin, L.; Cai, Q.; Wang, S.; Mondal, T.; Wang, J.; Quan, Z. Long noncoding RNA MEG3 regulates LATS2 by promoting the ubiquitination of EZH2 and inhibits proliferation and invasion in gallbladder cancer. *Cell Death Dis.* **2018**, *9*, 1017. [CrossRef]
101. Tian, J.; Hu, X.; Gao, W.; Zhang, J.; Chen, M.; Zhang, X.; Ma, J.; Yuan, H. Identification of the long non-coding RNA LET as a novel tumor suppressor in gastric cancer. *Mol. Med. Rep.* **2017**, *15*, 2229–2234. [CrossRef] [PubMed]
102. Gu, L.; Zhang, J.; Shi, M.; Zhan, Q.; Shen, B.; Peng, C. lncRNA MEG3 had anti-cancer effects to suppress pancreatic cancer activity. *Biomed. Pharm.* **2017**, *89*, 1269–1276. [CrossRef] [PubMed]
103. Sun, K.K.; Hu, P.P.; Xu, F. Prognostic significance of long non-coding RNA MALAT1 for predicting the recurrence and metastasis of gallbladder cancer and its effect on cell proliferation, migration, invasion, and apoptosis. *J. Cell Biochem.* **2018**, *119*, 3099–3110. [CrossRef] [PubMed]

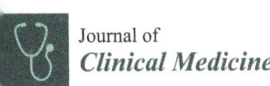

Journal of Clinical Medicine

Article

Investigation of the Indications for Endoscopic Papillectomy and Transduodenal Ampullectomy for Ampullary Tumors

Masanari Sekine [1,*], Fumiaki Watanabe [2], Takehiro Ishii [1], Takaya Miura [1], Yudai Koito [1], Hitomi Kashima [1], Keita Matsumoto [1], Hiroshi Noda [2], Toshiki Rikiyama [2] and Hirosato Mashima [1]

1. Saitama Medical Center, Department of Gastroenterology, Jichi Medical University, Saitama 330-8503, Japan; take3546@jichi.ac.jp (T.I.); tmiura0630@gmail.com (T.M.); koito0406@yahoo.co.jp (Y.K.); hitomi.19881206@gmail.com (H.K.); wrcr1007@gmail.com (K.M.); hmashima@jichi.ac.jp (H.M.)
2. Saitama Medical Center, Department of Surgery, Jichi Medical University, Saitama 330-8503, Japan; fwatanabe210@yahoo.co.jp (F.W.); noda164@omiya.jichi.ac.jp (H.N.); trikiyama@jichi.ac.jp (T.R.)
* Correspondence: msekine@jichi.ac.jp; Tel.: +81-48-647-2111; Fax: +81-48-648-5188

Abstract: Objective: The standard treatment for ampullary tumors is pancreaticoduodenectomy. However, minimally invasive procedures such as endoscopic papillectomy (EP) and transduodenal ampullectomy (TDA) have recently gained popularity. Therefore, we aimed to evaluate the effectiveness of these minimally invasive procedures for ampullary tumors. Methods: We conducted a retrospective study of 42 patients who underwent either EP or TDA for ampullary tumors between June 2011 and November 2020. Results: We found that in patients with significantly larger tumors, TDA was often selected. Patients who underwent EP had significantly shorter hospital stays. No significant differences were observed regarding procedural accidents, tumor size, and recurrence. Conclusion: No differences were observed regarding the treatment outcomes of EP and TDA except hospital stay. EP is less invasive and can be the initial choice of procedure. TDA is performed when EP is not technically feasible. No significant relationship was noted between tumor size and recurrence, and careful observation of the patient's postoperative course is required.

Keywords: endoscopic papillectomy; transduodenal ampullectomy; ampullary tumors; adenoma; adenocarcinoma

1. Introduction

Pancreaticoduodenectomy (PD) has been commonly performed to manage ampullary tumors regardless of malignancy status. However, PD is associated with the high degree of invasiveness. In 1983, the first report on endoscopic papillectomy (EP) by Suzuki et al. [1] was published. Subsequently, it was widely used despite a high-risk treatment, but it has not become the standard treatment yet. Contrastingly, the first report of transduodenal ampullectomy (TDA) was published in 1899 by Halsted. [2] However, consensus regarding its indications remain controversial due to its high recurrence rate.

The European Society of Gastrointestinal Endoscopy (ESGE) guidelines for ampullary tumors have recently been reported, which stipulates that the indication for EP is high-grade dysplasia with a size between 20 and 30 mm and bile or pancreatic duct progression measuring ≤20 mm [3]. Conversely, the indication for TDA includes Tis cancer, adenoma demonstrating bile or pancreatic duct progression measuring >20 mm, and adenoma wherein EP would present with technical difficulties due to diverticulum or a large size measuring ≥40 mm. Systematic review with meta-analysis reported an increased rate of complete resection in surgical interventions (PD, TDA), accompanied with a high risk of complications (PD), and no significance in recurrence between EP and TDA [4].

EP was reported to be associated with increased risk of remnants, but its outcome is improving with the progress of the equipment. TDA is a more radical treatment but is associated with a high degree of invasiveness. In a society where the population is aging

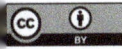

rapidly like Japan, it is important to evaluate whether less invasive EP or more radical TDA was more effective for ampullary adenomatous lesions. In this study, we compared and evaluated the effectiveness of EP and TDA for the treatment of ampullary tumors.

2. Methods

We conducted a retrospective study of 42 patients who underwent EP or TDA as the initial treatment for ampullary tumors at Saitama Medical Center, Jichi Medical University, between June 2011 and November 2020.

The information of patients was retrieved from medical records. Definition of mortality is 30 days mortality.

2.1. Preoperative Tests

All subjects were observed, and biopsies were performed using a rear oblique-view scope (JF260V, TJF260, TJF290, Olympus Corp, Tokyo, Japan). Endoscopic ultrasonography (EUS) and/or endoscopic retrograde cholangiopancreatography was used to observe and assess the T factor and superficial bile or pancreatic duct progression. Multidetector computed tomography (MD-CT) scan was used to assess N and M factors. During the study period, no clear guidelines regarding ampullary tumors have been detailed; therefore, the attending physicians discussed and determined the choice of EP or TDA. As a general rule, the target was adenoma lesions; however, a small number of patients with adenocarcinoma were included. PD was selected when the patient was positive for bile or pancreatic duct progression, T2 or deeper invasion, or positive N-factor.

2.2. Treatment Details

2.2.1. Endoscopic Papillectomy

All the procedures were performed under intravenous anesthesia. All patients underwent evaluation using rear oblique view scopes (JF260V, TJF260, TJFQ290V, Olympus Corp.). After confirming the presence of the ampullary tumor, a margin was established around the tumor from the oral protrusion to the frenulum, and snaring was performed. Resection was performed using a high-frequency device (ICC200 Erbe Elektromedizin, Tubingen, Germany. ENDO CUT® Effect3 cut 120 W coag 30 W, or ESG-100 Olympus Corp., Tokyo, Japan. Pulsecut-slow LEVEL30). The scope was removed temporarily. After collecting the specimen, the scope was reinserted, and the frenulum was sutured with clips. After bile and pancreatic duct cannulation, guidewire indwelling plastic stents (bile duct, 7 Fr., 5 or 7 cm; pancreatic duct, 5 Fr., 4, 7, or 9 cm) were installed in the bile and pancreatic ducts. Without conducting a second look, the rear oblique view scope was re-inserted 5–7 days after to evaluate the resection site; additionally, the stents were removed and a biopsy of the margin of the resected ulcer was performed.

2.2.2. Transduodenal Ampullectomy

TDA was performed in all patients under general anesthesia. A Kocher maneuver was performed with duodenal mobilization and exposure of the posterior wall of duodenum. After palpation of the duodenum for the identification of the ampullary lesion, a 2–4 cm longitudinal duodenotomy was performed and the ampullary lesion was visualized (Figure 1A). Stay sutures were placed around the circumference of the tumor and physiological saline (5 cc) was injected into the submucosa to lift the lesion. The duodenal mucosa was incised at least 5 mm from tumor and ampulla tumor was resected with careful identification of the sphincter of Oddi (Figure 1B). To repair the cavity of the lost mucosa, the mucosa and the sphincter of Oddi were radially sutured to prevent obstruction of the Wirsung duct and the common bile duct (CBD). The duodenum wall was sutured in the direction of the short axis using the Gambee suture pattern.

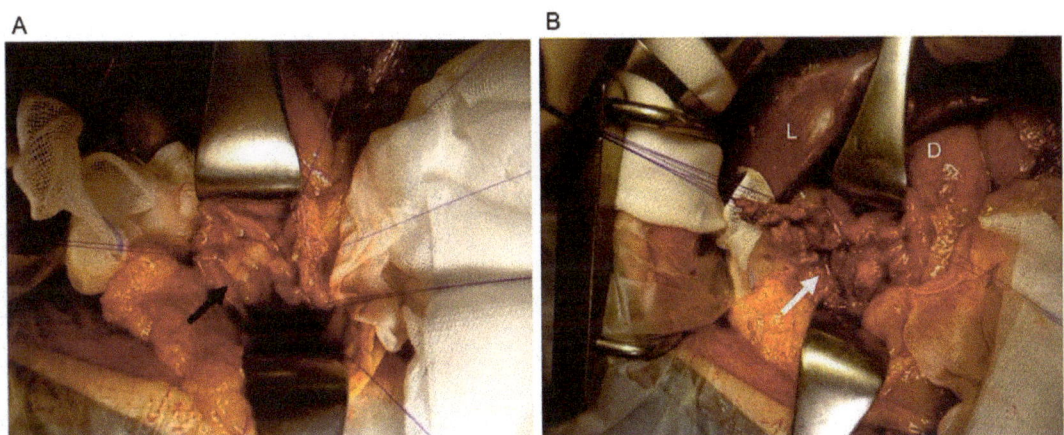

Figure 1. Intraoperative image of TDA. (**A**) After duodenotomy and before TDA, the ampullary tumor was visualized (black arrow). (**B**) The ampullary tumor was resected (white arrow). L: Liver, D: Duodenum.

2.2.3. Observation of Postoperative Progress

Postoperative observations were made every 6 months to 1 year using either direct or rear oblique view endoscopy. Biopsies were performed when necessary. Patients diagnosed with adenoma upon repeat biopsy were considered as recurrence.

During the study period, no clear guidelines regarding recurrence of ampullary tumors have been detailed; therefore, the attending physicians discussed and determined the choice of treatment.

2.3. Statistical Analysis

Data were analyzed using the statistical EZR software (version 1.54; 'EZR' (Easy R), Saitama, Japan) [5]. Student's *t*-test or Mann-Whitney U test was used to compare categorical and continuous variables within groups. The log rank-test was used to evaluate the cumulative recurrence free rate between EP and TDA group.

3. Results

Patients' background characteristics and therapeutic outcomes are shown in Tables 1 and 2, respectively. No significant difference was observed regarding the age and sex between the EP and TDA groups. Tumor size was significantly larger in the TDA group compared to the EP group. No significant difference was observed regarding the preoperative diagnoses between the two groups; however, a significantly higher percentage of final diagnoses of adenocarcinoma was observed in the TDA group. Additionally, two patients from the EP group were finally diagnosed as having "normal epithelium." Preoperative biopsies of these patients showed adenoma measuring 8 mm in one patient and adenocarcinoma (Tis) measuring 6 mm in the other. Both patients showed no recurrence during the follow-up period.

Investigation of the resected samples showed that all samples from the TDA group were en bloc resections, and two patients from the EP group had their samples split into two. No significant difference was observed regarding the positive results of the lateral and vertical margins between the two groups. Figure 2 shows the distribution of the tumor sizes as related to lateral and vertical margins for both EP and TDA patients. No significant difference was observed regarding negative and positive/unevaluable margins in the two groups.

Table 1. Patients' background characteristics.

	Total (42)	EP (33)	TDA (9)	p-Value
Gender				0.0805
Male	28	24	4	
Female	14	9	5	
Age (years median range)	67.7 (31–83)	67.9 (44–81)	66.8 (31–83)	0.975
Tumor size (mm median range)	14.6 (6–49)	11.5 (6–25)	26.3 (12–49)	0.0196
Preoperative diagnosis				0.347
Adenoma	39	32	7	
Adenocarcinoma	3	1	2	
Extensive intraepithelial progress in the common bile duct				0.195
Nagative	37	30	7	
Positive	1	0	1	
Unevaluable	4	3	1	
Extensive intraepithelial progress in the main pancreatic duct				0.374
Nagative	38	30	8	
Positive	0	0	0	
Unevaluable	4	3	1	

Table 2. Post-treatment outcomes.

	Total (42)	EP (33)	TDA (9)	p-Value
Postoperative diagnosis				0.0353
Adenoma	32	26	6	
Adenocarcinoma	8	5	3	
Normal epithelium	2	2	0	
En block resection				NA
Yes	40	31	9	
No	2	2	0	
Lateral margin				0.195
Negative	33	26	7	
Positive	3	2	1	
Unevaluable	6	5	1	
Vertical margin				0.195
Negative	30	23	7	
Positive	3	3	0	
Unevaluable	9	7	2	
Adverse event	6	7	3	0.594
Bleeding	3	3	0	
Mild pancreatitis	2	3	1	

Table 2. Cont.

	Total (42)	EP (33)	TDA (9)	p-Value
Bile duct stenosis	1	1	0	
Perforation	1	0	1	
Intra-abdominal abscess	1	0	1	
Mortality	0	0	0	
Duration of hospitalization (day, mean, range)	15.7 (8–52)	13.6 (8–28)	23.4 (13–52)	**0.0471**
Follow-up period (month, mean, range)	37.4 (1–114)	36.5 (1–114)	40.3 (6–96)	0.587
Recurrence	5	3	2	0.169
Time to recurrence (month, mean, range)	31.2 (3–56)	21.3 (3–53)	46 (36–56)	0.169

Bold: significant differences.

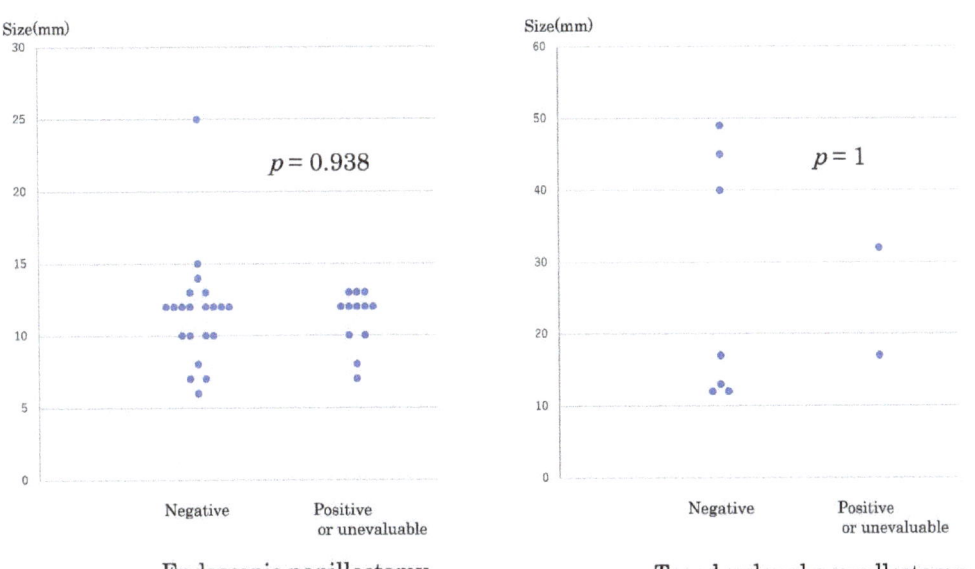

Figure 2. Distribution of tumor sizes related to negative and positive/unevaluable margins. EP (endoscopic papillectomy) (**left**), TDA (transduodenal ampullectomy) (**right**).

Adverse events that occurred in the EP group were bleeding (three patients), mild pancreatitis (three patients), and bile duct stenosis (one patient; Table 2). In the TDA group, adverse events included mild pancreatitis (one patient), perforation (one patient), and intra-abdominal abscess (one patient). No significant difference was noted regarding the number of adverse events between the two groups. However, long-term hospitalization (over 30days) was observed in 2 cases in the TDA group. One patient was hospitalized for 58 days due to perforation and intra-abdominal abscess, and another patient was hospitalized for 38 days due to acute pancreatitis. This significantly increased the length of hospital stay in the TDA group.

The mean follow-up time was 36.5 months (EP), and 40.3 months (TDA). No significant difference was observed regarding the recurrence rate and interval until recurrence between the two groups (Table 2, Figure 3A). Three and two patients from the EP and TDA group, respectively, developed recurrence. The characteristics of the patients who developed recurrence are shown in Table 3. Two patients and one patient from the EP and TDA group, respectively, demonstrated either positive or unevaluable resection margins. However, one patient each from the EP and TDA groups developed recurrence despite negative margins following en bloc resection. Recurrences occurred in 7.4% (2/27) of patients with negative margins. No significant difference was observed regarding the relationship of recurrence with tumor size between the two groups (Figure 3B). The attending physicians discussed and determined the choice of treatments for recurrence of ampullary tumors. Argon plasma coagulation (APC), hot biopsy, radiofrequency ablation (RFA), and/or EP were applied (Table 3).

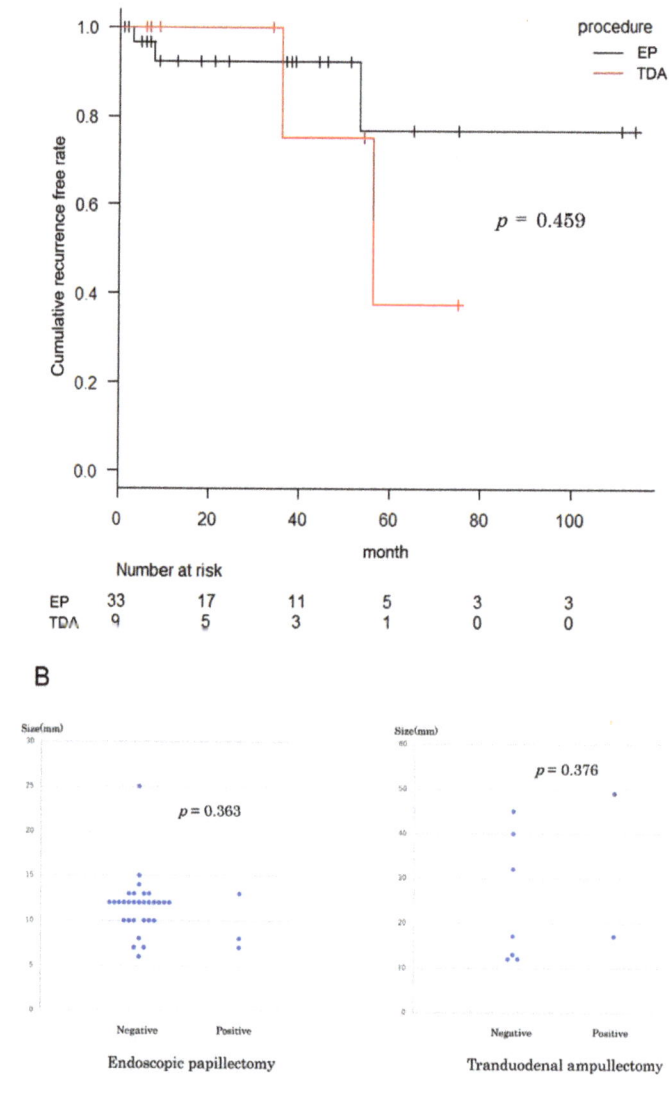

Figure 3. Comparison of recurrence between EP and TDA group. (A) Cumulative recurrence free rate. (B) Distribution of tumor sizes related to recurrence (positive vs. negative): EP (left), TDA (right).

Table 3. Characteristics of patients who developed recurrence.

Tumor Size (mm)	Preoperative Diagnosis	Extensive Intraepithelial Progress in the Common Bile Duct	Extensive Intraepithelial Progress in the Main Pancreatic Duct	En Block Resection	Postoperative Diagnosis	Lateral Margin	Vertical Margin	Time to Recurrence (Month)	Treatment for Recurrence
8	Adenoma	Negative	Negative	Yes	Adenoma	Unevaluable	Unevaluable	53	APC
17	Adenoma	Positive	Negative	Yes	Adenoma	Unevaluable	Negative	56	APC, RFA
13	Adenoma	Negative	Negative	No	Adenoma	Negative	Unevaluable	8	EP, Hot biopsy
7	Adenoma	Negative	Negative	Yes	Adenoma	Negative	Negative	3	EP
49	Adenoma	Negative	Negative	Yes	Adenoma	Negative	Negative	36	Hot biopsy

4. Discussion

In this study, we retrospectively compared the clinicopathological features and postoperative outcomes between EP and TDA groups. There were no significant differences in the therapeutic outcomes between the two groups except the shorter hospital stay in EP group.

The adenoma-carcinoma sequence is believed to be related to the malignant transformation of ampullary tumors, similarly observed in colorectal cancer [6–8]. A previous study found that the preoperative diagnostic accuracy is not high, particularly in its diagnosis of adenoma [9]. In the present study, the diagnostic accuracy rate was 83.3% (35/42). Therefore, EP and TDA implies a complete excision biopsy. Regarding cancer, lymph node metastasis does not occur in cases of Tis but occurs in pT1 in addition to microlymphatic invasion [10]. Lymph node metastasis is not rare in patients with T1b with sphincter of Oddi invasion, compared to T1a which are limited to ampullary mucosa. Trikudanathan et al. [11]. reported that the sensitivity (95%CI)/specificity (95%/CI) of EUS was 77% (0.69–0.83)/78% (0.72–0.84) for T1, 72% (0.65–0.80)/76% (0.71–0.83) for T2, 79% (0.71–0.85)/76% (0.71–0.83) for T3, and 84% (0.73–0.92)/74% (0.63–0.83) for T4, indicating poor diagnostic accuracy [12]. In EP and TDA indications, opinions regarding their sole indication for adenoma or the inclusion of Tis or T1a remain controversial. Difficulties in the preoperative diagnosis are expected. Previous studies have shown that tumors measuring until 50 mm are managed using EP [13,14]. However, perceptions regarding the correlation between tumor size and cancer remain controversial [15]. In the present study, no significance was observed regarding the relationship of tumor size and the final diagnosis of adenoma and adenocarcinoma (Figure 4). The TDA group had significantly larger tumors. This may be attributed to the concern regarding the difficult performance of EP when the tumor is laterally and widely spread or the endoscopic range of motion is restricted in the duodenum; in these cases, TDA was performed. Additionally, reports regarding the use of EP with hybrid-ESD in patients demonstrating superficial layer progress have recently been published [16]; we look forward to future research in this field.

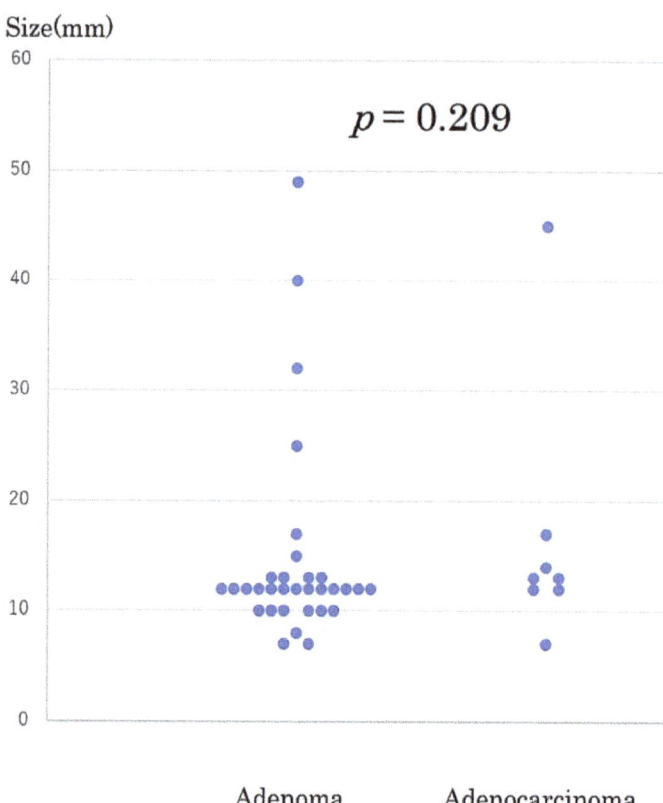

Figure 4. Distribution of tumor sizes according to final diagnoses of adenoma and adenocarcinoma. Adenoma (**left**), Adenocarcinoma (**right**).

Regarding the N and M factors, PD is indicated in patients with N1, and chemotherapy is indicated in patients with M1; MD-CT is the main diagnostic examination in both cases. Fong et al. found that among 41 patients with ampullary adenocarcinoma, MD-CT indicated lymphadenopathy in 10 patients, of whom, 5 were diagnosed lymph node metastases at pathology (50%). Furthermore, they found lymph node metastasis was found in 61.3% of the patients without lymphadenopathy on imaging [17]. Thus, even when the preoperative diagnosis is N0M0, in cases of T1a or deeper, the patient's course needs to be carefully observed and PD or other additional therapies need to be considered.

Heise et al. reported that the rate of complication was clearly higher in PD group than in EP and TDA groups [4]. Similarly, our investigation of treatment invasiveness indicated that there was no significant difference between EP and TDA regarding adverse events. The length of hospital stay was shorter, and the degree of invasiveness was lower in the EP group, which were consistent with those of a previous study [18].

A previous study observed that 33% of patients developed recurrence which was related to final diagnosis, intraluminal tumor presence, FAP complication, and experience of endoscopist [13]. Systematic review indicated that the recurrence rate was 13.0% in EP and 9.4% in TDA [4]. In the present study, we found that 9.1% (3/33) of the patients from the EP group and 22.2% (2/9) of those from the TDA group developed recurrence. Intraoperative frozen section was evaluated in only 2cases in the TDA group. This may be the reason for the relatively high recurrence rate in the TDA group, but there was no significance between the groups. No significant difference was noted in tumor size and recurrence (Figure 3B). All cases of recurrence were adenoma. Additionally, patients with negative margins in the resected samples suffered recurrence; particularly, in one patient, recurrence developed after 3 years. We believe that postoperative monitoring is essential even in patients with negative margins. Furthermore, careful monitoring and management are required since recurrence occurred after >4 years in one patient.

The limitations of this study include the single-center location, the relatively small number of patients in the TDA group, the non-standardization of pathologic sample processing, and insufficient evaluation of the bile and pancreatic ducts in resected specimens.

Regarding the issue of the treatment indicated for ampullary tumors, EP can be the first-line treatment for adenomatous lesions, because it is associated with less degree of invasiveness and does not have a poor clinical outcome. However, when performing EP with technical difficulties, such as in cases of large tumor size, we consider the use of TDA. This does not deviate from the ESGE guideline [3]. We believe that EP with hybrid-ESD should be considered in patients who are unable to tolerate surgery and general anesthesia.

5. Conclusions

In cases of ampullary tumors, it is prudent to consider the possibility of adenocarcinoma as the final diagnosis even if preoperative biopsy indicates adenoma, regardless of tumor size. No significant difference was observed in the therapeutic outcomes of EP and TDA, except hospital stay; therefore, minimally invasive EP is initially considered. TDA is considered as an option based on tumor size and other factors. Recurrence may occur even in patients with negative margins; therefore, careful monitoring during the postoperative course is necessary.

Author Contributions: M.S., T.R. and H.M. contributed to the conception and design of this study. M.S., F.W., T.I., T.M., Y.K., H.K., K.M. contributed to the acquisition of data. M.S. wrote the draft of the manuscript. F.W., H.N., T.R. and H.M. revised it critically. H.M. gave the final approval. All authors have read and agreed to the published version of the manuscript.

Funding: The research received no external funding.

Data Availability Statement: Data available in a publicly accessible repository.

Conflicts of Interest: The authors declare no conflict of interest.

References

1. Suzuki, K.; Kantou, U.; Murakami, Y. Two cases with ampullary cancer who underwent endoscopic excision. *Prog. Dig. Endosc.* **1983**, *23*, 236–239.
2. Halsted, W.S. Contributions to the surgery of the bile passages, especially of the common bile duct. *Boston Med. Surg. J.* **1899**, *141*, 645–654. [CrossRef]
3. Vanbiervliet, G.; Strijker, M.; Arvanitakis, M.; Aelvoet, A.; Arnelo, U.; Beyna, T.; Busch, O.; Deprez, P.H.; Kunovsky, L.; Larghi, A.; et al. Endoscopic management of ampullary tumors: European Society of Gastrointestinal Endoscopy (ESGE) Guideline. *Endoscopy* **2021**, *53*, 429–448. [PubMed]
4. Heise, C.; Abou Ali, E.; Hasenclever, D.; Auriemma, F.; Gulla, A.; Regner, S.; Gaujoux, S.; Hollenbach, M. Systematic Review with Meta-Analysis: Endoscopic and Surgical Resection for Ampullary Lesions. *J. Clin. Med.* **2020**, *9*, 3622. [CrossRef] [PubMed]
5. Kanda, Y. Investigation of the freely available easy-to-use software 'EZR' for medical statics. *Bone Marrow Transplant.* **2013**, *48*, 452–458. [CrossRef] [PubMed]
6. Fischer, H.-P.; Zhou, H. Pathogenesis of carcinoma of the papilla of Vater. *J. Hepatobiliary Pancreat. Surg.* **2004**, *11*, 301–309. [CrossRef] [PubMed]
7. Ruemmele, P.; Dietmaier, W.; Terracciano, L.; Tornillo, L.; Bataille, F.; Kaiser, A.; Wuensch, P.H.; Heinmoeller, E.; Homayounfar, K.; Luettges, J.; et al. Histopathologic features and microsatellite instability of cancers of the papilla of Vater and their precursor lesions. *Am. J. Surg. Pathol.* **2009**, *33*, 691–704. [CrossRef] [PubMed]
8. Wittekind, C.; Tannapfel, A. Adenoma of the papilla and ampulla—premalignant lesions? *Langenbeck's Arch. Surg.* **2001**, *20*, 172–175. [CrossRef] [PubMed]
9. Kim, J.; Choi, S.H.; Choi, D.W.; Heo, J.S.; Jang, K.T. Role of transduodenal ampullectomy for tumors of the ampulla of Vater. *J. Korean Surg. Soc.* **2011**, *81*, 250–256. [CrossRef] [PubMed]
10. Yoon, Y.S.; Kim, S.W.; Park, S.J.; Lee, H.S.; Jang, J.Y.; Choi, M.G.; Kim, W.H.; Lee, K.U.; Park, Y.H. Clinicopathologic analysis of early ampullary cancers with a focus on the feasibility of ampullectomy. *Ann. Surg.* **2005**, *242*, 92–100. [CrossRef] [PubMed]

11. Yoon, S.M.; Kim, M.-H.; Kim, M.J.; Jang, S.J.; Lee, T.Y.; Kwon, S.; Oh, H.-C.; Lee, S.S.; Seo, D.W.; Lee, S.K. Focal early stage cancer in ampullary adenoma: Surgery or endoscopic papillectomy? *Gastrointest. Endosc.* **2007**, *66*, 701–707. [CrossRef] [PubMed]
12. Trikudanathan, G.; Njei, B.; Attam, R.; Arain, M.; Shaukat, A. Staging accuracy of ampullary tumors by endoscopic ultrasound: Meta-analysis and systematic review. *Dig. Endosc.* **2014**, *26*, 617–626. [CrossRef] [PubMed]
13. Ardengh, J.C.; Kemp, R.; Lima-Filho, É.R.; Dos Santos, J.S. Endoscopic papillectomy: The limits of the indication, technique and results. *World J. Gastrointest. Endosc.* **2015**, *7*, 987–994. [CrossRef] [PubMed]
14. de Castro, S.M.; van Heek, N.T.; Kuhlmann, K.F.; Busch, O.R.; Offerhaus, G.J.; van Gulik, T.M.; Obertop, H.; Gouma, D.J. Surgical management of neoplasms of the ampulla of Vater: Local resection or pancreatoduodenectomy and prognostic factors for survival. *Surgery* **2004**, *136*, 994–1002. [CrossRef] [PubMed]
15. Askew, J.; Connor, S. Review of the investigation and surgical management of resectable ampullary adenocarcinoma. *HPB (Oxford)* **2013**, *15*, 829–838. [CrossRef] [PubMed]
16. Takahara, N.; Tsuji, Y.; Nakai, Y.; Suzuki, Y.; Inokuma, A.; Kanai, S.; Noguchi, K.; Sato, T.; Hakuta, R.; Ishigaki, K. A novel technique of endoscopic papillectomy with hybrid endoscopic submucosal dissection for ampullary tumors: A proof-of-concept study (with video). *J. Clin. Med.* **2020**, *9*, 2671. [CrossRef] [PubMed]
17. Fong, Z.V.; Tan, W.P.; Lavu, H.; Kennedy, E.P.; Mitchell, D.G.; Koniaris, L.G.; Sauter, P.K.; Rosato, E.L.; Yeo, C.J.; Winter, J.M. Preoperative imaging for resectable periampullary cancer: Clinicopathologic implications of reported radiographic findings. *J. Gastrointest. Surg.* **2013**, *17*, 1098–1106. [CrossRef] [PubMed]
18. Kim, A.L.; Choi, Y.I. Safety of duodenal ampullectomy for benign periampullary tumors. *Ann. Hepatobiliary Pancreat. Surg.* **2017**, *21*, 146–150. [CrossRef] [PubMed]

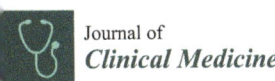

Review

Long-Term Outcomes of Endoscopic Gallbladder Drainage for Cholecystitis in Poor Surgical Candidates: An Updated Comprehensive Review

Tadahisa Inoue [1,*], Michihiro Yoshida [2], Yuta Suzuki [3], Rena Kitano [1], Fumihiro Okumura [3] and Itaru Naitoh [2]

1. Department of Gastroenterology, Aichi Medical University, 1-1 Yazakokarimata, Nagakute 480-1195, Japan; kitano.rena.035@mail.aichi-med-u.ac.jp
2. Department of Gastroenterology and Metabolism, Graduate School of Medical Sciences, Nagoya City University, 1 Kawasumi, Mizuho-cho, Mizuho-ku, Nagoya 467-8601, Japan; mityoshi@med.nagoya-cu.ac.jp (M.Y.); inaito@med.nagoya-cu.ac.jp (I.N.)
3. Department of Gastroenterology, Gifu Prefectural Tajimi Hospital, 5-161 Maehata-cho, Tajimi 507-8522, Japan; suzuki-yuta@tajimi-hospital.jp (Y.S.); okumura-fumihiro@tajimi-hospital.jp (F.O.)
* Correspondence: tinoue-tag@umin.ac.jp; Tel.: +81-561-62-3311; Fax: +81-561-63-3208

Abstract: Laparoscopic cholecystectomy is the standard and fundamental treatment of choice for acute cholecystitis; however, there are cases in which patients may be poor surgical candidates due to advanced age, comorbidities, and/or general condition. The rate of recurrent cholecystitis is high in patients who are not surgically treated; therefore, the prevention of recurrence in this patient population is an important subject of investigation in the management of cholecystitis. Although it has recently been reported that long-term stent placement by endoscopic gallbladder stenting or endoscopic ultrasound-guided gallbladder drainage may reduce the recurrence rate, its efficacy and safety remain controversial. Additionally, details surrounding the long-term stent management of these treatment methods should be further investigated. In this review, we summarize the updated evidence regarding the usefulness of long-term stent placement with endoscopic gallbladder stenting or endoscopic ultrasound-guided gallbladder drainage as a preventive measure for recurrence of cholecystitis and discuss issues that should be addressed in future studies.

Keywords: acute cholecystitis; recurrent cholecystitis; endoscopic gallbladder stenting; endoscopic ultrasound-guided gallbladder drainage

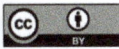

1. Introduction

Acute cholecystitis is a very common condition wherein approximately 90% of cases are caused by gallbladder stones [1,2]. The main pathogenic mechanisms of acute cholecystitis are cystic duct obstruction due to the impaction of the stones and intracholecystic cholestasis. Early cholecystectomy is the standard and definitive treatment of choice for acute cholecystitis, but patients who are unsuitable for emergency cholecystectomy are initially managed with gallbladder decompression [3,4]. There are two main approaches to gallbladder decompression [5]: percutaneous and endoscopic ones. The percutaneous approach includes percutaneous transhepatic gallbladder aspiration (PTGBA) and percutaneous transhepatic gallbladder drainage (PTGBD). The endoscopic approach includes endoscopic naso-gallbladder drainage (ENGBD), endoscopic gallbladder stenting (EGBS), and endoscopic ultrasound-guided gallbladder drainage (EUS-GBD). In recent years, the implementation of endoscopic drainage has been increasing with the progress of techniques and the advancement of devices. Additionally, EGBS and EUS-GBD avoid the use of external drainage catheters and thus provide a benefit to patient quality of life and obviate the risk to self-remove the drainage tubes. After achieving infection resolution and clinical improvement following initial gallbladder decompression, elective cholecystectomy is recommended to prevent recurrence [3].

However, there are cases where surgery is difficult or not indicated even in an elective setting after drainage and the improvement of infection due to the patient's advanced age and/or underlying disease. Recurrent cholecystitis frequently occurs if cholecystectomy is not performed in acute cholecystitis; the reported recurrence rate ranges from 22 to 47% in patients who did not undergo cholecystectomy after percutaneous gallbladder drainage [6–8]. These patients can experience frequent, repeated acute cholecystitis; therefore, the long-term management of cholecystitis in poor surgical candidates of cholecystectomy is a major concern. Recently, it has been suggested that long-term stent placement by EGBS or EUS-GBD may reduce the recurrence rate of cholecystitis. However, there is no clear consensus yet, and no detailed review article to date has explored the current state of knowledge pertaining to this subject. In this comprehensive narrative review, we provide an updated summary of the current evidence found on the PubMed database while discussing existing controversies and future prospects of the use of EGBS or EUS-GBD as a preventive measure for recurrent cholecystitis in poor surgical candidates.

2. EGBS vs. PTGBD for Long-Term Outcomes

ENGBD and EGBS are classified as transpapillary approaches; a naso-gallbladder tube is placed in ENGBD and a plastic stent extending from the gallbladder to the duodenum is placed in EGBS [9]. Since EGBS is an internal fistula method, the tube can be indwelling for a long period of time without impairing a patient's quality of life; in fact, long-term placement can be useful in preventing cholecystitis recurrence in patients with end-stage liver disease [10–12] and poor surgical candidates [13–26] (Figure 1). Based on research surrounding biliary stent placement for malignant or benign biliary strictures, it is unlikely that the stent will remain patent for years [27,28]. However, it appears that the stent not only facilitates bile drainage but also prevents gallstone impaction, thereby preventing recurrent cholecystitis. Additionally, even if stent occlusion were to occur, "wicking", which causes bile to flow along the outer surface of the stent, may effectively prevent recurrence [29].

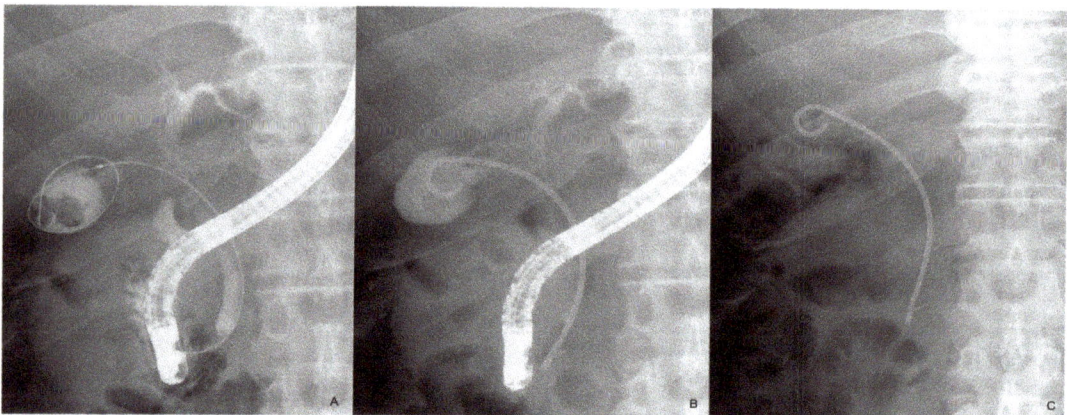

Figure 1. Endoscopic gallbladder stenting. The cystic duct is sought with a guidewire after biliary cannulation and the guidewire is inserted and placed in the gallbladder (**A**). A 7 Fr pigtail plastic stent is placed from the gallbladder to the duodenum (**B**). The stent remains in place 2 years after the procedure with no recurrent cholecystitis (**C**).

To date, three retrospective comparative studies [30–32] have investigated the usefulness of long-term stent placement via EGBS in poor surgical candidates with acute cholecystitis (Table 1). Kedia et al. [30] compared outcomes between patients who underwent EGBS (the study also includes some cases of EUS-GBD) and patients who underwent PTGBD followed by removal of the tube after clinical improvement. They reported that the mean durations of follow-up for each cohort were 9.4 months in the percutaneous drainage group and 8.8 months in the endoscopic drainage group ($p = 0.38$), and significantly more late adverse events, including recurrent cholecystitis, occurred in the percutaneous drainage group (27.9% vs. 0%, $p < 0.0001$). Inoue et al. [31] compared patients who underwent observation with tube removal after percutaneous drainage and those who underwent EGBS. Stents were kept without any stent exchange in the EGBS group. The median duration of follow-up was 485 days in the observation group and 473 days in the EGBS group, with no significant difference ($p = 0.649$). The recurrence rate of cholecystitis was significantly higher in the observation group (17.2% vs. 0%, $p = 0.043$), but the rate of overall biliary events, which not only include cholecystitis but also cholangitis, was not significantly different (24.1% vs. 9.1%, $p = 0.207$). Maruta et al. [32] compared the outcomes of patients with the removal of the gallbladder drainage tube after PTGBD or ENGBD and those with long-term stent placement by EGBS. Both the cumulative cholecystitis recurrence rate (16.0% vs. 5.0%, $p = 0.024$) and the cumulative late adverse event rate (22.1% vs. 5.0%, $p = 0.002$) were significantly higher in the removal group than in the EGBS group, with median follow-up periods of 307 days and 375 days, respectively ($p = 0.577$).

Based on the results of the three studies, long-term stent placement with EGBS is expected to have a preventive effect on the recurrence of cholecystitis, but the results were inconclusive regarding the overall adverse event rate such as cholangitis. There are also reported cases of stent–stone complex formation instigated by the presence of a biliary stent in the bile duct for an extended period, and cases of liver abscesses caused by cholestasis in the bile duct [18]. Therefore, the possibility of increased rates of adverse events other than cholecystitis, such as cholangitis and liver abscess formation with long-term stent placement, cannot be ruled out and warrants future investigation. In addition, there have been reports of rare side effects, such as a case of a migrated stent blocking the pancreatic duct orifice and causing pancreatitis [33] and a case of gallbladder perforation due to long-term contact with the stent [34]. Given that the median or mean observation period only lasts approximately 1 year in all the studies to date, the long-term safety and efficacy of stent placement are still unclear. In cases of extremely prolonged stent placement, it may be beneficial to replace or remove it as appropriate.

Furthermore, EGBS is a more technically difficult procedure than PTGBD; in fact, in previous studies, some patients underwent PTGBD after EGBS failed. The presence of cystic duct stones, dilatation of the common bile duct, and direction of the cystic duct were reported as risk factors affecting technical failure [35]. Although the success rate of the procedure has been increasing in recent years, owing to advances in both the procedural devices and techniques, the success rate remains at approximately 75–94.1% even in recent studies presenting results of cholangioscopic guidance by experienced endoscopists [36,37]. Moreover, patients need to be under conscious sedation for EGBS compared to local anesthesia for PTGBD, and the nature of early adverse events in EGBS and PTGBD are significantly different. There is a concern that the events associated with EGBS, such as pancreatitis, may be more severe than those associated with PTGBD. To establish and implement more widespread use of this treatment method, improving the success rate is crucial, and it is also necessary to verify whether the severity of early adverse events does not increase. In any case, given that there are only three retrospective studies to date, which were limited by selection and publication bias, further randomized controlled trials (RCT) are necessary.

Table 1. Studies comparing long-term outcomes of endoscopic gallbladder stenting and percutaneous drainage.

Author	Study Design	Drainage Method	No. of Patients	Drainage Tube/Stent	Technical Success	Clinical Success	Early Adverse Event	Follow-Up Period (Median/Mean)	Recurrent Cholecystitis	Late Adverse Event (Including Recurrent Cholecystitis)
Kedia et al., 2015 [30]	Retrospective	EGBS †	30 †	5 or 7 Fr pigtail	100% $p = 0.58$	86.7% $p = 0.08$	13.3% $p = 0.55$	8.8 m $p = 0.39$	-	0 $p < 0.0001$
		PTGBD	43	8 or 10 Fr	97.6%	97.6%	11.6%	9.4 m	-	27.9%
Inoue et al., 2016 [31]	Retrospective	EGBS	35	7 Fr pigtail	82.9%	82.9%	2.9%	15.6 m $p = 0.649$	0 $p = 0.043$	9.1% $p = 0.207$
		PTGBD/PTGBA	29	PTGBD: 7 or 8.5 Fr	-	-	-	16.0 m	17.2%	24.1%
Maruta et al., 2021 [32]	Retrospective	EGBS	40	5 or 6 Fr pigtail	78.9% ‡ $p < 0.0001$	94.6% ‡ $p = 1.000$	4.2% ‡ $p = 1.000$	12.3 m $p = 0.577$	5.0% $p = 0.024$	5.0% $p = 0.002$
		PTGBD/ENGBD	131	PTGBD: 8 or 8.5 Fr ENGBD: 5 or 6 Fr	100% ‡	93.5% ‡	4.5% ‡	10.1 m	16.0%	22.1%

EGBS, endoscopic gallbladder stenting; PTGBD, percutaneous transhepatic gallbladder drainage; PTGBA, percutaneous transhepatic gallbladder aspiration; ENGBD, endoscopic naso-gallbladder drainage. † Some cases of endoscopic ultrasound-guided gallbladder drainage were included. ‡ EGBS/ENGBD vs. PTGBD.

3. EUS-GBD vs. PTGBD for Long-Term Outcomes

EUS-GBD is a procedure that involves puncturing the gallbladder transgastrically or transduodenally under EUS guidance to place a naso-gallbladder drainage tube, double-pigtail plastic stent, or metal stent [38]. There are some specialized metal stents for use in EUS-GBD such as a metal stent with an anti-migration system, but there has recently been an increasing number of reports showing the usefulness of the lumen-apposing metal stent (LAMS) for EUS-GBD [39]. It is also suggested that long-term stent placement by EUS-GBD prevents the recurrence of cholecystitis [40–45] (Figure 2).

Three retrospective studies [46–48] and one RCT [49] have compared EUS-GBD and PTGBD and described the long-term outcomes of these methods (Table 2). Irani et al. [46] conducted a retrospective study to compare EUS-GBD using LAMS vs. PTGBD. Although there was no significant difference in the rate of adverse events, including cholecystitis recurrence, the EUS-GBD group had fewer repeat interventions ($p = 0.001$). Tyberg et al. [47] similarly reported that there was a significantly higher number of patients requiring repeat interventions in the percutaneous drainage group compared with the EUS-GBD group (27.78% vs. 9.52%, $p = 0.037$). However, in these two reports, nearly half of the study participants' cholecystitis was associated with a malignant biliary stricture, and the median or average observation period was brief, lasting less than 1 year. Their results should be interpreted in consideration of these limitations. Prognosis tends to be poor for cholecystitis associated with unresectable pancreato-biliary malignancy, and the time course of cholecystitis and long-term recurrence prevention may not be a priority in the care of these patients.

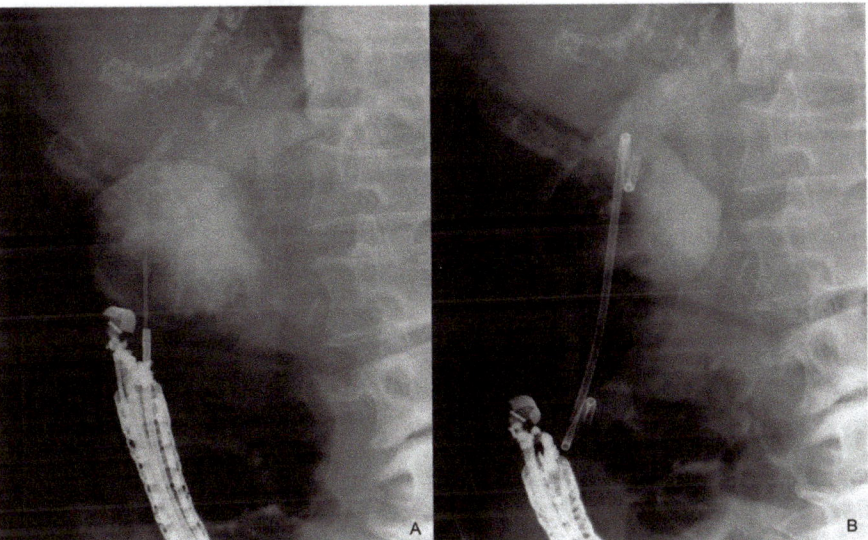

Figure 2. Endoscopic ultrasound-guided gallbladder drainage. After the gallbladder is punctured transduodenally (**A**), a guidewire is placed in the gallbladder. A 7 Fr double-pigtail plastic stent is placed after dilation of the fistula (**B**). The stent remains in place after the procedure without any stent exchange and removal.

Teoh et al. [48] conducted a retrospective comparative study that only examined calculous cholecystitis. They mentioned that although the rate of recurrent acute cholecystitis was similar between the percutaneous and EUS-GBD groups (6.8% vs. 0%, $p = 0.12$), the overall adverse event rates were significantly higher in patients who underwent percutaneous cholecystostomy (74.6% vs. 32.2%, $p < 0.001$). However, it should be noted that in the study, the mean duration of follow-up was 834.1 days in the percutaneous group and

450.7 days in the EUS-GBD group, showing a significant difference ($p < 0.001$). Teoh et al. later conducted an RCT [49] comparing EUS-GBD using LAMS and PTGBD in patients with calculous cholecystitis, as in their prior retrospective study. Patients who received EUS-GBD were scheduled for a follow-up for oral cholecystoscopy via the LAMS one month after the procedure, and if all gallstones were cleared, the LAMS was removed and replaced with a permanent 7 Fr double-pigtail plastic stent. All patients were followed-up for 1 year or until death. Significantly fewer patients in the EUS-GBD group had recurrent acute cholecystitis (20% vs. 2.6%, $p = 0.029$), and EUS-GBD significantly reduced adverse events by 1 year following the procedure (77.5% vs. 25.6%, $p < 0.001$). However, the total rate of recurrent biliary complication at 1 year was 20% in the PTGBD group and 10.3% in the EUS-GBD group, which was not statistically significant ($p = 0.227$).

From these research results, it can be said that long-term stent placement by EUS-GBD may be useful for reducing recurrent cholecystitis and further biliary events. However, there is no clear consensus yet in the existing literature. Even if EUS-GBD is useful for preventing cholecystitis recurrence, it is unclear whether LAMS/metal stents should be left to indwell for a long period of time, replaced with a plastic stent, or removed after symptom improvement. Long-term placement of LAMS can cause buried LAMS syndrome [41]. With the exception of cholecystitis associated with unresectable malignant biliary strictures, that is, as long as long-term survival is expected, it may be better to remove LAMS with or without plastic stent replacement. Alternatively, if a long-term placement is planned, the initial placement of a plastic stent may be an option. It is also unknown whether gallstone removal should be attempted when the stent is removed and replaced, although one retrospective study reported that EUS-GBD followed by the removal of gallstones had a rate of recurrent biliary events comparable to laparoscopic cholecystectomy, based on their one-year follow-up data [50]. More robust evidence regarding the utility and implications of EUS-GBD in preventing recurrent cholecystitis is necessary, and further long-term observation is warranted.

Table 2. Studies comparing long-term outcomes of endoscopic ultrasound-guided gallbladder drainage and percutaneous drainage.

Author	Study Design	Drainage Method	No. of Patients	Drainage Tube/Stent	Technical Success		Clinical Success		Early Adverse Event		Follow-Up Period (Median/Mean)		Recurrent Cholecystitis		Late Adverse Event (Including Recurrent Cholecystitis)	
Irani et al., 2017 [46]	Retrospective	EUS-GBD	45	LAMS	98%	$p = 0.98$	96%	$p = 0.12$	18% [†]	$p = 0.07$	7.1 m	$p = 0.25$	6.7%	-	-	-
		PTGBD£	45	8 or 10 Fr	100%		91%		31% [†]		8.7 m		8.9%		-	
Teoh et al., 2017 [48]	Retrospective	EUS-GBD	59	LAMS	96.6%	$p = 0.15$	89.8%	$p = 0.30$	28.8%	$p = 0.13$	14.9 m	$p < 0.001$	0	$p = 0.12$	32.2% [‡]	$p < 0.001$
		PTGBD	59	6–10 Fr	100%		94.9%		16.9%		27.5 m		6.8%		74.6% [‡]	
Tyberg et al., 2018 [47]	Retrospective	EUS-GBD	42	PS/CSEMS/LAMS	95.23%	$p = 0.179$	95.23%	$p = 0.157$	4.76%	$p = 0.613$	4.4 m	-	7.1%	-	16.67%	$p = 0.783$
		PTGBD	113	-	99.12%		88.18%		2.65%		7.6 m		8.0%		18.58%	
Teoh et al., 2020 [49]	RCT	EUS-GBD	39	LAMS	97.4%	$p = 0.494$	92.3%	$p = 1$	12.8%	$p = 0.001$	- [§]	-	2.6%	$p = 0.029$	10.3%	$p = 0.227$
		PTGBD	40	8.5 Fr	100%		92.5%		47.5%		- [§]		20%		20%	

RCT, randomized controlled trial; EUS-GBD, endoscopic ultrasound-guided gallbladder drainage; PTGBD, percutaneous transhepatic gallbladder drainage; LAMS, lumen-apposing metal stent; PS, plastic stent; CSEMS, covered self-expandable metal stent. [†] Late adverse events were also included. [‡] Early adverse events were also included. [§] Patients were followed-up until one year or death.

4. EGBS vs. EUS-GBD for Long-Term Outcomes

As mentioned above, long-term stent placement with EGBS and EUS-GBD are both considered treatment methods with the potential for preventing the recurrence of cholecystitis. Two retrospective studies [51,52] comparing the long-term outcomes of EGBS and EUS-GBD have been reported (Table 3). One was a study by Oh et al. [51], in which a 7 Fr double-pigtail stent was used for EGBS, and a covered metal stent was used for EUS-GBD. In both cases, patients were followed up without regular stent exchange or stent removal. After adjustment with the inverse probability of treatment weighting, both technical success (86.6% vs. 99.3%, $p < 0.01$) and clinical success (86.0% vs. 99.3%, $p < 0.01$) were significantly higher in the EUS-GBD group, while the procedure-related adverse event rate (19.3% vs. 7.1%, $p = 0.02$) was significantly lower in the EUS-GBD group. Regarding long-term outcomes, the recurrence rates of cholecystitis or cholangitis were 12.4% and 3.2% in the EGBS group and the EUS-GBD group, respectively, reflecting a significant difference ($p = 0.04$), with the mean follow-up periods of 20.7 months and 21.9 months, respectively ($p = 0.06$). Another study reported by Higa et al. [52] compared EGBS that used a 7 Fr double-pigtail stent and EUS-GBD that used LAMS. Clinical success rate was significantly higher in the EUS-GBD group (76.3% vs. 95.0, $p = 0.020$), and recurrent cholecystitis rate was lower in the EUS-GBD group (18.8% vs. 2.6%, $p = 0.023$). However, in the study, the median follow-up period was as short as 5 months in the EGBS group and 7 months in the EUS-GBD group, and 56.2% of the patients in the EGBS group and 10.3% in the EUS-GBD group eventually underwent surgical cholecystectomy. Therefore, it seems to be a slightly different study from the viewpoint of the usefulness of long-term stent placement for preventing recurrence. As a further note, both studies involved a considerable number of patients with cholecystitis associated with malignant biliary stricture with/without biliary stent placement.

Based on the results of available studies, EUS-GBD may be superior in terms of technical and clinical success, as well as in preventing recurrence, compared with EGBS. However, the fistula formation by EUS-GBD may have a negative effect if elective cholecystectomy becomes possible later (this has not been fully investigated yet). Moreover, calculous cholecystitis and cholecystitis associated with malignant biliary stricture differ in multiple aspects, including pathogenic mechanisms, long-term course, and treatment strategies. These should be considered separately, especially when considering long-term outcomes, including recurrence, which has not been done in studies to date. It is considered that the prevention of recurrent cholecystitis is more important in calculous cholecystitis cases and less so in cases of advanced malignancy with limited prognoses. Consequently, it will be difficult to directly apply the results of current studies to the long-term management of patients with cholecystitis who are poor surgical candidates for cholecystectomy. Future studies that compare the results of treatment via EGBS vs. EUS-GBD through better-controlled, standardized study designs may further help this field of research.

Table 3. Studies comparing long-term outcomes of endoscopic gallbladder stenting and endoscopic ultrasound-guided gallbladder drainage.

Author	Study Design	Drainage Method	No. of Patients	Stent	Technical Success		Clinical Success		Early Adverse Event		Follow-Up Period (Median/Mean)		Recurrent Cholecystitis		Late Adverse Event (Including Recurrent Cholecystitis)	
Oh et al., 2019 [51]	Retrospective	EGBS	96	7 Fr pigtail	86.6% [†]	$p < 0.01$	86.0% [†]	$p < 0.01$	19.3% [‡]	$p = 0.02$	20.7 m [†]	$p = 0.73$	10.5% [†]	-	12.4% [†]	$p = 0.04$
		EUS-GBD	83	CSEMS	99.3% [†]		99.3% [†]		7.1% [‡]		21.9 m [†]		3.2% [†]		3.2% [†]	
Higa et al., 2019 [52]	Retrospective	EGBS	38	7 Fr pigtail	84.2%	$p = 0.072$	76.3%	$p = 0.020$	9.4% [‡]	$p = 0.80$	5 m	$p = 0.80$	18.8%	$p = 0.023$	-	
		EUS-GBD	40	LAMS	97.5%		95.0%		17.9% [‡]		7 m		2.6%		-	

EGBS, endoscopic gallbladder stenting; EUS-GBD, endoscopic ultrasound-guided gallbladder drainage; CSEMS, covered self-expandable metal stent; LAMS, lumen-apposing metal stent.
[†] These were evaluated using inverse probability of treatment weighting. [‡] Late adverse events were also included.

5. Conclusions

In this review article, we discussed the current state of knowledge, shortcomings, and prospects of endoscopic management for preventing recurrent cholecystitis in patients unfit for cholecystectomy. It is particularly important to prevent recurrence in this patient population. Long-term stent placement with EGBS and EUS-GBD is a therapeutic method that may be a useful option for the prevention of recurrent cholecystitis. It is expected that the efficacy and safety of these procedures will be better established by future studies.

Author Contributions: T.I., conception and design, data acquisition, analysis and interpretation, and drafting and revision of the manuscript. M.Y., Y.S., R.K., F.O. and I.N., data interpretation, and revision of the manuscript. All authors have read and agreed to the published version of the manuscript.

Funding: This research received no external funding.

Institutional Review Board Statement: Not applicable.

Informed Consent Statement: Not applicable.

Conflicts of Interest: The authors declare no conflict of interest.

References

1. Gouma, D.J.; Obertop, H. Acute calculous cholecystitis. What is new in diagnosis and therapy? *HPB Surg.* **1992**, *6*, 69–78. [CrossRef] [PubMed]
2. Sharp, K.W. Acute cholecystitis. *Surg. Clin. North. Am.* **1988**, *68*, 269–279. [CrossRef]
3. Okamoto, K.; Suzuki, K.; Takada, T.; Strasberg, S.M.; Asbun, H.J.; Endo, I.; Iwashita, Y.; Hibi, T.; Pitt, H.A.; Umezawa, A.; et al. Tokyo Guidelines 2018: Flowchart for the management of acute cholecystitis. *J. Hepato-Biliary-Pancreat. Sci.* **2018**, *25*, 55–72, Correction in **2019**, *26*, 534. [CrossRef]
4. Serban, D.; Socea, B.; Balasescu, S.A.; Badiu, C.D.; Tudor, C.; Dascalu, A.M.; Vancea, G.; Spataru, R.I.; Sabau, A.D.; Sabau, D.; et al. Safety of Laparoscopic Cholecystectomy for Acute Cholecystitis in the Elderly: A Multivariate Analysis of Risk Factors for Intra and Postoperative Complications. *Medicina* **2021**, *57*, 230. [CrossRef]
5. Mori, Y.; Itoi, T.; Baron, T.H.; Takada, T.; Strasberg, S.M.; Pitt, H.A.; Ukai, T.; Shikata, S.; Noguchi, Y.; Teoh, A.Y.B.; et al. Tokyo Guidelines 2018: Management strategies for gallbladder drainage in patients with acute cholecystitis (with videos). *J. Hepato-Biliary-Pancreat. Sci.* **2018**, *25*, 87–95. [CrossRef]
6. McLoughlin, R.F.; Patterson, E.J.; Mathieson, J.R.; Cooperberg, P.L.; MacFarlane, J.K. Radiologically guided percutaneous cholecystostomy for acute cholecystitis: Long-term outcome in 50 patients. *Can. Assoc. Radiol. J.* **1994**, *45*, 455–459.
7. Andrén-Sandberg, A.; Haugsvedt, T.; Larssen, T.B.; Søndenaa, K. Complications and late outcome following percutaneous drainage of the gallbladder in acute calculous cholecystitis. *Dig. Surg.* **2001**, *18*, 393–398. [CrossRef]
8. Granlund, A.; Karlson, B.M.; Elvin, A.; Rasmussen, I. Ultrasound-guided percutaneous cholecystostomy in high-risk surgical patients. *Langenbecks Arch. Surg.* **2001**, *386*, 212–217. [CrossRef] [PubMed]
9. Itoi, T.; Kawakami, H.; Katanuma, A.; Irisawa, A.; Sofuni, A.; Itokawa, F.; Tsuchiya, T.; Tanaka, R.; Umeda, J.; Ryozawa, S.; et al. Endoscopic nasogallbladder tube or stent placement in acute cholecystitis: A preliminary prospective randomized trial in Japan (with videos). *Gastrointest. Endosc.* **2015**, *81*, 111–118. [CrossRef]
10. Shrestha, R.; Trouillot, T.E.; Everson, G.T. Endoscopic stenting of the gallbladder for symptomatic gallbladder disease in patients with end-stage liver disease awaiting orthotopic liver transplantation. *Liver Transpl. Surg.* **1999**, *5*, 275–281. [CrossRef]
11. Conway, J.D.; Russo, M.W.; Shrestha, R. Endoscopic stent insertion into the gallbladder for symptomatic gallbladder disease in patients with end-stage liver disease. *Gastrointest. Endosc.* **2005**, *61*, 32–36. [CrossRef]
12. Schlenker, C.; Trotter, J.F.; Shah, R.J.; Everson, G.; Chen, Y.K.; Antillon, D.; Antillon, M.R. Endoscopic gallbladder stent placement for treatment of symptomatic cholelithiasis in patients with end-stage liver disease. *Am. J. Gastroenterol.* **2006**, *101*, 278–283. [CrossRef]
13. Tamada, K.; Seki, H.; Sato, K.; Kano, T.; Sugiyama, S.; Ichiyama, M.; Wada, S.; Ohashi, A.; Tomiyama, G.; Ueno, A.; et al. Efficacy of endoscopic retrograde cholecystoendoprosthesis (ERCCE) for cholecystitis. *Endoscopy* **1991**, *23*, 2–3. [CrossRef] [PubMed]
14. Siegel, J.H.; Kasmin, F.E.; Cohen, S.A. Endoscopic retrograde cholangiopancreatography treatment of cholecystitis: Possible? Yes; practical? *Diagn. Endosc.* **1994**, *1*, 51–56. [CrossRef]
15. Pannala, R.; Petersen, B.T.; Gostout, C.J.; Topazian, M.D.; Levy, M.J.; Baron, T.H. Endoscopic transpapillary gallbladder drainage: 10-year single center experience. *Minerva Gastroenterol. Dietol.* **2008**, *54*, 107–113.
16. Mutignani, M.; Iacopini, F.; Perri, V.; Familiari, P.; Tringali, A.; Spada, C.; Ingrosso, M.; Costamagna, G. Endoscopic gallbladder drainage for acute cholecystitis: Technical and clinical results. *Endoscopy* **2009**, *41*, 539–546. [CrossRef]

7. Lee, T.H.; Park, D.H.; Lee, S.S.; Seo, D.W.; Park, S.H.; Lee, S.K.; Kim, M.H.; Kim, S.J. Outcomes of endoscopic transpapillary gallbladder stenting for symptomatic gallbladder diseases: A multicenter prospective follow-up study. *Endoscopy* **2011**, *43*, 702–708. [CrossRef] [PubMed]
8. Maekawa, S.; Nomura, R.; Murase, T.; Ann, Y.; Oeholm, M.; Harada, M. Endoscopic gallbladder stenting for acute cholecystitis: A retrospective study of 46 elderly patients aged 65 years or older. *BMC Gastroenterol.* **2013**, *13*, 65. [CrossRef]
9. McCarthy, S.T.; Tujios, S.; Fontana, R.J.; Rahnama-Moghadam, S.; Elmunzer, B.J.; Kwon, R.S.; Wamsteker, E.J.; Anderson, M.A.; Scheiman, J.M.; Elta, G.H.; et al. Endoscopic Transpapillary Gallbladder Stent Placement Is Safe and Effective in High-Risk Patients Without Cirrhosis. *Dig. Dis. Sci.* **2015**, *60*, 2516–2522. [CrossRef] [PubMed]
20. Widmer, J.; Alvarez, P.; Sharaiha, R.Z.; Gossain, S.; Kedia, P.; Sarkaria, S.; Sethi, A.; Turner, B.G.; Millman, J.; Lieberman, M.; et al. Endoscopic Gallbladder Drainage for Acute Cholecystitis. *Clin. Endosc.* **2015**, *48*, 411–420. [CrossRef]
21. Kamada, H.; Kobara, H.; Uchida, N.; Kato, K.; Fujimori, T.; Kobayashi, K.; Yamashita, T.; Ono, M.; Aritomo, Y.; Tsutsui, K.; et al. Long-Term Management of Recurrent Cholecystitis after Initial Conservative Treatment: Endoscopic Transpapillary Gallbladder Stenting. *Can. J. Gastroenterol. Hepatol.* **2018**, *2018*, 3983707. [CrossRef] [PubMed]
22. Nakahara, K.; Michikawa, Y.; Morita, R.; Suetani, K.; Morita, N.; Sato, J.; Tsuji, K.; Ikeda, H.; Matsunaga, K.; Watanabe, T.; et al. Endoscopic transpapillary gallbladder stenting using a newly designed plastic stent for acute cholecystitis. *Endosc. Int. Open* **2019**, *7*, E1105–E1114. [CrossRef]
23. Sagami, R.; Hayasaka, K.; Ujihara, T.; Nakahara, R.; Murakami, D.; Iwaki, T.; Suehiro, S.; Katsuyama, Y.; Harada, H.; Nishikiori, H.; et al. Endoscopic transpapillary gallbladder drainage for acute cholecystitis is feasible for patients receiving antithrombotic therapy. *Dig. Endosc.* **2020**, *32*, 1092–1099. [CrossRef]
24. Kim, T.H.; Park, D.E.; Chon, H.K. Endoscopic transpapillary gallbladder drainage for the management of acute calculus cholecystitis patients unfit for urgent cholecystectomy. *PLoS ONE* **2020**, *15*, e0240219. [CrossRef]
25. Storm, A.C.; Vargas, E.J.; Chin, J.Y.; Chandrasekhara, V.; Dayyeh, B.K.A.; Levy, M.J.; Martin, J.A.; Topazian, M.D.; Andrews, J.C.; Schiller, H.J.; et al. Transpapillary gallbladder stent placement for long-term therapy of acute cholecystitis. *Gastrointest. Endosc.* **2021**, *94*, 742–748.e1. [CrossRef]
26. Sobani, Z.A.; Sánchez-Luna, S.A.; Rustagi, T. Endoscopic Transpapillary Gallbladder Drainage for Acute Cholecystitis using Two Gallbladder Stents (Dual Gallbladder Stenting). *Clin. Endosc.* **2021**. [CrossRef]
27. Isayama, H.; Yasuda, I.; Ryozawa, S.; Maguchi, H.; Igarashi, Y.; Matsuyama, Y.; Katanuma, A.; Hasebe, O.; Irisawa, A.; Itoi, T.; et al. Results of a Japanese multicenter, randomized trial of endoscopic stenting for non-resectable pancreatic head cancer (JM-test): Covered Wallstent versus DoubleLayer stent. *Dig. Endosc.* **2011**, *23*, 310–315. [CrossRef]
28. Mukai, T. Ways to improve stenting in unresectable malignant distal biliary obstruction: Stent design, intraductal placement, and protective role of an intact papilla? *Dig. Endosc.* **2020**, *32*, 891–893. [CrossRef]
29. Elmunzer, B.J.; Novelli, P.M.; Taylor, J.R.; Piraka, C.R.; Shields, J.J. Percutaneous cholecystostomy as a bridge to definitive endoscopic gallbladder stent placement. *Clin. Gastroenterol. Hepatol.* **2011**, *9*, 18–20. [CrossRef] [PubMed]
30. Kedia, P.; Sharaiha, R.Z.; Kumta, N.A.; Widmer, J.; Jamal-Kabani, A.; Weaver, K.; Benvenuto, A.; Millman, J.; Barve, R.; Gaidhane, M.; et al. Endoscopic gallbladder drainage compared with percutaneous drainage. *Gastrointest. Endosc.* **2015**, *82*, 1031–1036. [CrossRef] [PubMed]
31. Inoue, T.; Okumura, F.; Kachi, K.; Fukusada, S.; Iwasaki, H.; Ozeki, T.; Suzuki, Y.; Anbe, K.; Nishie, H.; Mizushima, T.; et al. Long-term outcomes of endoscopic gallbladder stenting in high-risk surgical patients with calculous cholecystitis (with videos). *Gastrointest. Endosc.* **2016**, *83*, 905–913. [CrossRef]
32. Maruta, A.; Iwashita, T.; Iwata, K.; Yoshida, K.; Uemura, S.; Mukai, T.; Yasuda, I.; Shimizu, M. Permanent endoscopic gallbladder stenting versus removal of gallbladder drainage, long-term outcomes after management of acute cholecystitis in high-risk surgical patients for cholecystectomy: Multi-center retrospective cohort study. *J. Hepato-Biliary-Pancreat. Sci.* **2021**. [CrossRef]
33. Yane, K.; Katanuma, A.; Maguchi, H. Late onset pancreatitis 6 months after endoscopic transpapillary gallbladder stenting for acute cholecystitis. *Dig. Endosc.* **2014**, *26*, 494–495. [CrossRef] [PubMed]
34. Naitoh, I.; Nakazawa, T.; Miyabe, K.; Mizoguchi, K.; Kimura, M.; Takeyama, H.; Joh, T. A cholecystocolonic fistula caused by penetration of a double-pigtail plastic stent after endoscopic transpapillary gallbladder stenting. *Endoscopy* **2015**, *47* (Suppl. 1), E399–E400. [CrossRef] [PubMed]
35. Maruta, A.; Iwata, K.; Iwashita, T.; Mizoguchi, K.; Kimura, M.; Takeyama, H.; Joh, T. Factors affecting technical success of endoscopic transpapillary gallbladder drainage for acute cholecystitis. *J. Hepato-Biliary-Pancreat. Sci.* **2020**, *27*, 429–436. [CrossRef]
36. Ridtitid, W.; Piyachaturawat, P.; Teeratorn, N.; Angsuwatcharakon, P.; Kongkam, P.; Rerknimitr, R. Single-operator peroral cholangioscopy cystic duct cannulation for transpapillary gallbladder stent placement in patients with acute cholecystitis at moderate to high surgical risk (with videos). *Gastrointest. Endosc.* **2020**, *92*, 634–644. [CrossRef]
37. Yoshida, M.; Naitoh, I.; Hayashi, K.; Jinno, N.; Hori, Y.; Natsume, M.; Kato, A.; Kachi, K.; Asano, G.; Atsuta, N.; et al. Four-Step Classification of Endoscopic Transpapillary Gallbladder Drainage and the Practical Efficacy of Cholangioscopic Assistance. *Gut Liver* **2021**, *15*, 476–485. [CrossRef]
38. Park, S.W.; Lee, S.S. Current status of endoscopic management of cholecystitis. *Dig. Endosc.* **2021**. [CrossRef] [PubMed]
39. Jain, D.; Bhandari, B.S.; Agrawal, N.; Singhal, S. Endoscopic Ultrasound-Guided Gallbladder Drainage Using a Lumen-Apposing Metal Stent for Acute Cholecystitis: A Systematic Review. *Clin. Endosc.* **2018**, *51*, 450–462. [CrossRef]

40. Choi, J.H.; Lee, S.S.; Choi, J.H.; Park, D.H.; Seo, D.W.; Lee, S.K.; Kim, M.K. Long-term outcomes after endoscopic ultrasonography-guided gallbladder drainage for acute cholecystitis. *Endoscopy* **2014**, *46*, 656–661. [CrossRef]
41. Walter, D.; Teoh, A.Y.; Itoi, T.; Pérez-Miranda, M.; Larghi, A.; Sanchez-Yague, A.; Siersema, P.D.; Vleggaar, F.P. EUS-guided gall bladder drainage with a lumen-apposing metal stent: A prospective long-term evaluation. *Gut* **2016**, *65*, 6–8. [CrossRef]
42. Kamata, K.; Takenaka, M.; Kitano, M.; Omoto, S.; Miyata, T.; Minaga, K.; Yamao, K.; Imai, H.; Sakurai, T.; Watanabe, T.; et al. Endoscopic ultrasound-guided gallbladder drainage for acute cholecystitis: Long-term outcomes after removal of a self-expandable metal stent. *World J. Gastroenterol.* **2017**, *23*, 661–667. [CrossRef]
43. Cho, D.H.; Jo, S.J.; Lee, J.H.; Song, T.J.; Park, D.H.; Lee, S.K.; Kim, M.H.; Lee, S.S. Feasibility and safety of endoscopic ultrasound-guided gallbladder drainage using a newly designed lumen-apposing metal stent. *Surg. Endosc.* **2019**, *33*, 2135–2141. [CrossRef] [PubMed]
44. Cho, S.H.; Oh, D.; Song, T.J.; Park, D.H.; Seo, D.W.; Lee, S.K.; Kim, M.H.; Lee, Y.N.; Moon, J.H.; Lee, S.S. Comparison of the effectiveness and safety of lumen-apposing metal stents and anti-migrating tubular self-expandable metal stents for EUS-guided gallbladder drainage in high surgical risk patients with acute cholecystitis. *Gastrointest. Endosc.* **2020**, *91*, 543–550. [CrossRef]
45. Teoh, A.Y.B.; Kongkam, P.; Bapaye, A.; Ratanachu, T.; Reknimitr, R.; Lakthakia, S.; Chan, S.M.; Gadhikar, H.P.; Korrapati, S.K.; Lee, Y.N.; et al. Use of a novel lumen apposing metallic stent for drainage of the bile duct and gallbladder: Long term outcomes of a prospective international trial. *Dig. Endosc.* **2020**. [CrossRef]
46. Irani, S.; Ngamruengphong, S.; Teoh, A.; Will, U.; Nieto, J.; Abu Dayyeh, B.K.; Gan, S.I.; Larsen, M.; Yip, H.C.; Topazian, M.D.; et al. Similar Efficacies of Endoscopic Ultrasound Gallbladder Drainage with a Lumen-Apposing Metal Stent Versus Percutaneous Transhepatic Gallbladder Drainage for Acute Cholecystitis. *Clin. Gastroenterol. Hepatol.* **2017**, *15*, 738–745. [CrossRef]
47. Tyberg, A.; Saumoy, M.; Sequeiros, E.V.; Giovannini, M.; Artifon, E.; Teoh, A.; Nieto, J.; Desai, A.P.; Kumta, N.K.; Gaidhane, M.; et al. EUS-guided Versus Percutaneous Gallbladder Drainage: Isn't It Time to Convert? *J. Clin. Gastroenterol.* **2018**, *52*, 79–84. [CrossRef] [PubMed]
48. Teoh, A.Y.B.; Serna, C.; Penas, I.; Chong, C.C.N.; Perez-Miranda, M.; Ng, E.K.W.; Lau, J.Y.W. Endoscopic ultrasound-guided gallbladder drainage reduces adverse events compared with percutaneous cholecystostomy in patients who are unfit for cholecystectomy. *Endoscopy* **2017**, *49*, 130–138. [CrossRef]
49. Teoh, A.Y.B.; Kitano, M.; Itoi, T.; Pérez-Miranda, M.; Ogura, T.; Chan, S.M.; Serna-Higuera, C.; Omoto, S.; Torres-Yuste, R.; Tsuichiya, T.; et al. Endosonography-guided gallbladder drainage versus percutaneous cholecystostomy in very high-risk surgical patients with acute cholecystitis: An international randomised multicentre controlled superiority trial (DRAC 1). *Gut* **2020**, *69*, 1085–1091. [CrossRef]
50. Teoh, A.Y.B.; Leung, C.H.; Tam, P.T.H.; Yeung, K.K.Y.A.; Mok, R.C.Y.; Chan, D.L.; Chan, S.M.; Yip, H.C.; Chiu, P.W.Y.; Ng, E.K.W. EUS-guided gallbladder drainage versus laparoscopic cholecystectomy for acute cholecystitis: A propensity score analysis with 1-year follow-up data. *Gastrointest. Endosc.* **2021**, *93*, 577–583. [CrossRef] [PubMed]
51. Oh, D.; Song, T.J.; Cho, D.H.; Park, D.H.; Seo, D.W.; Lee, S.K.; Kim, M.H.; Lee, S.S. EUS-guided cholecystostomy versus endoscopic transpapillary cholecystostomy for acute cholecystitis in high-risk surgical patients. *Gastrointest. Endosc.* **2019**, *89*, 289–298. [CrossRef] [PubMed]
52. Higa, J.T.; Sahar, N.; Kozarek, R.A.; La Selva, D.; Larsen, M.C.; Gan, S.I.; Ross, A.S.; Irani, S.S. EUS-guided gallbladder drainage with a lumen-apposing metal stent versus endoscopic transpapillary gallbladder drainage for the treatment of acute cholecystitis (with videos). *Gastrointest. Endosc.* **2019**, *90*, 483–492. [CrossRef] [PubMed]

Practical Tips for Safe and Successful Endoscopic Ultrasound-Guided Hepaticogastrostomy: A State-of-the-Art Technical Review

Saburo Matsubara *, Keito Nakagawa, Kentaro Suda, Takeshi Otsuka, Masashi Oka and Sumiko Nagoshi

Department of Gastroenterology and Hepatology, Saitama Medical Center, Saitama Medical University, 1981, Kamoda, Kawagoe 350-8550, Japan; kate-ill@hotmail.co.jp (K.N.); leclearlshelly@gmail.com (K.S.); ohitoyosinokaze@yahoo.co.jp (T.O.); oka@dd.iij4u.or.jp (M.O.); snagoshi@saitama-med.ac.jp (S.N.)
* Correspondence: saburom@saitama-med.ac.jp; Tel.: +81-49-228-3400 (ext. 7839); Fax: +81-49-226-5284

Abstract: Currently, endoscopic ultrasound-guided hepaticogastrostomy (EUS-HGS) is widely performed worldwide for various benign and malignant biliary diseases in cases of difficult or unsuccessful endoscopic transpapillary cholangiopancreatography (ERCP). Furthermore, its applicability as primary drainage has also been reported. Although recent advances in EUS systems and equipment have made EUS-HGS easier and safer, the risk of serious adverse events such as bile leak and stent migration still exists. Physicians and assistants need not only sufficient skills and experience in ERCP-related procedures and basic EUS-related procedures such as fine needle aspiration and pancreatic fluid collection drainage, but also knowledge and techniques specific to EUS-HGS. This technical review mainly focuses on EUS-HGS with self-expandable metal stents for unresectable malignant biliary obstruction and presents the latest and detailed tips for safe and successful performance of the technique.

Keywords: hepaticogastrostomy; endoscopic ultrasound; endoscopic ultrasound-guided biliary drainage (EUS-BD); endoscopic ultrasound-guided hepaticogastrostomy (EUS-HGS)

1. Introduction

Endoscopic ultrasound-guided biliary drainage (EUS-BD) has become a promising alternative to percutaneous transhepatic biliary drainage (PTBD) after difficult or failed endoscopic retrograde cholangiopancreatography (ERCP) in patients with benign or malignant biliary obstruction [1–4]. Furthermore, its applicability as a primary drainage has also been reported [5–7]. The technique of EUS-BD is divided into rendezvous with ERCP, antegrade stenting, and bilioenterostomy, which includes EUS-guided hepaticogastrostomy (EUS-HGS) and EUS-guided choledochoduodenostomy (EUS-CDS) [8]. Among these techniques, EUS-HGS has the broadest indications, including duodenal stenosis [9], surgically altered anatomy [10], high-grade hilar stenosis [11,12] as well as failed biliary cannulation, and is therefore considered to be the most frequently performed technique in EUS-BD [13,14]. However, EUS-HGS can cause serious adverse events such as bleeding [15], bile leak leading to peritonitis or biloma/abscess, perforation, focal cholangitis, and stent migration [16].

Several guidelines or technical reviews on EUS-HGS have been reported [8,17,18]. However, techniques and devices are constantly evolving, and it is necessary to keep up to date with the latest advances. This latest technical review provides detailed tips and tricks for safe and successful EUS-HGS using many easy-to-understand illustrations and figures with reference to the recent literature.

2. Physician and Facility Requirements

EUS-HGS is a technically complex procedure with life-threatening risks and should be performed by a physician with extensive experience and skill in ERCP and basic EUS-guided procedures such as fine needle aspiration (FNA) and peripancreatic fluid collection drainage [8]. If a physician is performing EUS-HGS for the first time, the procedure should be performed under the supervision of an expert with adequate experience in EUS-HGS. Physicians and assistants must be familiar with endoscopic system and various accessories including FNA needles, guidewires, dilation devices, and stents. Furthermore, it is important that immediate support from interventional radiologists and surgeons are available in case of serious adverse events such as arterial bleeding or migration of the stent into the abdominal cavity [8].

3. Preparation for a Safe Procedure

Contrast-enhanced computed tomography (CT) prior to EUS-HGS is essential to evaluate not only the biliary tree but also ascites, collateral vessels, tumor location in the liver, and distance between the left hepatic lobe and the lesser curvature of the stomach. If ascites is present between the left hepatic lobe and the lesser curvature of the stomach, a fistula will not form after EUS-HGS, and even if a covered self-expandable metal stent (SEMS) is used, bile, gastric juice, and air may leak into the abdominal cavity over time, causing peritonitis. Therefore, EUS-HGS should not be performed in patients with uncontrollable ascites in this region [19,20]. Collateral vessels are often observed around the stomach due to tumor invasion of the portal vein or splenic vein. In such cases, the feasibility of EUS-HGS is not known until EUS observation is performed in Doppler mode, so an alternative drainage plan should be prepared before starting the procedure. Likewise, if there is a tumor in segment 2 or 3 of the liver, a backup plan should be discussed beforehand, as it is not known whether EUS-HGS can be carried out while avoiding the tumor until EUS observation is conducted. A long distance between the liver and stomach before EUS-HGS may increase the risk of migration of the gastric end of the stent into the abdominal cavity after EUS-HGS [21], so it is advisable to use a stent of sufficient length or a stent with an anti-migration system.

4. EUS System

The EUS system is comprised of an echoendoscope with a curved linear array transducer and a processor. Optically, the oblique-viewing echoendoscope is the most common type in ES-HGS, while some endoscopists prefer the forward-viewing type [22]. There are three types of EUS systems available worldwide (Table 1). EG-580UT (Fujifilm Medical Corp, Tokyo, Japan), GF-UCT260 (Olympus Medical Systems, Tokyo, Japan), and EG38-J10UT (Pentax medical, Tokyo, Japan) are oblique-viewing echoendoscopes that have large bore accessory channels. EG-580UT and EG38-J10UT have better maneuverability with greater vertical angle mobility than GF-UCT260. Meanwhile, GF-UCT260 has a greater range of the ultrasound view, which helps to identify intervening mucosa or vessels before advancing the needle into the gastric wall. EG-580UT and GF-UCT260 have dedicated ultrasound processors (SU-1; Fujifilm Medical Corp, EU-ME2; Olympus Medical Systems), which can be mounted on an endoscope trolley and have ancillary functions: Doppler mode and contrast harmonic mode. The former allows the needle to avoid vessels when puncturing. Contrast-enhanced EUS using the latter function facilitates the identification of bile ducts when they are obscured by echogenic lesions such as stones or sludge [23]. EG38-J10UT does not have a dedicated processor, so it needs to be connected to an external ultrasound platform (ARIETTA series; Fujifilm Medical Corp).

Table 1. Specifications of endoscopic ultrasound systems.

		EG-580UT (Fujifilm)	GF-UCT260 (Olympus)	EG38-J10UT (Pentax)
Endoscopic Functions	Viewing direction	Forward oblique viewing 40°	Forward oblique viewing 55°	Forward oblique viewing 45°
	Observation range	3–100 mm	3–100 mm	3–100 mm
	Field of view	140°	100°	120°
	Distal end diameter	13.9 mm	14.6 mm	14.3 mm
	Insertion tube diameter	12.4 mm	12.6 mm	12.8 mm
	Bending capacity up/down	150°/150°	130°/90°	160°/130°
	Bending capacity left/right	120°/120°	90°/90°	120°/120°
	Working channel diameter	3.8 mm	3.7 mm	4.0 mm
	Working length	1250 mm	1250 mm	1250 mm
	Total length	1550 mm	1555 mm	1566 mm
Ultrasound Functions	Dedicated processor	SU-1	EU-ME2	None
	Sound method	Electronic curved linear array	Electronic curved linear array	Electronic curved linear array
	Scanning area	150°	180°	150°
	Frequency	5–12 MHz	5–12 MHz	5–13 MHz
	Scanning mode	B-Mode, M-Mode, Color Doppler, Power Doppler, Pulse Doppler	B-Mode, Color Flow Mode, Power Flow Mode	Depends on ultrasound-platforms (ARIETTA series)

5. Step-by-Step Tutorial on EUS-HGS Procedure including Devise Selection

In EUS-HGS, the left lateral branch of the intrahepatic bile duct is first punctured from the stomach or jejunum (in the case of post-gastrectomy) with an FNA needle, followed by injection of contrast medium and insertion of a guidewire. After the needle is removed, a dilation device is inserted into the bile duct to dilate the tract. Next, an introducer of a SEMS or plastic stent (PS) is inserted into the bile duct. Finally, a stent is deployed between the bile duct and the stomach or jejunum (Figure 1).

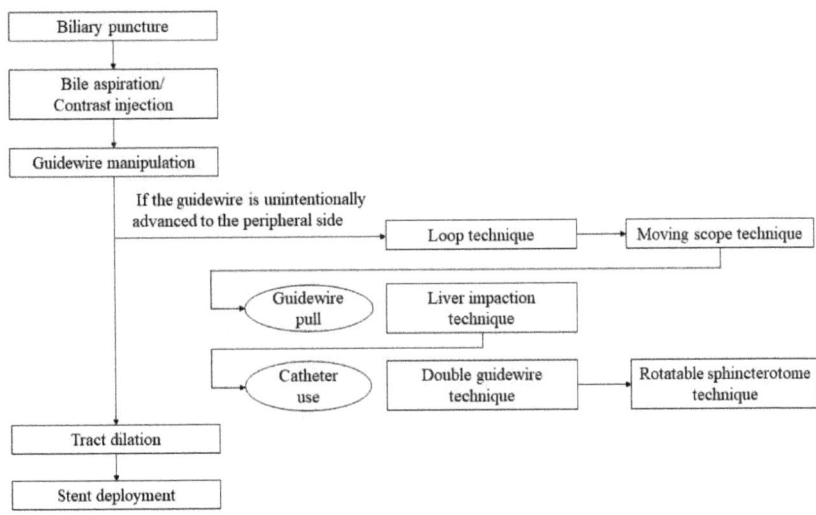

Figure 1. A flow diagram of step-by-step procedures in EUS-HGS.

5.1. Selection of Bile Duct Puncture Site and Scope Position

The intrahepatic bile ducts (B2 or B3) in the left lateral lobe of the liver are candidates for the puncture. On EUS imaging, B2 is directed from the B2/B3 junction to the right superiorly, and B3 is directed to the left superiorly [24]. Therefore, the B2 puncture is easier for inserting the guidewire into the bile duct because the trajectory of the needle and the direction of the bile duct are similar. However, most experts prefer to puncture B3 rather than B2 because puncturing B2 can be a transesophageal puncture, which may result in the risk of mediastinitis [8,25]. Because the position of the segment 2 of the liver is more cephalad than the segment 3, the position of the scope when puncturing B2 is shallower than that of B3, and even if the transducer is in the stomach, the exit of the accessory channel is often in the esophagus.

Before starting B3 puncture, it is desirable to adjust the position of the scope and the direction of the needle. For easy and reliable manipulation of the guidewire toward the hilum, the angle formed by the needle and the bile duct on the hilar side should be obtuse. When the scope is in a shallow position, that angle is often acute, making it difficult to manipulate the guidewire toward the hilum (Figure 2A,B); pushing the scope while turning the large wheel upward rotates the EUS image clockwise and makes that angle obtuse (Figure 3A,B). In fact, Ogura et al. reported in a retrospective multivariate analysis that strongly applying the up-angle of the scope to make the angle between the scope and the needle less than 135 degrees was a positive predictive factor of successful guidewire manipulation toward the hilum [26]. However, this bent scope shape reduces the forward push force during device insertion, and in the worst case, the scope may be pushed back, and the guidewire may be dislodged from the bile duct. Shiomi et al. [27] and Nakai et al. [28] reported the usefulness of the "Double guidewire technique" using a double lumen catheter (Uneven Double Lumen Cannula [UDLC]; Piolax Medical Device, Kanagawa, Japan), which allows a second 0.035 inch guidewire to be inserted adjacent to the first 0.025 inch guidewire (Figure 4). This technique improves the stability of the scope during device insertion and allows the use of the stiffer second guidewire if necessary. In addition, the second guidewire can be used to perform another stent insertion in case of a failed stent insertion, ensuring a safe procedure.

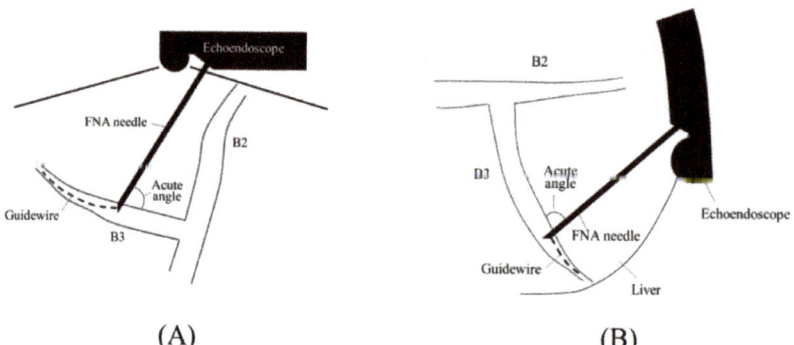

Figure 2. Too shallow echoendoscope position in B3 puncture. In a shallow scope position, the angle formed by a needle and the bile duct on the hilar side is often acute, and a guidewire can easily go to the peripheral side ((**A**); ultrasound image, (**B**); fluoroscopic image).

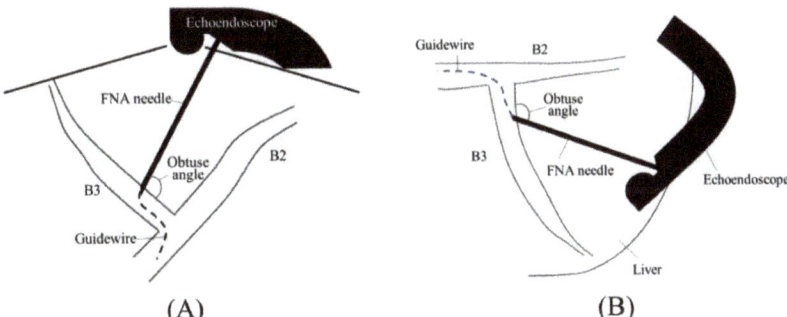

Figure 3. Optimal echoendoscope position in B3 puncture. Pushing a scope while turning the large wheel upward rotates the EUS image clockwise and makes the angle between a needle and the bile duct on the hilar side obtuse, making a guidewire manipulation toward the hilar region easy (**A**). Fluoroscopic image (**B**).

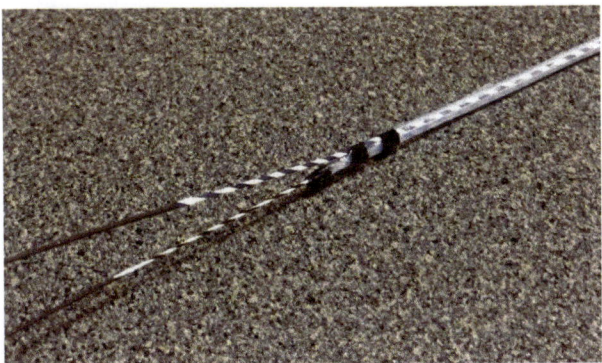

Figure 4. Uneven Double Lumen Cannula (Piolax Medical Device). The double lumen catheter allows a second 0.035 inch guidewire to be inserted adjacent to the first 0.025 inch guidewire. (Courtesy of Piolax Medical Device).

The choice of puncture site is important; Oh et al. reported that a bile duct diameter >5 mm and a distance ≤3 cm from the hepatic surface to the punctured bile duct at the puncture site were associated with technical success [29]. On the other hand, Yamamoto et al. reported that bile peritonitis was more likely to occur when the distance between the hepatic surface and the punctured bile duct was less than 2.5 cm [30]. Taking these factors into consideration, we believe that puncture at B3 close to the B2/3 bifurcation is the best choice. This is because the bile duct diameter is large, which makes puncture easy; the liver parenchyma is sufficiently intervened to avoid bile leakage; and the angle between the needle and the bile duct on the hilar side is obtuse, which facilitates successful insertion of the guidewire into the hilar bile duct (Figure 3A,B). If the biliary stricture is close to the B2/3 bifurcation, the puncture point must be on the peripheral side in order to secure the space in the bile duct for stent placement.

When performing a B2 puncture, it is of paramount importance to avoid transesophageal puncture. There are several methods to achieve this, such as confirming the needle puncture position under direct endoscopic view, clipping the esophagogastric junction and confirming it under fluoroscopy [25], or confirming the diaphragmatic crus by ultrasound. If the scope is shallow, the needle and B2 are parallel to each other, making puncture difficult and increasing the risk of transesophageal puncture (Figure 5A,B); therefore, slightly pushing the scope while turning the large wheel upward facilitates transgastric and reliable bile duct puncture (Figure 6A,B).

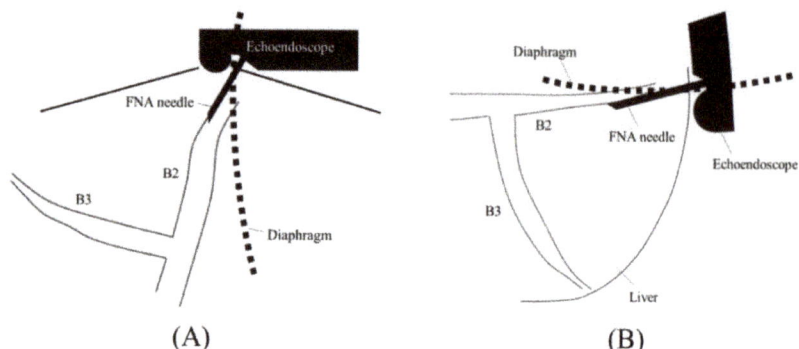

Figure 5. Too shallow echoendoscope position in B2 puncture. In a shallow scope position, a needle and B2 are parallel to each other, making puncture difficult and increasing the risk of transesophageal puncture ((**A**); ultrasound image, (**B**); fluoroscopic image).

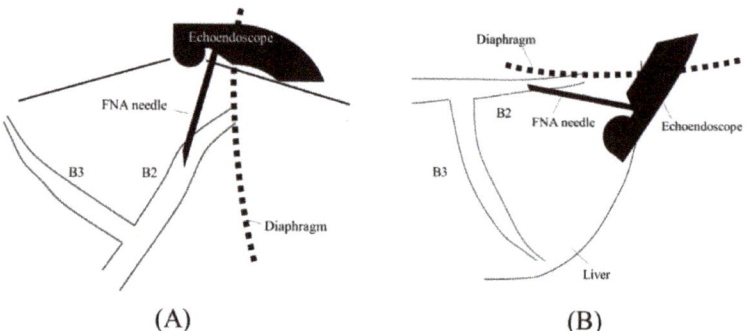

Figure 6. Optimal echoendoscope position in B2 puncture. Pushing a scope while turning the large wheel upward facilitates transgastric and reliable bile duct puncture ((**A**); ultrasound image, (**B**); fluoroscopic image).

5.2. Biliary Puncture

There are various types of FNA needles, each with a different tip shape and different materials for the needle and sheath. Nitinol needles are more flexible and less prone to bending than steel needles. Additionally, the coil sheath has a higher lumen retention when bent than the plastic sheath. These properties are useful for performing EUS-HGS. The EZ-shot 3 plus (Olympus Medical Systems) (Figure 7A) is the only commercially available nitinol needle with a coil sheath. In EUS-HGS, one of the most difficult steps is the manipulation of the guidewire through the needle [31]. The main issue is guidewire shearing, which in turn created a risk of leaving a tip of the guidewire in the patient. The EchoTip Access Needle (Cook Medical, Winston Salem, NC, USA) is a dedicated needle for interventional EUS, which has a sharp stylet for puncture, and the needle tip becomes blunt when the stylet is removed, thus avoiding guidewire shearing [17,32] (Figure 7B).

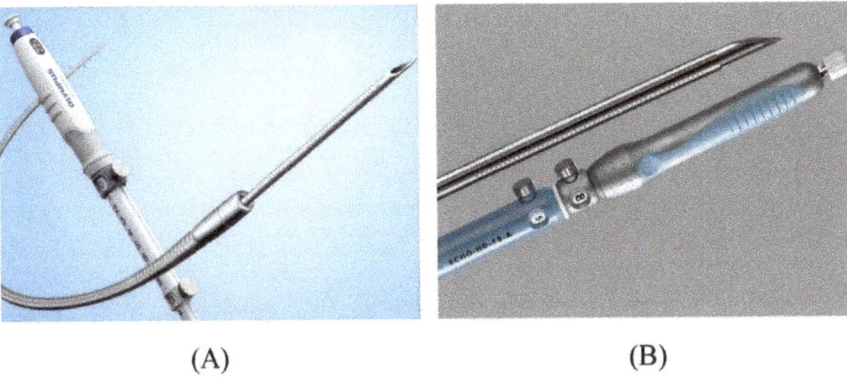

Figure 7. Needles suitable for EUS-HGS. EZ shot 3 plus (Olympus Medical Systems) has a nitinol needle with a coil sheath (Courtesy of Olympus Medical Systems) (**A**). EchoTip Access Needle (Cook Medical) has a sharp stylet and blunt-tipped needle (Courtesy of Cook Medical) (**B**).

As for the needle size, a 19-gauge needle is preferable to a 22-gauge needle because a 0.025 inch guidewire can be used, which performs better than a 0.018 inch guidewire. Usually, a 22-gauge needle is used with a 0.018 inch guidewire for thin bile ducts.

Prior to inserting the needle into the accessory channel of the scope, remove the biopsy valve from its socket and attach it to a dilation device (Figure 8A). Before puncture, remove the stylet of the needle and place a syringe filled with contrast medium to pre-fill the lumen with contrast medium (Figure 8B).

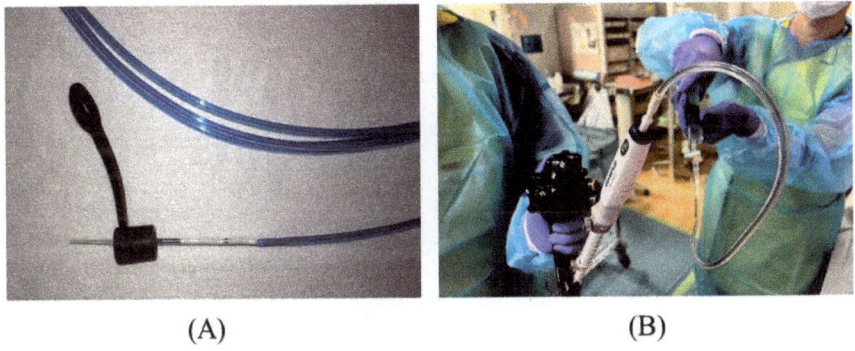

Figure 8. Preparation for puncture. The biopsy valve is attached to a dilation device (**A**). The needle stylet is removed, and a syringe filled with contrast medium is attached to the needle to pre-fill the lumen with contrast medium (**B**).

Unlike PTBD, in EUS-HGS, the scope moves with the liver and stomach due to respiration, and thus the fluctuations of the liver on the ultrasound image are small. Therefore, rapid puncture is usually not necessary, and careful puncture is advisable to avoid intervening vessels. However, if the bile duct wall is stiffened due to fibrosis (due to prior biliary drainage or cholangitis), a slow puncture speed will not allow the needle to be inserted into the bile duct. In such cases, the needle should be punctured quickly and strongly, once penetrating the bile duct wall completely. After penetration, the needle is slowly withdrawn while applying suction pressure (Seldinger method) [33,34]. The success of the bile duct puncture is confirmed by aspiration of bile usually, but it is not possible to aspirate bile if the bile duct is narrow. In such cases, when the needle enters the bile duct, the air drawn from the stomach by the aspiration enters the bile duct and is recognized as a moving strong echo. This is a useful finding to determine the success of the puncture.

If a favorable biliary puncture line cannot be obtained due to the intervening vessels or tumors, or due to the alignment of the liver and stomach, pressing the scope after advancing the needle into the liver parenchyma can move the liver to the right and rotate it counterclockwise on ultrasound image using the liver access point as a fulcrum, thereby can alter the trajectory of the needle (Figure 9A,B). Ishiwatari et al. also reported the "Bent needle technique" in which a manually pre-bent needle is used to puncture in such a case [35].

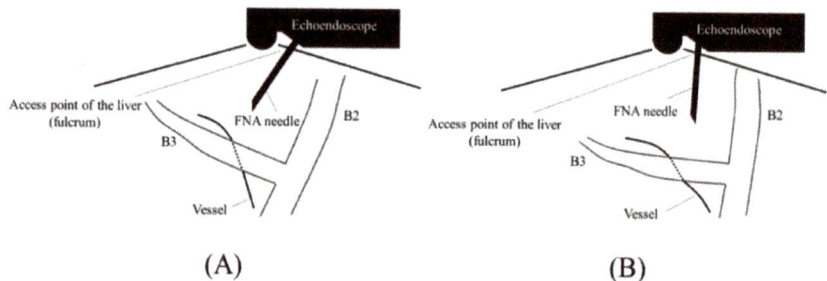

Figure 9. Changing a needle trajectory during biliary puncture. If a favorable biliary puncture line cannot be obtained due to the intervening vessels (**A**), pushing a scope after advancing a needle into the liver parenchyma to change the needle direction using the liver access point as a fulcrum (**B**).

5.3. Contrast Injection

If contrast medium is injected directly after bile duct access, the intraductal pressure will increase. The increased intraductal pressure may not only cause bile leak but also cause cholangio-venous reflux, which may lead to bacteremia in case of cholangitis. Therefore, it is necessary to aspirate as much bile as possible before injecting the contrast medium. Ishiwatari et al. reported in a retrospective study that bile aspiration of 10 mL or more was a significant factor in reducing the occurrence of adverse events associated with bile leak [36]. In this study, a catheter was inserted into the bile duct to aspirate bile prior to tract dilation, which requires more steps in the procedure; therefore, bile aspiration with an FNA needle seems preferable. Following bile aspiration, contrast medium is injected to depict the biliary tract. In order to improve the handling of the guidewire through the needle and the visibility of the guidewire under fluoroscopy, it is recommended to use a contrast medium diluted to half its concentration in saline. The amount of contrast medium injected should be limited to the minimum amount that will allow the hilar region to be visualized to avoid increased intraductal pressure.

5.4. Guidewire Manipulation

When using a 19-gauge needle, a 0.035 inch or 0.025 inch guidewire can be used. However, the 0.025 inch guidewire is preferable because there is less risk of the guidewire being sheared by the needle tip and it is easier to manipulate. In recent years, a number of 0.025 inch guidewires have been released, such as VisiGlide2 (Olympus Medical Systems), EndoSelector (Boston Scientific Corp, Natick, MA, USA), M-Through (Medicos Hirata, Osaka, Japan), and INAZUMA (Kaneka Medix, Osaka, Japan), which have a hydrophilic coating on the tip, a stiff shaft, and excellent torque and supportability. When using a 22-gauge needle, a 0.021 inch or 0.018 inch guidewire can be used, but the performance of these conventional guidewires has not been sufficient. Most recently, a new 0.018 inch guidewire (Fielder 18; Olympus Medical Systems) has been released, which has a high performance similar to that of the 0.025 inch guidewire [22,37,38].

The guidewire is advanced through the needle, and once it enters the bile duct, it is slowly and carefully advanced with gentle rotation to guide it toward the hilar region. If the guidewire is unintentionally advanced to the peripheral side, the "Loop technique" should be attempted first. Push the guidewire with rotation, and when the tip of the guidewire is caught on a lateral branch (Figure 10A), push the guidewire further. Since the tip of the guidewire is fixed, the body of the guidewire will bend with the pushing force and form a loop (Figure 10B). If the loop is facing the hilar region, the guidewire can be advanced to the hilum by pushing further (Figure 10C,D). If the "Loop technique" fails, the "Moving scope technique" is an alternative to change the direction of the guidewire, where pushing the scope while turning the large wheel upward may change the direction of the needle to the cranial side, allowing the guidewire to proceed toward the hilum [39] (Figure 11A–C).

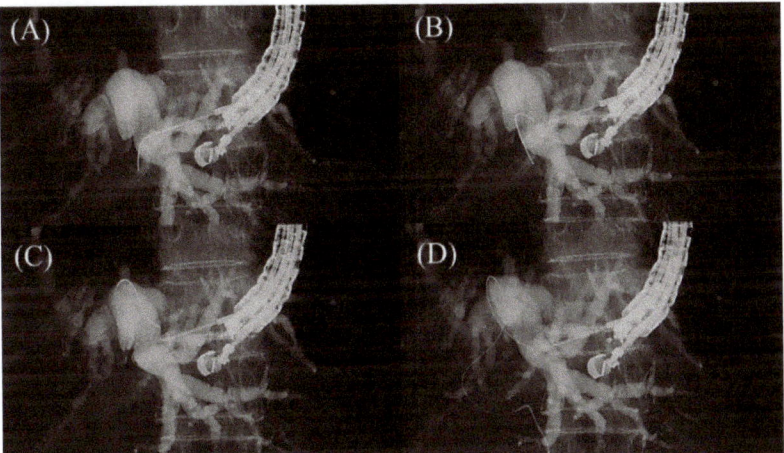

Figure 10. Loop technique for redirection of a guidewire. If a guidewire is unintentionally advanced to the peripheral side, push the guidewire with rotation. When the tip of the guidewire is caught on a lateral branch (**A**), the guidewire will bend and form a loop by pushing force (**B**). If the loop is facing the hilar region, the guidewire can be advanced to the hilum by pushing further (**C,D**).

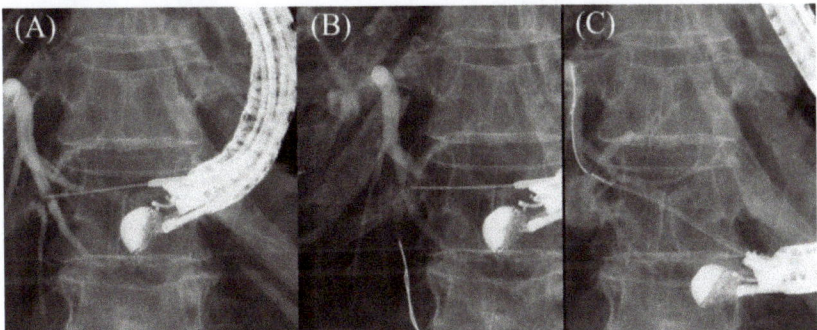

Figure 11. Moving scope technique for redirection of a guidewire. If a guidewire is unintentionally advanced to the peripheral side (**A,B**), push the scope while turning the large wheel upward to change the needle direction to the cranial side, allowing the guidewire to proceed toward the hilum (**C**).

When these methods are unsuccessful, the guidewire must be pulled out and reoriented toward the hilar region. However, if there is any resistance while pulling, the guidewire should not be pulled out forcibly because the tip of the guidewire may be sheared off and remain as a foreign body. In such a case, it is recommended to pull the guidewire out while slowly moving it back and forth with rotation. If this does not work, Ogura et al. reported the usefulness of the "Liver impaction technique" [40]. By pulling the needle tip slightly into the hepatic parenchyma, the angle between the guidewire and the needle is loosened, and the tip of the needle is covered by the hepatic parenchyma to prevent shearing the guidewire (Figure 12A–D). The aforementioned dedicated needle (EchoTip Access Needle; Cook Medical) is expected to prevent shearing of the guidewire [17,32], but is not yet widely available in the world.

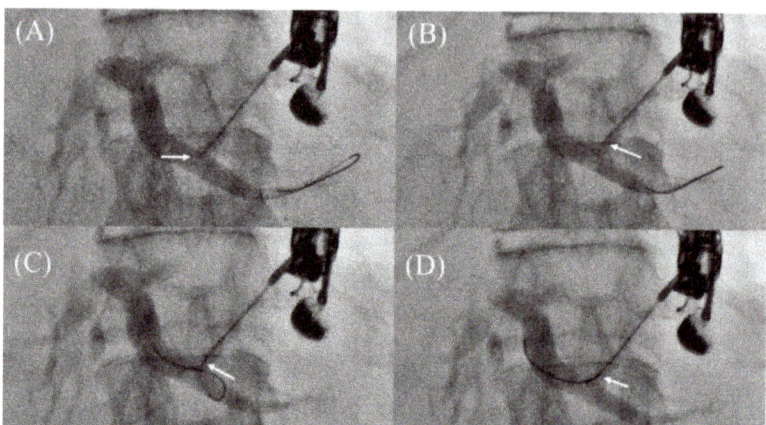

Figure 12. Liver impaction technique for redirection of a guidewire. If a guidewire is unintentionally advanced to the peripheral side (**A**), pull the needle tip slightly into the hepatic parenchyma (**B**). The guidewire can be pulled without shearing because the tip of the needle is covered by the hepatic parenchyma (**C**). The guidewire is successfully manipulated toward hilum (**D**). Arrows indicate the tip of the needle.

If changing the direction of the guidewire is not successful even using these techniques, it is necessary to change the needle to a catheter to improve the manipulation of the guidewire. However, the guidewire and catheter may become dislodged from the bile duct while struggling to change the direction of the guidewire by pulling the tip of the catheter back to the shallowest part of the bile duct. In order to avoid such an eventuality, the aforementioned "Double guidewire technique" using UDLC is effective. While securing the bile duct with the first guidewire, the second guidewire is manipulated to advance to the hilar region [41]. Although UDLC is a double-lumen catheter, the second guidewire is located away from the tip, allowing the tip to be thin enough to be inserted directly into the bile duct without pre-dilation.

In cases where the guidewire cannot be redirected using UDLC, a rotatable sphincterotome (TRUEtome; Boston Scientific Corp) may be of assistance. After two guidewires are implanted in the peripheral bile duct and removal of UDLC, TRUEtome is inserted into the bile duct over the guidewire. Then, the guidewire is directed to the hilar region by rotating and bending the tip of TRUEtome while securing the bile duct with another guidewire (Figure 13A–C) [42].

If all else fails, the only option is to withdraw the needle completely and re-puncture the bile duct. The recently developed "steerable access device", which has a bendable needle tip, allows the guidewire to direct the hilar region easily and reliably [43,44]. However, this device has not yet been made widely commercially available in the world.

Once the guidewire has passed through the stricture, it must remain in place as long as possible to prevent dislodgement by the assistant's pulling during subsequent insertion of the device.

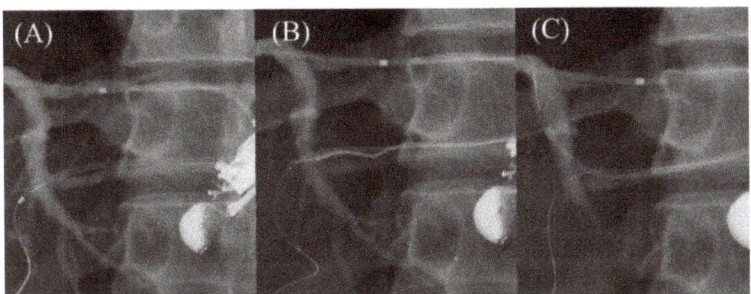

Figure 13. Redirection of a guidewire using a rotatable sphincterotome. In cases where the guidewire cannot be advanced toward hilum even using double guidewire technique (**A**), the guidewire is manipulated with a rotatable sphincterotome by rotating and bending the tip of the catheter while securing the bile duct with another guidewire (**B**). The catheter is successfully advanced toward the hilar region (**C**).

5.5. Tract Dilation

After a sufficient length of guidewire is placed, the needle is replaced with a dilatation device. In ERCP, the elevator is usually raised completely after device removal to prevent guidewire dislodgement. However, in EUS-HGS, the elevator should not be raised further after the needle is removed, because it is most critical to maintain ultrasound visualization of the puncture line to ensure subsequent device insertion. The more skilled the physician is in ERCP, the more likely it is that he or she will do this unconsciously, so care must be taken.

The dilatation of the tract is carried out using a mechanical dilator such as a bougie dilator or balloon dilator, or a diathermic dilator. The bougie dilator is the safest, but insertion of an introducer of covered SEMS is often difficult because the size of the hole opened on the bile duct is the smallest, usually only 7 Fr. The balloon dilator can make the largest hole, but it is associated with the risk of bile leak. The diathermic dilator is the most reliable in penetrating the bile duct wall, but the burning effect can cause bleeding from the surrounding liver parenchyma and hepatic artery. Therefore, the bougie dilator is appropriate for stents with small caliber introducers (7 Fr or less), such as plastic stents and some kinds of covered SEMS, while the balloon dilator is suitable for conventional covered SEMS where the introducer is usually 8 Fr or more. The diathermic dilator had better be used as a rescue when the bile duct wall is too hard to be breached by other dilators [8].

In the initial era of EUS-HGS, mechanical dilation was accomplished gradually: the ERCP catheter was inserted first after the needle removal, followed by sequential dilatation with a bougie dilator or balloon dilator [45–47]. Recently, however, the properties of mechanical dilators have been improved so that they can be inserted directly without dilation by the ERCP catheter. Balloon dilators include Hurricane RX (Boston Scientific Corp), which has a rigid shaft with a stylet (Figure 14A) [46], and REN (Kaneka Medics), which has an ultra-thin tip of 3 Fr (Figure 14B) [48]. ES dilator (Zeon Medical, Tokyo, Japan) is a 7 Fr bougie dilator which has an ultra-thin tip of 2.5 Fr (Figure 14C) [49–51]. REN and ES dilator are dedicated dilation devices for EUS-HGS that are adapted to 0.025 inch guidewires, and the gap between the tip of these devices and the 0.025 inch guidewire is extremely small.

Balloon dilation is usually performed with a 4 mm or 3 mm diameter balloon, which creates a larger tract than a bougie dilator or diathermic dilator and is therefore more prone to bile leak. The "Segmental dilation method" may be beneficial in preventing bile leak. As previously stated, it has been reported that a short distance of intervening liver parenchyma (≤ 2.5 cm) is more likely to cause biliary peritonitis, and in this study, balloon dilation was performed in in around two-thirds of cases [30]. Usually, balloon dilation is performed by first dilating the bile duct wall and then the gastric wall, but since the balloon is as long as

4 cm or 3 cm, the dilated portions on both sides partially overlap each other, creating a thick path from the bile duct to the extrahepatic area, causing bile to flow out. This phenomenon is especially likely to occur when the distance of the hepatic parenchyma is short and is thought to be one of the reasons for the results of the aforementioned study that biliary peritonitis is more likely to occur when the distance of the hepatic parenchyma is short. To avoid this phenomenon, the balloon catheter should be pushed into the bile duct as deeply as possible when dilating the bile duct wall and pulled into the scope channel as long as possible when dilating the gastric wall to prevent overlap of the two dilated areas (Figure 15A,B). The hepatic parenchyma left un-dilated is thought to prevent bile leakage due to the tamponade effect.

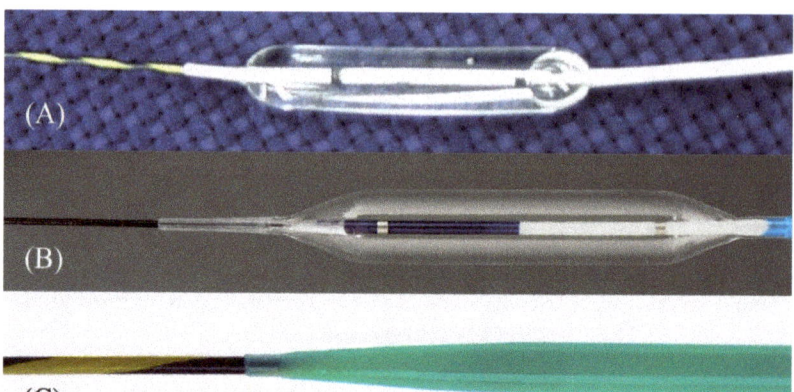

Figure 14. One-step mechanical dilation devices. Hurricane (Boston Scientific) is a balloon dilator with a rigid shaft and stylet (Courtesy of Boston Scientific) (**A**). REN (Kaneka Medics) is a balloon dilator with an ultra-tapered tip adapted to a 0.025 inch guidewire (Courtesy of Kaneka Medics) (**B**). ES dilator (Zeon Medical) is a bougie dilator with an ultra-tapered tip adapted to a 0.025 inch guidewire. (Courtesy of Zeon Medical) (**C**).

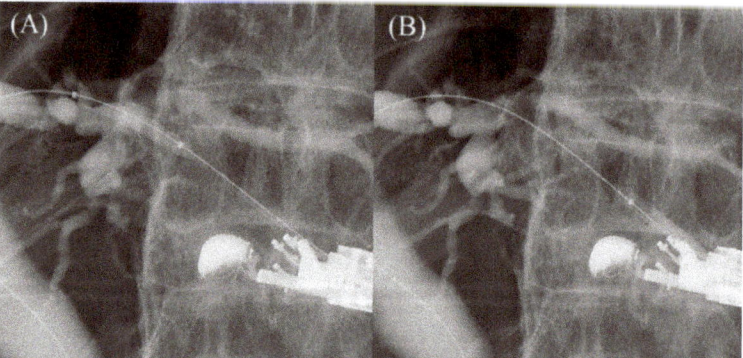

Figure 15. Segmental dilation method for prevention of bile leak during balloon dilation. A balloon catheter is pushed into the bile duct as deeply as possible when dilating the bile duct wall (**A**) and pulled into the scope channel as long as possible when dilating the gastric wall to prevent overlap of the two dilated areas (**B**). The hepatic parenchyma left un-dilated is thought to prevent bile leakage due to the tamponade effect.

Regarding the diathermic dilation, a wire-guided needle knife was initially used in EUS-HGS. Although this type of catheter could be advanced over the guidewire, the axis of the needle was misaligned with the guidewire at the site of bending, which could cause bleeding from the surrounding organs [52,53]. In fact, Park et al. reported that the use of the needle knife was significantly associated with post-procedure adverse events compared to gradual dilation using a mechanical dilator [52]. To address this major concern, a fine diameter (6 Fr) coaxial diathermic dilator (Cysto-Gastro set; Endo-flex, Voerde, Düsseldorf, Germany) was developed to allow for safer dilation [53]. However, even with this coaxial dilator, the risk of bleeding appears to be higher than with mechanical dilators [50]. Honjo et al. reported that in EUS-HGS, bleeding occurred in 5/23 (21.7%) patients with 6 Fr Cysto-Gastro set and 0/26 patients with the bougie dilator ($p = 0.04$) [50]. Since all bleeding cases used plastic stents and spontaneous hemostasis was achieved with conservative therapy alone without interventional radiology (IVR), the bleeding was not arterial but from the surrounding hepatic parenchyma due to the burning effect. Recently, Ogura et al. reported a pilot study using a new coaxial diathermic dilator (Fine025; Medicos Hirata) with a smaller diathermic ring at the tip and less burning effect on the surrounding tissues than the Cysto-Gastro set [54]. In this pilot study, 12 patients had no adverse events. Since this dilator has a thinner tip and thicker shaft than Cysto-Gastro set, it does not need to cauterize the liver parenchyma and only needs to cauterize the gastric and bile duct walls, which may reduce bleeding. However, since the burning effect on the surrounding tissues cannot be completely eliminated, arterial bleeding might be caused from the interlobular artery in the Glisson's sheath when cauterizing the bile duct wall.

5.6. Stent Deployment

In the early days of EUS-HGS, plastic stents were predominantly used [55–58]. Although plastic stents are inexpensive and easy to place, they are prone to stent clogging due to their small caliber and bile leakage due to their lack of self-expandability. Therefore, conventional biliary-covered SEMS with a length of 6 cm or 8 cm have come into use in the expectation of preventing bile leaks by closing the fistula with self-expandability and prolonging the stent patency period with a large diameter [59,60]. In fact, the adverse events of EUS-HGS with a covered SEMS have been reported to be lower than with a plastic stent [53]. However, the migration of the gastric end of the stent into the abdominal cavity leading to fatal biliary peritonitis has been recognized as a major problem with a covered SEMS. For this reason, some experts initially recommended the use of a plastic stent for EUS-HGS and its replacement with a covered SEMS after fistula maturation [61,62]. However, recent advances in methodology and instrumentation have made it possible to prevent migration.

Migration can occur in two situations: early migration, when the stent detaches from the scope [63–66], and delayed migration, after successful deployment [16,62,67–70]. In EUS-HGS, the stomach and liver are initially brought in closer together by pushing the echoendoscope against the gastric wall. However, the distance between the liver and stomach becomes increased because the scope must be moved away from the gastric wall to eventually release the stent. This event and the shortening of the SEMS can cause early migration, in which the gastric end of the SEMS is pulled into the abdominal cavity. Recently, early migration can be avoided by using the "Intra-channel (conduit) release method" (see below), which can ensure that the end of the SEMS is placed in the stomach while minimizing the distance between the liver and stomach. However, since the stomach will eventually return to its original position, delayed migration may occur if the initial distance between the liver and stomach is long [21]. To prevent delayed migration, a long (≥ 10 cm) SEMS is recommended to ensure sufficient intragastric stent length [8,71,72]. Nakai et al. [71] and Ogura et al. [72] reported that sufficient intragastric length (>30–35 mm on CT the next day) may not only prevent delayed migration but also prolong stent patency by reducing the reflux of gastric juice and food. Nevertheless, even in cases with long intragastric stent length, the stent may be migrated by sudden gastric movements such as hiccups or vomiting [71]. Therefore, long stents with anti-migration properties may be optimal [21].

Currently, various types of SEMS are available for EUS-HGS with respect to stent design (braided or laser-cut type), coverage (partial or full), presence or absence of anti-migration properties at the gastric end, and size of the introducer. As a dedicated device for EUS-HGS, several partially covered braided SEMSs with anti-migration properties have been released by Korean companies (Figure 16A–D) [17,73–79]. In Japan, the most common SEMS for EUS-HGS is Niti-S S-type stent (modified Giobor stent; Taewoong Medical, Seoul, Korea), which is a partially covered SEMS with a 1 cm uncovered portion at the hepatic end [71,80]. Since this stent is a braided SEMS with a cross-wire structure, it gradually expands in the stomach from the non-expanded part in the gastric wall to form a smooth and gently sloping stent surface. Therefore, the effect of holding down the gastric wall is weak. Furthermore, the shortening rate of the stent is large, which tends to cause delayed migration of the gastric end into the peritoneal cavity (Figure 17A–C). In order to prevent this, the stent length should be longer than 10 cm, but even a long stent cannot prevent it completely as mentioned above. For this reason, Niti-S Spring Stopper Stent (Taewoong Medical) was developed with a spring-type stopper at the gastric end to prevent migration (Figure 18). This stent can reliably prevent delayed migration of the gastric end. Meanwhile, pre-dilation of the tract is usually required for these SEMSs insertion because the diameter of the introducer is 8.5 Fr.

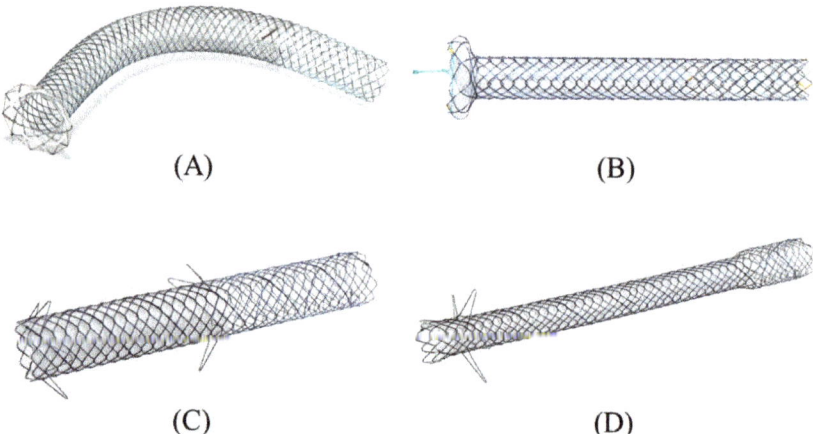

Figure 16. Partially covered SEMSs with anti-migration properties dedicated for EUS-HGS developed by Korean companies. GIOBOR stent (Taewoong medical) (**A**). HANARO stent BPD (M.I.Tech, Seoul, Korea) (**B**). Hybrid BONA stent (Standard Sci. Tech, Seoul, Korea) (**C**). DEUS (Standard Sci. Tech) (**D**). Courtesy of each company.

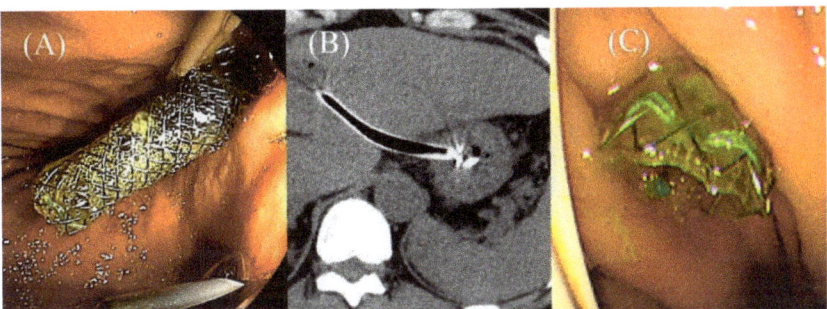

Figure 17. Impending delayed migration in Niti-S S-type stent (Taewoong Medical). A sufficient length of the gastric end of the stent is seen after the procedure (**A**). The next day's CT shows that the intragastric stent length has shortened (**B**). Urgent endoscopy reveals impending migration of the gastric end of the stent (**C**).

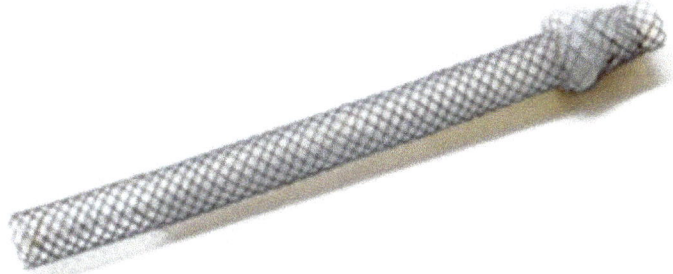

Figure 18. Spring Stopper Stent (Taewoong Medical), which has a spring-type stopper as an anti-migration system at the gastric end. (Courtesy of Taewoong Medical).

There are several SEMSs with a slim introducer allowing direct insertion without prior tract dilation. From Korea, HANAROSTENT Benefit (M.I.Tech, Seoul, Korea) [22,81,82] and EGIS Braided 6 (S&G Biotech, Seongnam, Korea) [83], which are fully covered SEMSs with a 6 Fr introducer for a 0.025 inch guidewire, have been released. In most cases, these SEMS can be inserted without prior dilation. Nevertheless, since these SEMS are of the fully covered type without any anti-migration properties, migration of both sides is feared. In addition, since the bile ducts on the peripheral side of the access point are dead spaces, these SEMS are not only unsuitable for hilar biliary obstruction but may also cause focal cholangitis in the dead spaces [84]. Most recently, Covered BileRush Advance (Piolax Medical Devices), a partially covered SEMS with a 2 cm uncovered portion at the hepatic end, has been launched (Figure 19A). This stent has an introducer compatible with a 0.025 inch guidewire that has a 2.4 Fr tip and a 7 Fr shaft and can be inserted directly without dilation in most cases (Figure 19B). Because this stent is a laser-cut type, the stent expands rapidly in the stomach from a non-expanded area in the gastric wall, resulting in a steep stent surface. This incised shape and jagged struts inhibit gastric wall return to its original position (Figure 20A,B); furthermore, there is almost no shortening of the stent, which results in little delayed migration [85]. One-step EUS-HGS without prior tract dilation has the potential to reduce adverse events and procedure time compared to conventional methods, and further studies are warranted.

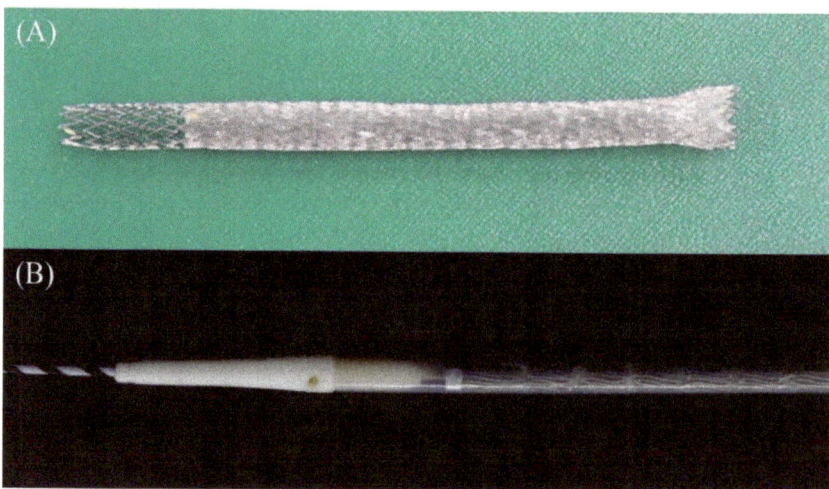

Figure 19. Covered BileRush Advance (Piolax Medical Device). The partially covered laser-cut stent of 8 × 120 mm in size with a 2 cm uncovered portion on the hepatic end (**A**). The slim introducer with a 7 Fr shaft and 2.4 Fr tip (**B**). (Courtesy of Piolax Medical Device).

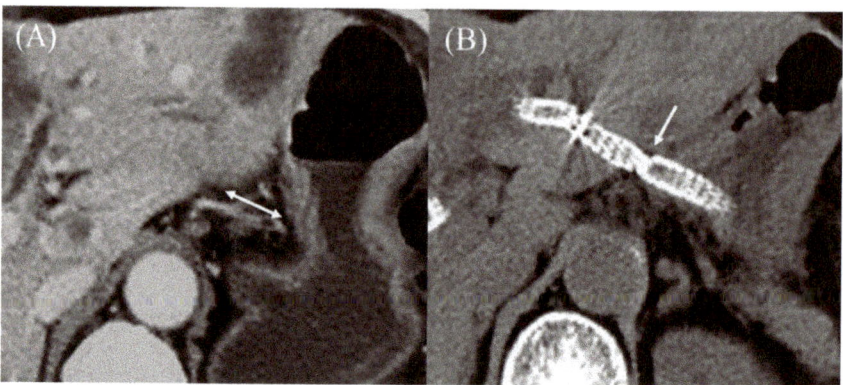

Figure 20. Endoscopic ultrasound-guided hepaticogastrostomy with a Covered BileRush Advance. Pre-procedure contrast-enhanced CT showed a long distance between the gastric body and left hepatic lobe (double arrow) (**A**). Post-procedure CT showed the Covered BileRush Advance fixed the gastric body near the left hepatic lobe by its jagged surface (arrow) (**B**).

The process of partially covered SEMS deployment is as follows. First, proper positioning of the stent introducer is performed. When the introducer is inserted into the bile duct, the scope is pushed back by the counteraction and the distance between the liver and stomach is increased. Stent deployment must not be started at this point, as the stent end may fall into the abdominal cavity. The introducer should be inserted deeply once and then pulled to adjust its position so that only the uncovered portion enters the bile duct. This pulling motion will shorten the distance between the liver and stomach. The next step is to detach the SEMS from the introducer. After positioning the introducer, the assistant pulls on the outer sheath to gradually release the SEMS. At this time, the introducer is retracted into the scope channel due to the counteraction, and the stent is advanced. The physician must pull the introducer as the assistant works, while watching the fluoroscopic view to ensure that the tip position of the stent remains the same. Once the uncovered area is fully expanded, the stent is fixed to the liver, and the physician's pulling force draws the liver into the scope, bringing the liver and stomach even closer together. The last step is SEMS implantation, which requires the scope to be pulled away from the gastric wall in order to bring the SEMS out of the channel. If the scope is simply pulled back, the pushing force of the scope will be lost, and the gastric wall will be moved away from the liver. As a result, the stent length in the abdominal cavity becomes longer while the stent length in the stomach becomes shorter, and the end of the stent may migrate into the abdominal cavity. To avoid this problem, "Intra-channel (conduit) release method [86,87]" is essential. The physician pulls the introducer as the assistant moves to deploy the stent but stops the deployment once the fluoroscopy shows that the tip of the outer sheath has been pulled about 1 to 2 cm inside the channel. At this point, the physician pushes the introducer in the opposite direction, and the expanded portion of the stent emerging from the channel is pressed strongly against the gastric wall (Figure 21A). This action creates a gap between the scope and the gastric wall, and stent deployment across the gastric wall can be directly confirmed (Figure 21B). Afterwards, the assistant resumes pulling the outer sheath, and the released stent pushes the gastric wall forward, and the counteraction pushes the scope back. By gradually loosening the push of the introducer and the up angle of the scope while feeling the counteraction force, the scope can be released from the gastric wall while keeping the stomach and liver close together, and finally the stent is completely released in the stomach. The trick of this method is to push the expanded part of the stent, which has been partially released in the channel, against the gastric wall; pushing without intra-channel release will only cause the introducer to enter the fistula.

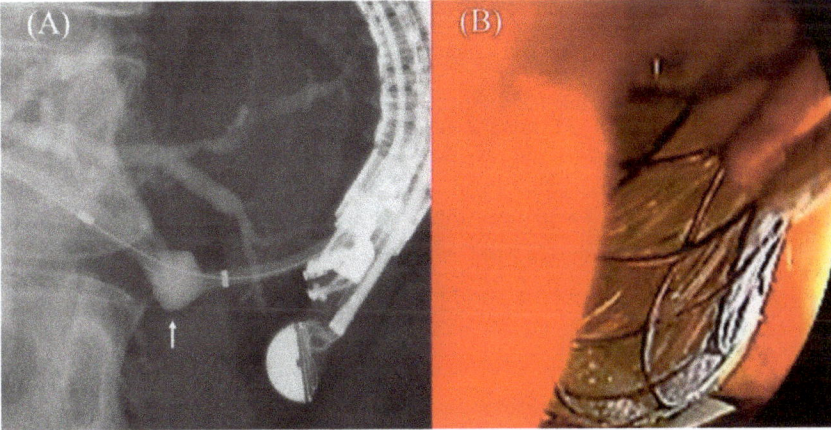

Figure 21. Intra-channel (conduit) release method. After pulling the introducer until 1 to 2 cm release inside the channel, push the expanded part of the stent (arrow) to strongly press the gastric wall for keeping the stomach and liver close together (**A**). Stent deployment across the gastric wall can be directly confirmed by endoscopic view (**B**).

6. Post-Procedure Management

If abnormal findings are found on laboratory tests or physical examination the day after the procedure, or if sufficient intragastric stent length is not obtained during the procedure, a CT should be performed to check for possible abnormalities such as stent migration, pneumoperitoneum, or fluid collection. If the intragastric stent length is no longer sufficient due to stent shortening or gastric movement (impending migration; Figure 14B,C), there is a risk of migration of the gastric end of the stent into the abdominal cavity. In such cases, immediate endoscopic reintervention using various technique such as Crisscross anchoring technique [88], Clip-flap technique [89], and Stent-in-stent technique [90] should be performed to prevent stent migration. Pneumoperitoneum or fluid collection with new-onset abdominal pain or fever suggests bile leak, and antibiotics should be continued.

If melena or an unexpected drop in hemoglobin is seen, a contrast-enhanced CT is necessary. When bleeding from hepatic artery is suspected, angiography should be performed urgently. The results of the pooled analysis of early adverse events of EUS-HGS described in the Japanese clinical practice guidelines are summarized in Table 2.

Table 2. Adverse events of EUS-HGS.

Adverse Event	Incidence
Overall	18.2%
Bleeding	3.7%
Bile leak	2.8%
Biloma	2.6%
Stent migration	1.6%
Stent misplacement	1.2%
Intrahepatic hematoma	1.2%
Sepsis	1.2%

7. Conclusions

This review describes the technical tips for safe and successful EUS-HGS, in particular the method using a covered SEMS for palliative drainage purposes. Recent advances and innovation in EUS systems, equipment, and methods have made EUS-HGS an easier and safer procedure, but the risk of serious adverse events such as stent migration and bile leak still remains. The techniques described in this article are all practical and should be readily available, especially for physicians who are just starting EUS-HGS. It is hoped that further advances in instrumentation will make EUS-HGS safer and more reliable.

Author Contributions: Conceptualization, S.M.; methodology, S.M.; software, S.M.; validation, S.M., S.N., K.N., K.S., T.O. and M.O.; formal analysis, S.M.; investigation, S.M.; writing—original draft preparation, S.M.; writing—review and editing, S.N.; visualization, S.M.; supervision, S.N.; project administration, S.M. All authors have read and agreed to the published version of the manuscript.

Funding: This review received no external funding.

Institutional Review Board Statement: Not applicable.

Informed Consent Statement: Not applicable.

Data Availability Statement: Data sharing not applicable.

Acknowledgments: We would like to thank Hiroyuki Isayama for his useful advice.

Conflicts of Interest: All authors declare no conflict of interest.

References

1. Lee, T.H.; Choi, J.H.; Park do, H.; Song, T.J.; Kim, D.U.; Paik, W.H.; Hwangbo, Y.; Lee, S.S.; Seo, D.W.; Lee, S.K.; et al. Similar Efficacies of Endoscopic Ultrasound-guided Transmural and Percutaneous Drainage for Malignant Distal Biliary Obstruction. *Clin. Gastroenterol. Hepatol.* **2016**, *14*, 1011–1019.e1013. [CrossRef]
2. Sharaiha, R.Z.; Kumta, N.A.; Desai, A.P.; DeFilippis, E.M.; Gabr, M.; Sarkisian, A.M.; Salgado, S.; Millman, J.; Benvenuto, A.; Cohen, M.; et al. Endoscopic ultrasound-guided biliary drainage versus percutaneous transhepatic biliary drainage: Predictors of successful outcome in patients who fail endoscopic retrograde cholangiopancreatography. *Surg. Endosc.* **2016**, *30*, 5500–5505. [CrossRef] [PubMed]
3. Sharaiha, R.Z.; Khan, M.A.; Kamal, F.; Tyberg, A.; Tombazzi, C.R.; Ali, B.; Tombazzi, C.; Kahaleh, M. Efficacy and safety of EUS-guided biliary drainage in comparison with percutaneous biliary drainage when ERCP fails: A systematic review and meta-analysis. *Gastrointest. Endosc.* **2017**, *85*, 904–914. [CrossRef] [PubMed]
4. Nakai, Y.; Kogure, H.; Isayama, H.; Koike, K. Endoscopic Ultrasound-Guided Biliary Drainage for Benign Biliary Diseases. *Clin. Endosc.* **2019**, *52*, 212–219. [CrossRef] [PubMed]
5. Paik, W.H.; Lee, T.H.; Park, D.H.; Choi, J.H.; Kim, S.O.; Jang, S.; Kim, D.U.; Shim, J.H.; Song, T.J.; Lee, S.S.; et al. EUS-Guided Biliary Drainage Versus ERCP for the Primary Palliation of Malignant Biliary Obstruction: A Multicenter Randomized Clinical Trial. *Am. J. Gastroenterol.* **2018**, *113*, 987–997. [CrossRef]

8. Park, J.K.; Woo, Y.S.; Noh, D.H.; Yang, J.I.; Bae, S.Y.; Yun, H.S.; Lee, J.K.; Lee, K.T.; Lee, K.H. Efficacy of EUS-guided and ERCP-guided biliary drainage for malignant biliary obstruction: Prospective randomized controlled study. *Gastrointest. Endosc.* **2018**, *88*, 277–282. [CrossRef]
9. Bang, J.Y.; Navaneethan, U.; Hasan, M.; Hawes, R.; Varadarajulu, S. Stent placement by EUS or ERCP for primary biliary decompression in pancreatic cancer: A randomized trial (with videos). *Gastrointest. Endosc.* **2018**, *88*, 9–17. [CrossRef]
10. Isayama, H.; Nakai, Y.; Itoi, T.; Yasuda, I.; Kawakami, H.; Ryozawa, S.; Kitano, M.; Irisawa, A.; Katanuma, A.; Hara, K.; et al. Clinical practice guidelines for safe performance of endoscopic ultrasound/ultrasonography-guided biliary drainage: 2018. *J. Hepatobil. Pancreat. Sci.* **2019**, *26*, 249–269. [CrossRef]
11. Hamada, T.; Isayama, H.; Nakai, Y.; Kogure, H.; Yamamoto, N.; Kawakubo, K.; Takahara, N.; Uchino, R.; Mizuno, S.; Sasaki, T.; et al. Transmural biliary drainage can be an alternative to transpapillary drainage in patients with an indwelling duodenal stent. *Dig. Dis. Sci.* **2014**, *59*, 1931–1938. [CrossRef]
12. Khashab, M.A.; El Zein, M.H.; Sharzehi, K.; Marson, F.P.; Haluszka, O.; Small, A.J.; Nakai, Y.; Park, D.H.; Kunda, R.; Teoh, A.Y.; et al. EUS-guided biliary drainage or enteroscopy-assisted ERCP in patients with surgical anatomy and biliary obstruction: An international comparative study. *Endosc. Int. Open* **2016**, *4*, E1322–E1327. [CrossRef]
13. Nakai, Y.; Kogure, H.; Isayama, H.; Koike, K. Endoscopic Ultrasound-Guided Biliary Drainage for Unresectable Hilar Malignant Biliary Obstruction. *Clin. Endosc.* **2019**, *52*, 220–225. [CrossRef]
14. Kongkam, P.; Tasneem, A.A.; Rerknimitr, R. Combination of endoscopic retrograde cholangiopancreatography and endoscopic ultrasonography-guided biliary drainage in malignant hilar biliary obstruction. *Dig. Endosc.* **2019**, *31* (Suppl. S1), 50–54. [CrossRef] [PubMed]
15. Poincloux, L.; Rouquette, O.; Buc, E.; Privat, J.; Pezet, D.; Dapoigny, M.; Bommelaer, G.; Abergel, A. Endoscopic ultrasound-guided biliary drainage after failed ERCP: Cumulative experience of 101 procedures at a single center. *Endoscopy* **2015**, *47*, 794–801. [CrossRef] [PubMed]
16. Paik, W.H.; Park, D.H. Outcomes and limitations: EUS-guided hepaticogastrostomy. *Endosc. Ultrasound* **2019**, *8*, S44–S49. [CrossRef] [PubMed]
17. Prachayakul, V.; Thamtorawat, S.; Siripipattanamongkol, C.; Thanathanee, P. Bleeding left hepatic artery pseudoaneurysm: A complication of endoscopic ultrasound-guided hepaticogastrostomy. *Endoscopy* **2013**, *45* (Suppl. S2), E223–E224. [CrossRef]
18. Martins, F.P.; Rossini, L.G.; Ferrari, A.P. Migration of a covered metallic stent following endoscopic ultrasound-guided hepaticogastrostomy: Fatal complication. *Endoscopy* **2010**, *42* (Suppl. S2), E126–E127. [CrossRef]
19. Giovannini, M. EUS-guided hepaticogastrostomy. *Endosc. Ultrasound* **2019**, *8*, S35–S39. [CrossRef]
20. Ogura, T.; Higuchi, K. Endoscopic Ultrasound-Guided Hepaticogastrostomy: Technical Review and Tips to Prevent Adverse Events. *Gut Liver* **2021**, *15*, 196–205. [CrossRef]
21. Chantarojanasiri, T.; Ratanachu-Ek, T.; Pausawasdi, N. What You Need to Know Before Performing Endoscopic Ultrasound-guided Hepaticogastrostomy. *Clin. Endosc.* **2021**, *54*, 301–308. [CrossRef]
22. Okuno, N.; Hara, K.; Mizuno, N.; Kuwahara, T.; Iwaya, H.; Tajika, M.; Tanaka, T.; Ishihara, M.; Hirayama, Y.; Onishi, S.; et al. Infectious peritonitis after endoscopic ultrasound-guided biliary drainage in a patient with ascites. *Int. J. Gastrointest. Interv.* **2018**, *7*, 40–43. [CrossRef]
23. Ochiai, K.; Fujisawa, T.; Ishii, S.; Suzuki, A.; Saito, H.; Takasaki, Y.; Ushio, M.; Takahashi, S.; Yamagata, W.; Tomishima, K.; et al. Risk Factors for Stent Migration into the Abdominal Cavity after Endoscopic Ultrasound-Guided Hepaticogastrostomy. *J. Clin. Med.* **2021**, *10*, 3111. [CrossRef] [PubMed]
24. Hara, K.; Okuno, N.; Haba, S.; Kuwahara, T.; Koda, H.; Mizuno, N.; Miyano, A. How to perform EUS-guided hepaticogastrostomy easier and safer. *J. Hepatobil. Pancreat. Sci.* **2020**, *27*, 563–564. [CrossRef] [PubMed]
25. Minaga, K.; Kitano, M.; Yoshikawa, T.; Omoto, S.; Kamata, K.; Yamao, K.; Kudo, M. Hepaticogastrostomy guided by real-time contrast-enhanced harmonic endoscopic ultrasonography: A novel technique. *Endoscopy* **2016**, *48* (Suppl. S1), E228–E229. [CrossRef] [PubMed]
26. Tsujino, T.; Samarasena, J.B.; Chang, K.J. EUS anatomy of the liver segments. *Endosc. Ultrasound* **2018**, *7*, 246–251. [CrossRef]
27. Okuno, N.; Hara, K.; Mizuno, N.; Hijioka, S.; Kuwahara, T.; Tajika, M.; Tanaka, T.; Ishihara, M.; Hirayama, Y.; Onishi, S.; et al. Risks of transesophageal endoscopic ultrasonography-guided biliary drainage. *Int. J. Gastrointest. Interv.* **2017**, *6*, 82–84. [CrossRef]
28. Ogura, T.; Nishioka, N.; Ueno, S.; Yamada, T.; Yamada, M.; Imoto, A.; Hakoda, A.; Higuchi, K. Effect of echoendoscope angle on success of guidewire manipulation during endoscopic ultrasound-guided hepaticogastrostomy. *Endoscopy* **2021**, *53*, 369–375. [CrossRef]
29. Minaga, K.; Ogura, T.; Shiomi, H.; Imai, H.; Hoki, N.; Takenaka, M.; Nishikiori, H.; Yamashita, Y.; Hisa, T.; Kato, H.; et al. Comparison of the efficacy and safety of endoscopic ultrasound-guided choledochoduodenostomy and hepaticogastrostomy for malignant distal biliary obstruction: Multicenter, randomized, clinical trial. *Dig. Endosc.* **2019**, *31*, 575–582. [CrossRef]
30. Nakai, Y.; Oyama, H.; Kanai, S.; Noguchi, K.; Sato, T.; Hakuta, R.; Ishigaki, K.; Saito, K.; Saito, T.; Hamada, T.; et al. Double Guidewire Technique Using an Uneven Double Lumen Catheter for Endoscopic Ultrasound-Guided Interventions. *Dig. Dis. Sci.* **2021**, *66*, 1540–1547. [CrossRef]
31. Oh, D.; Park, D.H.; Song, T.J.; Lee, S.S.; Seo, D.W.; Lee, S.K.; Kim, M.H. Optimal biliary access point and learning curve for endoscopic ultrasound-guided hepaticogastrostomy with transmural stenting. *Ther. Adv. Gastroenterol.* **2017**, *10*, 42–53. [CrossRef]

30. Yamamoto, Y.; Ogura, T.; Nishioka, N.; Yamada, T.; Yamada, M.; Ueno, S.; Higuchi, K. Risk factors for adverse events associated with bile leak during EUS-guided hepaticogastrostomy. *Endosc. Ultrasound* **2020**, *9*, 110–115. [CrossRef]
31. Vila, J.J.; Perez-Miranda, M.; Vazquez-Sequeiros, E.; Abadia, M.A.; Perez-Millan, A.; Gonzalez-Huix, F.; Gornals, J.; Iglesias-Garcia, J.; De la Serna, C.; Aparicio, J.R.; et al. Initial experience with EUS-guided cholangiopancreatography for biliary and pancreatic duct drainage: A Spanish national survey. *Gastrointest. Endosc.* **2012**, *76*, 1133–1141. [CrossRef] [PubMed]
32. Committee, A.T.; Hwang, J.H.; Aslanian, H.R.; Thosani, N.; Goodman, A.; Manfredi, M.; Navaneethan, U.; Pannala, R.; Parsi, M.A.; Smith, Z.L.; et al. Devices for use with EUS. *VideoGIE* **2017**, *2*, 35–45. [CrossRef]
33. Seldinger, S.I. Catheter Replacement of the Needle in Percutaneous Arteriography: A new technique. *Acta Radiol.* **2010**, *39*, 368–376. [CrossRef] [PubMed]
34. Tyberg, A.; Karia, K.; Gabr, M.; Desai, A.; Doshi, R.; Gaidhane, M.; Sharaiha, R.Z.; Kahaleh, M. Management of pancreatic fluid collections: A comprehensive review of the literature. *World J. Gastroenterol.* **2016**, *22*, 2256–2270. [CrossRef]
35. Ishiwatari, H.; Satoh, T.; Sato, J.; Fujie, S.; Kaneko, J.; Matsubayashi, H.; Ono, H. Bent needle technique as a rescue for bile duct puncture in endoscopic ultrasonography-guided intrahepatic biliary drainage. *Endoscopy* **2019**, *51*, E103–E104. [CrossRef]
36. Ishiwatari, H.; Satoh, T.; Sato, J.; Kaneko, J.; Matsubayashi, H.; Yabuuchi, Y.; Kishida, Y.; Yoshida, M.; Ito, S.; Kawata, N.; et al. Bile aspiration during EUS-guided hepaticogastrostomy is associated with lower risk of postprocedural adverse events: A retrospective single-center study. *Surg. Endosc.* **2021**, *35*, 6836–6845. [CrossRef]
37. Kanno, Y.; Ito, K.; Sakai, T.; Okano, H. Novel combination of a 0.018-inch guidewire, dedicated thin dilator, and 22-gauge needle for EUS-guided hepaticogastrostomy. *VideoGIE* **2020**, *5*, 355–358. [CrossRef]
38. Ogura, T.; Ueno, S.; Okuda, A.; Nishioka, N.; Higuchi, K. EUS-guided hepaticogastrostomy for hepaticojejunostomy stricture using a 22G needle and a mechanical dilator (with video). *J. Hepatobil. Pancreat. Sci.* **2021**. [CrossRef]
39. Ueno, S.; Ogura, T.; Higuchi, K. Moving scope technique for guidewire insertion during endoscopic ultrasound-guided hepaticogastrostomy. *Dig. Endosc.* **2021**, *33*, e109–e110. [CrossRef]
40. Ogura, T.; Masuda, D.; Takeuchi, T.; Fukunishi, S.; Higuchi, K. Liver impaction technique to prevent shearing of the guidewire during endoscopic ultrasound-guided hepaticogastrostomy. *Endoscopy* **2015**, *47*, E583–E584. [CrossRef]
41. Kawakami, H.; Kubota, Y.; Makiyama, H.; Sato, S.; Ban, T. Uneven double-lumen cannula for rescue guidewire technique in endoscopic ultrasonography-guided hepaticogastrostomy. *Endoscopy* **2017**, *49*, E264–E265. [CrossRef] [PubMed]
42. Matsubara, S.; Oka, M.; Nagoshi, S. Rotatable sphincterotome as a salvage for guidewire manipulation in endoscopic ultrasound-guided hepaticogastrostomy. *Dig. Endosc.* **2021**, *33*, e119–e120. [CrossRef] [PubMed]
43. Ryou, M.; Benias, P.C.; Kumbhari, V. Initial clinical experience of a steerable access device for EUS-guided biliary drainage. *Gastrointest. Endosc.* **2020**, *91*, 178–184. [CrossRef] [PubMed]
44. Marrache, M.K.; Al-Sabban, A.; Itani, M.; Farha, J.; Fayad, L.; Khashab, M.A.; Kumbhari, V. Endoscopic ultrasound-guided rendezvous ERCP using a steerable access device. *Endoscopy* **2020**, *52*, E355–E356. [CrossRef]
45. Prachayakul, V.; Aswakul, P. A novel technique for endoscopic ultrasound-guided biliary drainage. *World J. Gastroenterol.* **2013**, *19*, 4758–4763. [CrossRef]
46. Paik, W.H.; Park, D.H.; Choi, J.H.; Choi, J.H.; Lee, S.S.; Seo, D.W.; Lee, S.K.; Kim, M.H.; Lee, J.B. Simplified fistula dilation technique and modified stent deployment maneuver for EUS-guided hepaticogastrostomy. *World J. Gastroenterol.* **2014**, *20*, 5051–5059. [CrossRef]
47. Park, D.H.; Jeong, S.U.; Lee, B.U.; Lee, S.S.; Seo, D.W.; Lee, S.K.; Kim, M.H. Prospective evaluation of a treatment algorithm with enhanced guidewire manipulation protocol for EUS-guided biliary drainage after failed ERCP (with video). *Gastrointest. Endosc.* **2013**, *78*, 91–101. [CrossRef]
48. Amano, M.; Ogura, T.; Onda, S.; Takagi, W.; Sano, T.; Okuda, A.; Miyano, A.; Masuda, D.; Higuchi, K. Prospective clinical study of endoscopic ultrasound-guided biliary drainage using novel balloon catheter (with video). *J. Gastroenterol. Hepatol.* **2017**, *32*, 716–720. [CrossRef]
49. Kanno, Y.; Ito, K.; Koshita, S.; Ogawa, T.; Masu, K.; Masaki, Y.; Noda, Y. Efficacy of a newly developed dilator for endoscopic ultrasound-guided biliary drainage. *World J. Gastrointest. Endosc.* **2017**, *9*, 304–309. [CrossRef]
50. Honjo, M.; Itoi, T.; Tsuchiya, T.; Tanaka, R.; Tonozuka, R.; Mukai, S.; Sofuni, A.; Nagakawa, Y.; Iwasaki, H.; Kanai, T. Safety and efficacy of ultra-tapered mechanical dilator for EUS-guided hepaticogastrostomy and pancreatic duct drainage compared with electrocautery dilator (with video). *Endosc. Ultrasound* **2018**, *7*, 376–382. [CrossRef]
51. Kawakami, H.; Kubota, Y. Novel wire-guided fine-gauge bougie dilator for transpapillary or endoscopic ultrasonography-guided biliary drainage. *Endoscopy* **2017**, *49*, E75–E77. [CrossRef] [PubMed]
52. Park, D.H.; Jang, J.W.; Lee, S.S.; Seo, D.W.; Lee, S.K.; Kim, M.H. EUS-guided biliary drainage with transluminal stenting after failed ERCP: Predictors of adverse events and long-term results. *Gastrointest. Endosc.* **2011**, *74*, 1276–1284. [CrossRef] [PubMed]
53. Khashab, M.A.; Messallam, A.A.; Penas, I.; Nakai, Y.; Modayil, R.J.; De la Serna, C.; Hara, K.; El Zein, M.; Stavropoulos, S.N.; Perez-Miranda, M.; et al. International multicenter comparative trial of transluminal EUS-guided biliary drainage via hepatogastrostomy vs. choledochoduodenostomy approaches. *Endosc. Int. Open* **2016**, *4*, E175–E181. [CrossRef] [PubMed]
54. Ogura, T.; Nakai, Y.; Iwashita, T.; Higuchi, K.; Itoi, T. Novel fine gauge electrocautery dilator for endoscopic ultrasound-guided biliary drainage: Experimental and clinical evaluation study (with video). *Endosc. Int. Open* **2019**, *7*, E1652–E1657. [CrossRef]
55. Burmester, E.; Niehaus, J.; Leineweber, T.; Huetteroth, T. EUS-cholangio-drainage of the bile duct: Report of 4 cases. *Gastrointest. Endosc.* **2003**, *57*, 246–251. [CrossRef]

56. Giovannini, M.; Dotti, M.; Bories, E.; Moutardier, V.; Pesenti, C.; Danisi, C.; Delpero, J.R. Hepaticogastrostomy by echo-endoscopy as a palliative treatment in a patient with metastatic biliary obstruction. *Endoscopy* **2003**, *35*, 1076–1078. [CrossRef]
57. Ramirez-Luna, M.A.; Tellez-Avila, F.I.; Giovannini, M.; Valdovinos-Andraca, F.; Guerrero-Hernandez, I.; Herrera-Esquivel, J. Endoscopic ultrasound-guided biliodigestive drainage is a good alternative in patients with unresectable cancer. *Endoscopy* **2011**, *43*, 826–830. [CrossRef]
58. Attasaranya, S.; Netinasunton, N.; Jongboonyanuparp, T.; Sottisuporn, J.; Witeerungrot, T.; Pirathvisuth, T.; Ovartlarnporn, B. The Spectrum of Endoscopic Ultrasound Intervention in Biliary Diseases: A Single Center's Experience in 31 Cases. *Gastroenterol. Res. Pract.* **2012**, *2012*, 680753. [CrossRef]
59. Fabbri, C.; Luigiano, C.; Fuccio, L.; Polifemo, A.M.; Ferrara, F.; Ghersi, S.; Bassi, M.; Billi, P.; Maimone, A.; Cennamo, V.; et al. EUS-guided biliary drainage with placement of a new partially covered biliary stent for palliation of malignant biliary obstruction: A case series. *Endoscopy* **2011**, *43*, 438–441. [CrossRef]
60. Artifon, E.L.; Marson, F.P.; Gaidhane, M.; Kahaleh, M.; Otoch, J.P. Hepaticogastrostomy or choledochoduodenostomy for distal malignant biliary obstruction after failed ERCP: Is there any difference? *Gastrointest Endosc.* **2015**, *81*, 950–959. [CrossRef]
61. Horaguchi, J.; Fujita, N.; Noda, Y.; Kobayashi, G.; Ito, K.; Koshita, S.; Kanno, Y.; Ogawa, T.; Masu, K.; Hashimoto, S.; et al. Metallic stent deployment in endosonography-guided biliary drainage: Long-term follow-up results in patients with bilio-enteric anastomosis. *Dig. Endosc.* **2012**, *24*, 457–461. [CrossRef] [PubMed]
62. Bories, E.; Pesenti, C.; Caillol, F.; Lopes, C.; Giovannini, M. Transgastric endoscopic ultrasonography-guided biliary drainage: Results of a pilot study. *Endoscopy* **2007**, *39*, 287–291. [CrossRef] [PubMed]
63. Hamada, T.; Nakai, Y.; Isayama, H.; Koike, K. Tandem stent placement as a rescue for stent misplacement in endoscopic ultrasonography-guided hepaticogastrostomy. *Dig. Endosc.* **2013**, *25*, 340–341. [CrossRef]
64. Okuno, N.; Hara, K.; Mizuno, N.; Hijioka, S.; Imaoka, H.; Yamao, K. Stent migration into the peritoneal cavity following endoscopic ultrasound-guided hepaticogastrostomy. *Endoscopy* **2015**, *47* (Suppl. S1), E311. [CrossRef] [PubMed]
65. Kamata, K.; Takenaka, M.; Minaga, K.; Omoto, S.; Miyata, T.; Yamao, K.; Imai, H.; Kudo, M. Stent migration during EUS-guided hepaticogastrostomy in a patient with massive ascites: Troubleshooting using additional EUS-guided antegrade stenting. *Arab J. Gastroenterol.* **2017**, *18*, 120–121. [CrossRef] [PubMed]
66. Sodarat, P.; Luangsukrerk, T.; Kongkam, P.; Seabmuangsai, O.; Wachiramatharuch, C. Surgical hepaticogastrostomy as a method for resolving stent migration in endoscopic ultrasound-guided hepaticogastrostomy. *Endoscopy* **2021**, *53*, E350–E351. [CrossRef]
67. Wang, S.; Guo, J.; Sun, S.; Liu, X.; Wang, S.; Ge, N.; Wang, G. Endoscopic ultrasound-guided repositioning of a migrated metal hepatogastrostomy stent using foreign body forceps. *Endoscopy* **2016**, *48* (Suppl. S1), E28–E29. [CrossRef]
68. Minaga, K.; Kitano, M.; Yamashita, Y.; Nakatani, Y.; Kudo, M. Stent migration into the abdominal cavity after EUS-guided hepaticogastrostomy. *Gastrointest. Endosc.* **2017**, *85*, 263–264. [CrossRef]
69. van Geenen, E.J.M.; Siersema, P.D. Stent migration into the abdominal cavity after EUS-guided hepaticogastrostomy. *Gastrointest. Endosc.* **2018**, *87*, 617–618. [CrossRef]
70. Yang, M.J.; Kim, J.H.; Kim, D.J.; Hwang, J.C.; Yoo, B.M. Hepatobiliary and Pancreatic: EUS-guided reintervention for extraluminal stent migration after EUS-guided hepaticogastrostomy. *J. Gastroenterol. Hepatol.* **2018**, *33*, 772. [CrossRef]
71. Nakai, Y.; Sato, T.; Hakuta, R.; Ishigaki, K.; Saito, K.; Saito, T.; Takahara, N.; Hamada, T.; Mizuno, S.; Kogure, H.; et al. Long-term outcomes of a long, partially covered metal stent for EUS-guided hepaticogastrostomy in patients with malignant biliary obstruction (with video). *Gastrointest. Endosc.* **2020**, *92*, 623–631.e621. [CrossRef] [PubMed]
72. Ogura, T.; Yamamoto, K.; Sano, T.; Onda, S.; Imoto, A.; Masuda, D.; Takagi, W.; Fukunishi, S.; Higuchi, K. Stent length is impact factor associated with stent patency in endoscopic ultrasound-guided hepaticogastrostomy. *J. Gastroenterol. Hepatol.* **2015**, *30*, 1748–1752. [CrossRef] [PubMed]
73. Lee, T.H.; Choi, J.H.; Lee, S.S.; Cho, H.D.; Seo, D.W.; Park, S.H.; Lee, S.K.; Kim, M.H.; Park, D.H. A pilot proof-of-concept study of a modified device for one-step endoscopic ultrasound-guided biliary drainage in a new experimental biliary dilatation animal model. *World J. Gastroenterol.* **2014**, *20*, 5859–5866. [CrossRef] [PubMed]
74. Song, T.J.; Lee, S.S.; Park, D.H.; Seo, D.W.; Lee, S.K.; Kim, M.H. Preliminary report on a new hybrid metal stent for EUS-guided biliary drainage (with videos). *Gastrointest. Endosc.* **2014**, *80*, 707–711. [CrossRef]
75. Park, D.H.; Lee, T.H.; Paik, W.H.; Choi, J.H.; Song, T.J.; Lee, S.S.; Seo, D.W.; Lee, S.K.; Kim, M.H. Feasibility and safety of a novel dedicated device for one-step EUS-guided biliary drainage: A randomized trial. *J. Gastroenterol. Hepatol.* **2015**, *30*, 1461–1466. [CrossRef]
76. Cho, D.H.; Lee, S.S.; Oh, D.; Song, T.J.; Park, D.H.; Seo, D.W.; Lee, S.K.; Kim, M.H. Long-term outcomes of a newly developed hybrid metal stent for EUS-guided biliary drainage (with videos). *Gastrointest. Endosc.* **2017**, *85*, 1067–1075. [CrossRef]
77. De Cassan, C.; Bories, E.; Pesenti, C.; Caillol, F.; Godat, S.; Ratone, J.P.; Delpero, J.R.; Ewald, J.; Giovannini, M. Use of partially covered and uncovered metallic prosthesis for endoscopic ultrasound-guided hepaticogastrostomy: Results of a retrospective monocentric study. *Endosc. Ultrasound* **2017**, *6*, 329–335. [CrossRef]
78. Leung Ki, E.L.; Napoleon, B. EUS-specific stents: Available designs and probable lacunae. *Endosc. Ultrasound* **2019**, *8*, S17–S27. [CrossRef]
79. Park, S.W.; Lee, S.S. Which Are the Most Suitable Stents for Interventional Endoscopic Ultrasound? *J. Clin. Med.* **2020**, *9*, 3595. [CrossRef]

80. Nakai, Y.; Isayama, H.; Yamamoto, N.; Matsubara, S.; Ito, Y.; Sasahira, N.; Hakuta, R.; Umefune, G.; Takahara, N.; Hamada, T.; et al. Safety and effectiveness of a long, partially covered metal stent for endoscopic ultrasound-guided hepaticogastrostomy in patients with malignant biliary obstruction. *Endoscopy* **2016**, *48*, 1125–1128. [CrossRef]
81. Ogura, T.; Okuda, A.; Higuchi, K. Endoscopic ultrasound-guided hepaticogastrostomy for hepaticojejunostomy stricture using a one-step stent deployment technique (with video). *J. Hepatobil. Pancreat. Sci.* **2021**, *28*, e34–e35. [CrossRef] [PubMed]
82. Ogura, T.; Yamada, M.; Nishioka, N.; Yamada, T.; Higuchi, K. One-step stent deployment of EUS-guided hepaticogastrostomy using a novel covered metal stent with a fine-gauge stent delivery system (with video). *Endosc. Ultrasound* **2020**, *9*, 267–269. [CrossRef] [PubMed]
83. Maehara, K.; Hijioka, S.; Nagashio, Y.; Ohba, A.; Maruki, Y.; Suzuki, H.; Sone, M.; Okusaka, T.; Saito, Y. Endoscopic ultrasound-guided hepaticogastrostomy or hepaticojejunostomy without dilation using a stent with a thinner delivery system. *Endosc. Int. Open* **2020**, *8*, E1034–E1038. [CrossRef] [PubMed]
84. Okuno, N.; Hara, K.; Mizuno, N.; Kuwahara, T.; Iwaya, H.; Ito, A.; Kuraoka, N.; Matsumoto, S.; Polmanee, P.; Niwa, Y. Efficacy of the 6-mm fully covered self-expandable metal stent during endoscopic ultrasound-guided hepaticogastrostomy as a primary biliary drainage for the cases estimated difficult endoscopic retrograde cholangiopancreatography: A prospective clinical study. *J. Gastroenterol. Hepatol.* **2018**, *33*, 1413–1421. [CrossRef]
85. Ogura, T.; Kitano, M.; Okuda, A.; Itonaga, M.; Ueno, S.; Yamashita, Y.; Nishioka, N.; Ashida, R.; Miyano, A.; Higuchi, K. Endoscopic ultrasonography-guided hepaticogastrostomy using a novel laser-cut type partially covered self-expandable metal stent (with video). *Dig. Endosc.* **2021**, *33*, 1188–1193. [CrossRef]
86. Miyano, A.; Ogura, T.; Yamamoto, K.; Okuda, A.; Nishioka, N.; Higuchi, K. Clinical Impact of the Intra-scope Channel Stent Release Technique in Preventing Stent Migration During EUS-Guided Hepaticogastrostomy. *J. Gastrointest. Surg.* **2018**, *22*, 1312–1318. [CrossRef]
87. Uchida, D.; Kawamoto, H.; Kato, H.; Goto, D.; Tomoda, T.; Matsumoto, K.; Yamamoto, N.; Horiguchi, S.; Tsutsumi, K.; Okada, H. The intra-conduit release method is useful for avoiding migration of metallic stents during EUS-guided hepaticogastrostomy (with video). *J. Med. Ultrason* **2018**, *45*, 399–403. [CrossRef]
88. Shima, Y.; Isayama, H.; Ito, Y.; Hamada, T.; Nakai, Y.; Tsujino, T.; Nakata, R.; Koike, K. Crisscross anchor-stents to prevent metal stent migration during endoscopic ultrasound-guided hepaticogastrostomy. *Endoscopy* **2014**, *46* (Suppl. S1), E563. [CrossRef]
89. Fujisawa, T.; Isayama, H.; Ishii, S. "ClipFlap" anchoring method for endoscopic ultrasonography-guided hepaticogastrostomy with a covered self-expandable metallic stent. *Dig. Endosc.* **2020**, *32*, 628. [CrossRef]
90. Fine, C.; Rivory, J.; Forestier, J.; Saurin, J.C.; Sosa-Valencia, L.; Ponchon, T.; Pioche, M. Endoscopic management of gastric wall bleeding and stent blood clot occlusion after endoscopic ultrasound-guided hepaticogastrostomy. *Endoscopy* **2016**, *48*, E351–E352. [CrossRef]

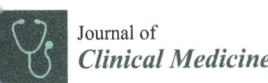

Article

Antibiotic Administration within Two Days after Successful Endoscopic Retrograde Cholangiopancreatography Is Sufficient for Mild and Moderate Acute Cholangitis

Sakue Masuda [1,*], Kazuya Koizumi [1], Makomo Makazu [1], Haruki Uojima [2], Jun Kubota [1], Karen Kimura [1], Takashi Nishino [1], Chihiro Sumida [1], Chikamasa Ichita [1], Akiko Sasaki [1] and Kento Shionoya [1]

[1] Department of Gastroenterology Medicine Center, Shonan Kamakura General Hospital, 1370-1 Okamoto, Kamakura 247-8533, Japan; kizm2010@gmail.com (K.K.); gonmarota@gmail.com (M.M.); kubojun090@gmail.com (J.K.); lion19930314@gmail.com (K.K.); tkshnshn8@gmail.com (T.N.); ycxcn117@yahoo.co.jp (C.S.); ichikamasa@yahoo.co.jp (C.I.); akikomontblanc@yahoo.co.jp (A.S.); kentosh0812@gmail.com (K.S.)

[2] Department of Gastroenterology, Internal Medicine, School of Medicine, Kitasato University, Sagamihara 252-0375, Japan; kiruha555@yahoo.co.jp

* Correspondence: sakue.masuda@tokushukai.jp; Tel.: +81-467-46-1717

Abstract: To prevent the increase of resistant bacteria, it is important to minimize the use of antimicrobial agents. Studies have found that administration for ≤3 days after successful endoscopic retrograde cholangiopancreatography (ERCP) is appropriate. Therefore, the present study aimed to verify if administration of antimicrobial agents can be further shortened to ≤2 days after ERCP. We divided 390 patients with mild and moderate cholangitis who underwent technically successful ERCP from January 2018 to June 2020 and had positive blood or bile cultures into two groups: antibiotic therapy within two days of ERCP (short-course therapy, SCT; n = 59, 15.1%), and for >3 days (long-course therapy, LCT; n = 331, 84.9%). The increased severity after admission and other outcomes were compared between the two groups, and the risk factors for increased severity were verified. There were no between-group differences in patient characteristics. Total length of hospital stay was shorter in SCT than in LCT, and other outcomes in SCT were not significantly different from those in LCT. Being 80 or older was a risk factor for increased severity; however, SCT was not associated with increased severity. Antimicrobial therapy for ≤2 days after successful ERCP is adequate in patients with mild and moderate acute cholangitis.

Keywords: antibiotics; antimicrobial stewardship; short-course antimicrobials; cholangitis; endoscopic retrograde cholangiopancreatography

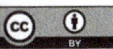

1. Introduction

At present, the incidence of antibiotic-resistant infections is increasing and represents a threat to global health care. One possible reason for this increase in antibiotic resistance is increased antibiotic exposure due to overuse, misuse, or even appropriate use. Prolonged antibiotic treatment can also lead to the development and increase of antibiotic-resistant bacteria [1]. Therefore, it is important to minimize the use of antibiotics in order to reduce the increase in resistant bacteria and the side effects of antibiotics. Furthermore, longer durations of antibiotic treatment are associated with longer hospital stay [2]. This exposes patients at risk to several well-documented complications of prolonged hospitalization, including pneumonia, venous thromboembolism, and muscle loss (especially in elderly patients) [3,4].

Acute cholangitis is a bacterial infection of the bile ducts that can be life-threatening if not diagnosed and treated on time. It is the second most common cause of community-acquired bacteremia and bacteremia in older patients [5,6]. Cholangitis-related mortality rates are relatively high (5–10%) [7,8], and the mortality rate of cholangitis patients who underwent successful endoscopic retrograde cholangiopancreatography (ERCP) is 0–7.2% [9]. The treatment for acute cholangitis mainly includes antimicrobial therapy and biliary decompression according to disease severity, and absence of treatment is associated with a high mortality risk [10]. The most up-to-date and widely used guideline on the subject is the 2018 Tokyo Guidelines (TG18) [9]. TG18 recommends four to seven days of antimicrobial therapy for patients with acute cholangitis once the source of infection has been controlled. However, the evidence level for this recommendation has been graded as low [10]. The national sepsis guideline in the Netherlands is the most progressive on antimicrobial therapy duration in cholangitis, with a recommended therapy duration of ≤3 days after successful biliary drainage [11]. Moreover, recent studies on acute cholangitis suggest that antimicrobial therapy for three days after successful ERCP is sufficient for treatment [11,12]. A large randomized controlled trial on patients with intra-abdominal infections demonstrated that a fixed four-day course of antimicrobial therapy was as effective as a longer, symptom-based treatment duration [13]. For mild or moderate acute cholecystitis, antimicrobial therapy for one day has also been reported to be sufficient after successful cholecystectomy [14,15]. Thus, there is a growing number of reports supporting that short-term administration of antimicrobial therapy is sufficient. In addition, several reports suggest that that even when antimicrobial therapy is ineffective, outcomes for patients with acute cholangitis are not worse if ERCP is successful [16,17].

Therefore, the purpose of this study was to verify whether the duration of antibiotic therapy for patients with mild and moderate acute cholangitis after ERCP can be shortened to ≤2 days.

2. Materials and Methods

2.1. Study Population

This retrospective observational cohort study was conducted at the Shonan Kamakura General Hospital in Japan. We searched the hospital records of patients treated at the hospital from January 2018 to June 2020 and identified 390 patients with mild and moderate cholangitis who had positive blood or bile cultures and had undergone technically successful ERCP. In principle, blood cultures were collected before antibiotic administration, and bile cultures were collected immediately after the start of the ERCP. We divided the 390 patients into two groups: antibiotic therapy within two days of ERCP (short-course antibiotic therapy, SCT) and antibiotic therapy for ≥3 days (long-course antibiotic therapy, LCT).

Patients who had suffered multiple episodes of cholangitis were included multiple times if the minimum interval between episodes was three months. Patients who had died within 2 days after the initial ERCP, or who were lost to follow-up within 30 days after the initial ERCP, were excluded. Patients who had died within 2 days after the initial ERCP were excluded because they did not have the chance to be treated with antibiotics for more than 2 days (Figure 1).

In our hospital, ampicillin/sulbactam, cefmetazole, ceftriaxone, piperacillin/tazobactam, meropenem, and ciprofloxacin are typically used for the initial treatment. Mild cases were primarily treated with cefmetazole, and other antibiotics were administered based on renal function and previous cultures.

In principle, the dose of each antibacterial agent was as follows: ampicillin/sulbactam (6.0 g/day), piperacillin/tazobactam (13.5 g/day), ceftriaxone (2.0 g/day), cefmetazole (3.0 g/day), meropenem (3.0 g/day), ciprofloxacin (0.6 g/day), levofloxacin (0.5 g/day), and vancomycin (30 mg/body weight kg/day); moreover, the dose of each antibiotic was reduced as needed in patients with reduced GFR.

This was a retrospective study, and there were no criteria for determining the duration of antimicrobial therapy; each physician in charge made the decision.

In cases where plastic stent implantation was needed in ERCP, a single 7-Fr stent was implanted as a rule. When implanting self-expandable metallic stents, stents with diameters of 10 and 8 mm were implanted in the common bile duct and hilar region, respectively.

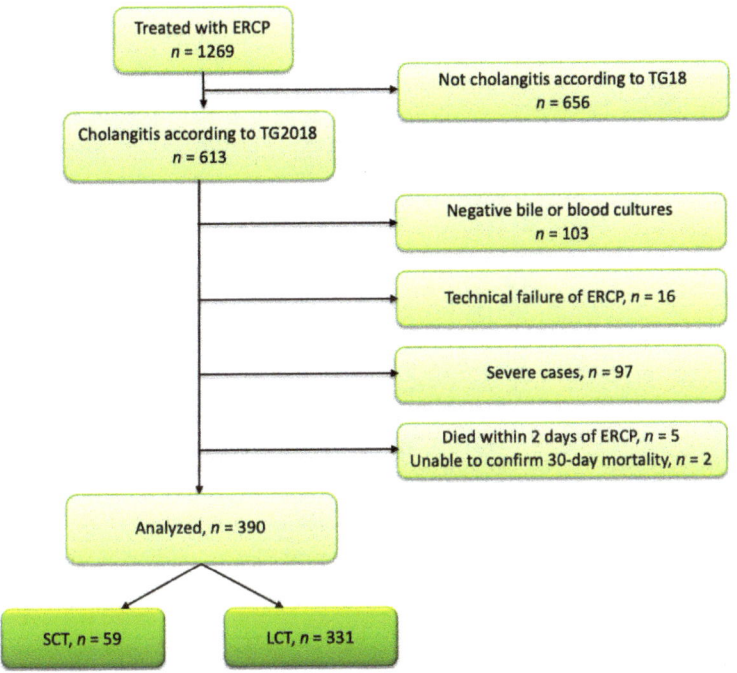

Figure 1. Study population. SCT: short course antibiotic therapy; LCT: long course antibiotic therapy; ERCP: endoscopic retrograde cholangiopancreatography; TG18: Tokyo Guidelines 2018.

2.2. Ethical Information

All procedures were performed in accordance with the ethical standards established in the 1964 Declaration of Helsinki and its later amendments. The study was reviewed and approved by the institutional review board of the Future Medical Research Center Ethical Committee (IRB no. TGE01849-024, date of approval was 25 November 2021). Due to the retrospective study design, informed consent was obtained from all participants by the opt-out method on our hospital website and in-hospital posting.

2.3. Study Outcomes

The primary outcome was an increase in disease severity after hospitalization. Secondary outcomes included national early warning score (NEWS), in-hospital mortality, 30 day mortality, total length of hospital stay, and three-month recurrence—defined as the recurrence of symptoms after complete recovery within 3 months of the disease onset. We reported the results per episode of cholangitis. The three-month recurrence included recurrent cholangitis, cholecystitis, and liver abscess, that could be related to the primary cholangitis episode.

The NEWS was developed by the United Kingdom's National Early Warning Score Development and Implementation Group in 2012 to assess deteriorating conditions in hospitalized patients, and to predict inpatient death or ICU admission [18]. NEWS measures physiological parameters (systolic blood pressure, pulse rate, respiratory rate, temperature, oxygen saturation), level of consciousness, and oxygen supplementation, all of which are simple and easily accessible [18,19]. NEWS is now widespread in many countries because of its greater ability compared to other early warning scores to identify patients at risk for the composite outcome of cardiac arrest, unexpected ICU admission, and death within 24 h. Most reports place the low-risk group for NEWS at 4 points or less, although one report places it at 3 points or less [20].

For reference, we confirmed the following items: number of days required to break the fever after ERCP, and complications of infective endocarditis within 3 months.

2.4. Definitions

The diagnosis and severity of cholangitis were based on the TG18 [21]. An increase in severity was defined as a change from mild to moderate or from moderate to severe, according to the TG18 criteria. Hospital stay was defined as the number of days from the day of admission to the day of discharge or date of death.

Pathogen resistance to the initial antibiotics was defined as a pathogen that was resistant to the initial antibiotics in vitro. Cholangitis is often caused by polymicrobial infections. Blood cultures have low sensitivity and may not detect the causative organism; moreover, bile cultures have low specificity and may detect enteric bacteria that are not the causative organism. This makes it difficult to accurately identify the causative organisms in cholangitis. Therefore, in this study, all the detected bacteria were treated equally as causative organisms.

Clinical success of ERCP was defined as a 50% decrease in the level of total bilirubin or alanine aminotransferase, or normalization within 1 week of ERCP.

Recurrent cholangitis was defined as recurrence of symptoms or laboratory tests after the complete cure of the disease within 3 months after the ERCP. ERCP was performed again in almost all cases of recurrent cholangitis.

The days required to break the fever after ERCP was determined when the temperature remained below 37 °C for 24 h [22].

2.5. Statistical Analyses

The Mann-Whitney U-test was used to compare non-normally distributed continuous variables, and the χ^2 test or Fisher's exact test was used to compare categorical variables. The Kolmogorov-Smirnov test and the Shapiro–Wilk normality test were used to test the normality of distribution. Multivariate analysis was performed using logistic regression. Variables that were clinically significant or reported in previous studies to be clinically significant were included in the multivariate analysis. Two-tailed p-values < 0.05 were considered significant. All statistical analyses were performed using EZR (Saitama Medical Center, Jichi Medical University, Saitama, Japan), which is a graphical user interface for the R statistical software (The R Foundation for Statistical Computing, Vienna, Austria). More precisely, it is a modified version of the R commander, designed to allow additional biostatistical functions [23].

3. Results

3.1. Patient Characteristics

Table 1 summarizes the patient characteristics. We retrospectively analyzed the data of 390 patients with positive blood or bile cultures who were treated with ERCP. Of these, 59 patients (15.1%) received short-course antibiotic treatment (SCT, ≤2 days) and 331 (84.9%) received long-course antibiotic treatment (LCT, ≥3 days). There were no significant between-group differences in age, sex, cause of cholangitis, disease severity, hyperbilirubinemia, abnormal white blood cells, hypoalbuminemia, NEWS (on admission, just before ERCP), positive blood culture, underlying disease, or patient background. This study included patients with mild and moderate cholangitis, and therefore, did not include patients with severe renal impairment or coagulation abnormalities.

Table 1. Patient characteristics.

	SCT, n = 59 (15.1%)	LCT, n = 331 (84.9%)	p-Value
Age (median) (range)	81 (26–100)	81 (25–102)	0.837
Sex (male:female)	28:31	172:159	0.579
Cause of cholangitis			
Malignant stricture	17 (28.8%)	85 (25.7%)	0.631
Bile duct stone	36 (61.0%)	216 (65.3%)	0.556
Benign bile duct stricture	3 (5.1%)	8 (2.4%)	0.223
Chronic pancreatitis	1 (1.7%)	4 (1.2%)	0.562
Mirizzi syndrome	0 (0.0%)	9 (2.7%)	0.366
Autoimmune pancreatitis	1 (1.7%)	1 (0.3%)	0.28
Others	1 (1.7%)	8 (2.4%)	>0.99
Severity			
Mild	32 (54.2%)	151 (45.6%)	0.258
Moderate	27 (45.8%)	180 (54.4%)	0.258
Bil ≥ 5.0 (mg/dL)	11 (18.6%)	72 (21.8%)	0.73
WBC < 4000, 12,000 < WBC (/μL)	14 (23.7%)	111 (33.5%)	0.173
Alb < 3.0 (g/dL)	18 (30.5%)	100 (30.2%)	>0.99
NEWS (median) (range)			
On admission	1 (0–7)	1 (0–13)	0.096
Just before ERCP	1 (0–7)	1 (0–13)	0.159
48 h after ERCP	0 (0–5)	0 (0–6)	0.429
Underlying disease			
CKD	5 (8.5%)	26 (7.9%)	0.797
CHF	2 (3.4%)	34 (10.3%)	0.139
LC	3 (5.1%)	15 (4.5%)	0.743
DM	8 (13.6%)	62 (18.7%)	0.461
Malignant tumor	18 (30.5%)	92 (27.8%)	0.642
Patient background			
Nursing home	7 (11.9%)	70 (21.1%)	0.112
Hemodialysis	0 (0.0%)	8 (2.4%)	0.613
Gastrostomy	1 (1.7%)	1 (0.3%)	0.28
Constant placement of urinary catheter	0 (0%)	2 (0.6%)	>0.99
Aspiration pneumonia	0 (0%)	7 (2.1%)	0.601
Immunosuppressant	0 (0%)	6 (1.8%)	0.597
Re-intervention to bile duct stent	11 (18.6%)	65 (19.6%)	>0.99

Some cases overlapped. SCT: short-course antibiotic therapy; LCT: long-course antibiotic therapy; Bil: bilirubin; WBC; white blood cells; Alb: albumin; NEWS: national early warning score; ERCP: endoscopic retrograde cholangiopancreatography; CKD: chronic kidney disease; CHF: chronic heart failure; LC: liver cirrhosis; DM: diabetes mellitus.

3.2. ERCP Findings

Table 2 summarizes the ERCP findings of the study population. The median time from first patient–physician contact to ERCP was longer in the SCT group than in the LCT group (SCT: median, 24 h; range 2–250 h; LCT: median, 10 h; range, 1–120 h; $p < 0.001$). The clinical success rates of ERCP were 94.3 and 95.3% in the SCT and LCT groups, respectively. No significant between-group differences were found with regard to the rate of prior ERCP, clinical success rate of biliary drainage, ERCP drainage procedure, or complications.

Table 2. ERCP findings.

	SCT, n = 59 (15.1%)	LCT, n = 331 (84.9%)	p-Value
Median time from first physician contact to ERCP * (hours) (range)	24 (2–250)	10 (1–120)	<0.001
Prior ERCP	22 (37.3%)	137 (41.4%)	0.666
Clinical success of ERCP*1	51/54 (94.3%)	302/317 (95.3%)	0.734
ERCP drainage procedure			
Stent replacement			
Self-expandable metallic stent	10 (16.9%)	37 (11.2%)	0.2
Plastic stent	14 (23.7%)	109 (32.9%)	0.174
ENBD	1 (1.7%)	20 (6.0%)	0.224
Lithotripsy	35 (59.3%)	177 (53.3%)	0.479
Others	1 (1.7%)	2 (0.6%)	0.389
Complications			
Pancreatitis	0 (0.0%)	10 (3.0%)	0.371
Bleeding	2 (3.4%)	8 (2.4%)	0.652
Perforation	0 (0.0%)	2 (0.6%)	>0.99
Cholecystitis	1 (1.7%)	9 (2.7%)	>0.99
Stent migration/early stent obstruction	0 (0.0%)	3 (0.9%)	>0.99
Others	0 (0.0%)	2 (0.6%)	>0.99
Total †	3 (5.1%)	31 (9.4%)	0.45

SCT: short-course antibiotic therapy; LCT: long-course antibiotic therapy; ERCP: endoscopic retrograde cholangiopancreatography; ENBD: endoscopic nasobiliary drainage. * Cases in which the efficacy of ERCP could not be determined were excluded † Some cases overlapped.

3.3. Microbiological Data

The laboratory findings of microbial cultures from the patients are summarized in Table 3. The positive rates of blood and bile cultures were 46.4% (13/28) and 100.0% (58/58) in the SCT group, and 49.2% (123/250) and 98.8% (321/325) in the LCT group, respectively. There were no significant differences in the positive rates of blood or bile cultures. A total of 210 patients (53.8%) had polymicrobial infections, for which *Escherichia coli*, *Klebsiella* sp., *Enterococcus* sp., and *Enterobacter* sp. were the most common pathogens.

Table 3. The laboratory findings of microbial cultures.

	SCT, n = 59 (15.1%)	LCT, n = 331 (84.9%)	p-Value
Blood culture			
Positive rate	13/28 (46.4%)	123/250 (49.2%)	0.153
Escherichia coli	7 (11.9%)	59 (17.8%)	0.346
Klebsiella sp.	2 (3.4%)	33 (10.0%)	0.137
Enterococcus sp.	0 (0.0%)	12 (3.6%)	0.227
Enterobacter sp.	1 (1.7%)	8 (2.4%)	>0.99
Citrobacter sp.	1 (1.7%)	3 (0.9%)	0.483
Staphylococcus sp.	0 (0.0%)	7 (2.1%)	0.601
Streptococcus sp.	1 (1.7%)	6 (1.8%)	>0.99
Pseudomonas sp.	0 (0.0%)	3 (0.9%)	>0.99
Aeromonas sp.	1 (1.7%)	13 (3.9%)	0.704
Others	1 (1.7%)	7 (2.1%)	>0.99
Negative	15 (25.4%)	128 (38.7%)	0.057
No culture	31 (52.5%)	81 (24.5%)	<0.001
Bile culture			
Positive rate	58/58 (100.0%)	321/325 (98.8%)	>0.99
Escherichia coli	18 (30.5%)	124 (37.5%)	0.378
Klebsiella sp.	16 (27.1%)	117 (35.3%)	0.237
Enterococcus sp.	29 (49.2%)	123 (37.2%)	0.085
Enterobacter sp.	9 (15.3%)	55 (16.6%)	>0.99
Citrobacter sp.	8 (13.6%)	22 (6.6%)	0.105
Staphylococcus sp.	0 (0.0%)	9 (2.7%)	0.366
Streptococcus sp.	7 (11.9%)	40 (12.1%)	>0.99
Pseudomonas sp.	2 (3.4%)	22 (6.6%)	0.555
Aeromonas sp.	6 (10.2%)	30 (9.1%)	0.807
Others	7 (11.9%)	24 (7.3%)	0.291
Negative	0 (0.0%)	4 (1.2%)	>0.99
No culture	1 (1.7%)	6 (1.8%)	>0.99

Some cases overlapped. SCT: short-course antibiotic therapy; LCT: long-course antibiotic therapy.

3.4. Antibiotic Therapy

Table 4 summarizes the findings related to antibiotics in the present study. Cefmetazole, ampicillin/sulbactam, and piperacillin/tazobactam were the most commonly used antibiotics. There were no significant differences in the rate of use of each antibiotic. Two patients in the SCT group (3.4%) did not receive any antibiotics.

The median times from the first patient–physician contact to antibiotic administration were 5 and 4 h in the SCT and LCT groups, respectively. The median total duration of antibiotic therapy—including pre-ERCP—was shorter in the SCT than in the LCT group (SCT: median, 2 days; range, 0–12 days; LCT: median, 5 days; range, 3–49; $p < 0.001$).

In the SCT and LCT groups, 23 (39.0%) and 72 (21.8%) patients, respectively, exhibited only pathogens resistant to the initial antibiotics. Of these patients, 38 (52.8%) in the LCT group changed the initial antibiotics to appropriate definitive antibiotic therapy, while those in the SCT group remained on inappropriate antibiotics and completed antimicrobial therapy.

Table 4. Antibiotic therapy.

	SCT, n = 59 (15.1%)	LCT, n = 331 (84.9%)	p-Value
Initial antimicrobial therapy			
Ampicillin/sulbactam	8 (13.6%)	60 (18.1%)	0.461
Piperacillin/tazobactam	8 (13.6%)	47 (14.2%)	>0.99
Ceftriaxone	3 (5.1%)	17 (5.1%)	>0.99
Cefmetazole	38 (64.4%)	189 (57.1%)	0.319
Meropenem	0 (0.0%)	8 (2.4%)	0.613
Ciprofloxacin	0 (0.0%)	9 (2.7%)	0.366
Levofloxacin	0 (0.0%)	1 (0.3%)	>0.99
Vancomycin	0 (0.0%)	1 (0.3%)	>0.99
Others	0 (0.0%)	1 (0.3%)	>0.99
No antibiotics	2 (3.4%)	0 (0.0%)	0.023
Median time from first physician contact to antibiotic administration (range)	5.0 h (0–96)	4.0 h (0–53)	0.039
Median total duration of antimicrobial therapy (range)	2 days (0–12)	5 days (3–49)	<0.001
Only pathogens resistant to the initial antibiotics	23 (39.0%)	72 (21.8%)	0.008

SCT: short-course antibiotic therapy; LCT: long-course antibiotic therapy.

3.5. Clinical Outcomes

Table 5 summarizes the clinical outcomes in the present study. Increased severity occurred in 23.7% (14 cases) in the SCT group and in 20.8% (69 cases) in the LCT group. We did not find any significant between-group differences in the increased severity, NEWS (96 h after ERCP, five points or more at five to seven days after ERCP), in-hospital mortality, 30 day mortality, and three-month recurrence.

The median duration of hospitalization was seven days (range, 3–39 days) in the SCT group and eight days (range, 3–120 days) in the LCT group. The duration of hospitalization was significantly shorter in the SCT group compared to the LCT group ($p = 0.009$).

The days required to break the fever after ERCP was significantly longer in the LCT group compared to the SCT group ($p < 0.001$).

No complications of infective endocarditis were identified within three months.

Table 5. Clinical outcomes.

	SCT, n = 59 (15.1%)	LCT, n = 331 (84.9%)	p-Value
Duration of hospitalization (days)	7 days (3–34)	7 days (3–120)	0.009
Increased severity	14 (23.7%)	69 (20.8%)	0.607
NEWS			
96 h after ERCP	0 (0–3)	1 (0–15)	0.45
5 points or more at 5 to 7 days after ERCP	1/29 (3.4%)	11/226 (4.9%)	>0.99
In-hospital mortality due to cholangitis	0 (0.0%)	5 (1.5%)	>0.99
Thirty-day mortality	1 (1.7%)	11 (3.3%)	>0.99
Three-month recurrence	4/57 (7.0%)	36/313 (11.5%)	0.485
Days required to break the fever after ERCP	0 (0–8)	1 (0–23)	<0.001

SCT: short-course antibiotic therapy; LCT: long-course antibiotic therapy; NEWS: national early warning score; ERCP: endoscopic retrograde cholangiopancreatography.

3.6. Multivariate Analysis for Increased Severity after Admission

Table 6 summarizes the multivariate analysis for increased severity. Multivariate analysis showed that an age of 80 or more independently predicted the increased severity (odds ratio [OR], 2.16; 95% confidence interval [CI], 1.16–4.05: $p = 0.016$), whereas SCT was not a risk factor. No significant differences were noted in other parameters, including residence in a nursing home, malignant biliary stricture, ERCP within 24 h of first physician contact, diabetes, pathogens resistant to the initial antibiotics, and positive blood culture.

Table 6. Multivariate analysis for increased severity after admission.

	Increased Severity, n = 83	No Change in Severity, n = 307	Univariate Analysis, p-Value	Multivariate Analysis, p-Value	Odds Ratio	95%CI
Aged 80 years or more	56 (67.5%)	158 (51.6%)	0.0126	0.016	2.16	1.16–4.05
Nursing home	15 (18.1%)	62 (20.2%)	0.757	0.166		
Malignant biliary stricture	22 (26.5%)	80 (26.1%)	>0.99	0.998		
ERCP within 24 h of first physician contact	65 (78.3%)	231 (75.2%)	0.665	0.116		
Diabetes	14 (16.9%)	56 (18.2%)	0.872	0.779		
Antimicrobials within 2 days of ERCP (SCT)	14 (16.9%)	45 (14.7%)	0.607	0.371		
Only resistant pathogens to the initial antibiotics	15 (18.1%)	80 (26.1%)	0.151	0.345		
Positive blood culture	35/66 (53.0%)	101/211 (47.9%)	0.484	0.742		

Area under the receiver operating characteristic curve: 0.636. ERCP: endoscopic retrograde cholangiopancreatography. SCT: short-course antibiotic therapy.

3.7. Clinical Outcomes in Positive Blood Culture Group

Table 7 summarizes the clinical outcomes in positive blood culture group. We performed a subgroup analysis focused on blood culture-positive patients and did not find any significant between-group differences in the increased severity, NEWS (96 h after ERCP, 5 points or more at 5 to 7 days after ERCP), in-hospital mortality, 30 day mortality, and three-month recurrence.

Table 7. Clinical outcomes in positive blood culture group.

	SCT, n = 13 (9.6%)	LCT, n = 123 (90.4%)	p-Value
Duration of hospitalization (days)	6 days (4–13)	8 days (3–120)	0.03
Increased severity	4 (30.8%)	31 (25.2%)	0.74
NEWS			
96 h after ERCP	1 (0–2)	0 (0–15)	0.913
5 or more at 4 to 7 days after ERCP	0/5 (0.0%)	4/88 (4.5%)	>0.99
In-hospital mortality due to cholangitis	0 (0.0%)	3 (2.4%)	>0.99
Thirty-day mortality	0 (0.0%)	4 (3.3%)	>0.99
Three-month recurrence	0 (0.0%)	11 (9.6%)	0.602

SCT: short-course antibiotic therapy; LCT: long-course antibiotic therapy; NEWS: national early warning score; ERCP: endoscopic retrograde cholangiopancreatography.

4. Discussion

In this study, there were no significant differences in the outcomes between the two groups with regard to increased severity, in-hospital mortality, thirty-day mortality, and three-month recurrence. The duration of hospitalization was shorter in the SCT group (≤2 days) than in the LCT group (≥3 days). This result on the duration of hospitalization may be because the duration of the antibiotics treatment itself led to an increased duration of hospitalization. However, the SCT was not associated with worsening of the cholangitis or prolongation of hospital stay. These findings suggest that SCT was not inferior to LCT in patients who underwent successful biliary drainage. Furthermore, the duration of hospitalization was lower in the SCT group. This observation, although statistically significant, may not be clinically meaningful; however, it may suggest that SCT may be useful for preventing complications associated with prolonged hospitalization, such as pneumonia, venous thromboembolism, and muscle loss in the elderly [3,4]. Multivariate analysis showed that an age of 80 or more increased the risk of increased severity, whereas SCT did not make outcomes worse. Several recent studies have acknowledged that SCT does not worsen outcomes—such as mortality and recurrence rates—in patients with successful ERCP. Similar results were reported by Satake et al. in a retrospective study on mild and moderate acute cholangitis and by Haal et al. in a retrospective study on acute cholangitis due to common bile duct stones [11,12]. Van Lent et al. concluded that short-duration (three days) antibiotic treatment for acute cholangitis following adequate biliary duct drainage appeared to be sufficient for treatment [24]. A recent systematic review has reported that short-course antibiotic therapy seems adequate for the treatment of acute cholangitis following successful biliary drainage. However, the review also described that the quality of evidence remains very low due to the low number of patients included, the differences in study design, and the heterogeneity of the definitions used for long- and short-course treatment [9]. The results of these studies suggest that once the source of infection is controlled with biliary drainage, bacteremia is likely to resolve, and the patient may not need further antibiotic therapy [25]. In the present study, we used data from 390 cases, and we conducted a detailed study of short-term prognosis, including not only increased severity of disease, but also NEWS (a new, simple, and easily accessible score for assessing deteriorating conditions and predicting increasing severity of disease). We also conducted long-term prognosis, including the rate of recurrence after three months and the complications of infective endocarditis. Using these data, we showed that SCT is non-inferior to LCT in acute cholangitis, even if the patient had a positive blood culture.

In the present study, more days were required to break the fever in the LCT group than in the SCT group; however, NEWS, the overall score of physical findings including fever, did not differ between the two groups. Although this may seem to indicate that severe cases were more common in LCT, it is possible that clinicians may be overly influenced by only a single item, i.e., fever, to prescribe antibiotics for a longer duration. Van Lent et al. stated that the fear of complications of acute cholangitis drives clinicians to prescribe antibiotics for longer periods of time [24]. Traditionally, physicians have administered antimicrobial therapy to patients with infections until the infection is cured based on clinical and laboratory evidence. This was because they believed that persistent sepsis indicated continued replication of the pathogen. However, recent experimental data suggest that prolonged SIRS may be a reflection of host immune activity rather than an indication of the presence of viable microorganisms. Efforts have therefore begun to shorten the duration of antimicrobial therapy. These efforts have already been successful in other severe infections, such as ventilator-associated pneumonia [13]. Thus, several recent studies have shown that antibiotics can be terminated in the short term, without clinical and laboratory evidence.

Although the level of evidence is low, the TG18 recommends two weeks of antibiotic therapy for cases with Gram-positive cocci (GPC)-positive blood cultures because of concerns about infected endocarditis (IE). However, Gomi et al. validated 6433 patients with cholangitis and found 243 cases with GPC-positive blood cultures, but no complications of IE were observed in those cases. In that study, the overall incidence of IE was 0.26%

(17 cases) [26]. In the present study, there were no complications of IE within three months among 40 patients with GPC-positive blood cultures. Although two weeks of antibiotic therapy may be appropriate in patients at risk for IE—such as patients with valvular disease and chronic poor oral hygiene—complications of IE are rare in patients with cholangitis. Therefore, SCT may be appropriate for cholangitis patients, even if their blood cultures are positive for GPC. Doi et al. showed that for acute cholangitis with bacteremia and successful biliary drainage, a shortened total duration (seven days) of antibiotic treatment may be a reasonable option [27]. However, it is still unknown whether the risk of complications from long-term antibiotic therapy should be prioritized over the risk of IE, or vice versa.

The aforementioned results should be interpreted with caution, taking into account some uncertainties. First, this was a single-center retrospective study, and the duration of antimicrobial therapy was determined by each physician in charge. Therefore, patients who were possibly considered to have a severe condition may have been categorized into the LCT group. This means that although there was no significant difference in the severity of the condition according to the TG18 and NEWS between the SCT and LCT groups, potentially severe cases may have been included in the LCT group. Second, because this was a retrospective study, we consider that there are confounding factors that are not included in this study. In addition, because of the small number of patients in the SCT group, rare complications such as IE and liver abscesses have not been adequately evaluated. In particular, data on complications of IE were not examined in detail and should be considered only as a reference. Furthermore, malignant biliary stricture accounted for 102 cases (26.2% of all cases) in this study, and further studies are needed to determine whether SCT is effective for malignant biliary stricture. Third, the rate of pathogen resistance to initial antibiotics was 21.8% in the LCT group. The inefficacy of antibiotics can be approximated as a short duration of antibiotic treatment; therefore, the proportion of patients with pathogen resistance to initial antibiotics (21.8%) in the LCT group may have influenced the results of the present study. However, pathogen resistance to initial antibiotics was also not associated with increased severity in the multivariate analysis. In view of these limitations, we believe that a new randomized controlled study on the duration of antibiotic treatment in acute cholangitis can provide high-quality evidence on the topic. The results of the present study provide a foundation for a future randomized controlled trial, which we plan to conduct to satisfy the need for high-quality evidence.

5. Conclusions

This retrospective study indicates that antimicrobial therapy for ≤2 days is sufficient after successful ERCP in patients with mild and moderate acute cholangitis. Prospective studies are needed to confirm our results and to ensure evidence-based recommendations of antibiotic therapy duration in patients with cholangitis. This could ultimately help reduce the unnecessary administration of antibiotics, duration of hospital stays, and associated adverse events.

Author Contributions: Conceptualization, S.M. and K.K. (Kazuya Koizumi); Methodology, S.M.; Software, S.M.; Validation, S.M., K.K. (Kazuya Koizumi), M.M., H.U., J.K., K.K. (Karen Kimura), T.N., C.S., C.I., A.S. and K.S.; Formal analysis, S.M.; Investigation, S.M.; Resources, S.M.; Data curation, S.M.; Writing—original draft preparation, S.M.; Writing—review and editing, S.M.; Visualization, S.M.; Supervision, S.M. and K.K. (Kazuya Koizumi); Project administration, S.M.; Funding acquisition, not applicable. All authors have read and agreed to the published version of the manuscript.

Funding: This research received no external funding.

Institutional Review Board Statement: The study was conducted in accordance with the Declaration of Helsinki and approved by the Institutional Review Board (or Ethics Committee) of FUTURE MEDICAL RESEARCH CENTER (IRB no. TGE01849-024).

Informed Consent Statement: As this is a retrospective study using information contained in medical charts and computerized records, informed consent was obtained from all individual participants included in the study through the opt-out method on our hospital website and in-hospital posting. The ethics committee approved this.

Data Availability Statement: The data that support the findings of this study are available from the corresponding author, SM, upon reasonable request. The technical appendix, statistical code, and dataset are available from the corresponding author upon request. No additional data are available.

Acknowledgments: We would like to thank Ayumu Sugitani for help in statistical analysis.

Conflicts of Interest: The authors declare no conflict of interest.

References

1. Spellberg, B.; Guidos, R.; Gilbert, D.; Bradley, J.; Boucher, H.W.; Scheld, W.M.; Bartlett, J.G.; Edwards, J.; Infectious Diseases Society of America. The Epidemic of Antibiotic-Resistant Infections: A Call to Action for the Medical Community from the Infectious Diseases Society of America. *Clin. Infect. Dis.* **2008**, *46*, 155–164. [CrossRef]
2. Uno, S.; Hase, R.; Kobayashi, M.; Shiratori, T.; Nakaji, S.; Hirata, N.; Hosokawa, N. Short-Course Antimicrobial Treatment for Acute Cholangitis with Gram-Negative Bacillary Bacteremia. *Int. J. Infect. Dis.* **2017**, *55*, 81–85. [CrossRef] [PubMed]
3. Heit, J.A.; Melton, L.J., 3rd; Lohse, C.M.; Petterson, T.M.; Silverstein, M.D.; Mohr, D.N.; O'Fallon, W.M. Incidence of Venous Thromboembolism in Hospitalized Patients vs Community Residents. *Mayo Clin. Proc.* **2001**, *76*, 1102–1110. [CrossRef] [PubMed]
4. Welch, C.; Hassan-Smith, Z.K.; Greig, C.A.; Lord, J.M.; Jackson, T.A. Acute Sarcopenia Secondary to Hospitalisation—an Emerging Condition Affecting Older Adults. *Aging Dis.* **2018**, *9*, 151–164. [CrossRef]
5. Melzer, M.; Toner, R.; Lacey, S.; Bettany, E.; Rait, G. Biliary Tract Infection and Bacteraemia: Presentation, Structural Abnormalities, Causative Organisms and Clinical Outcomes [Presentation]. *Postgrad. Med. J.* **2007**, *83*, 773–776. [CrossRef] [PubMed]
6. Esposito, A.L.; Gleckman, R.A.; Cram, S.; Crowley, M.; McCabe, F.; Drapkin, M.S. Community-Acquired Bacteremia in the Elderly: Analysis of One Hundred Consecutive Episodes. *J. Am. Geriatr. Soc.* **1980**, *28*, 315–319. [CrossRef]
7. Lai, E.C.; Mok, F.P.; Tan, E.S.; Lo, C.M.; Fan, S.T.; You, K.T.; Wong, J. Endoscopic Biliary Drainage for Severe Acute Cholangitis. *N. Engl. J. Med.* **1992**, *326*, 1582–1586. [CrossRef] [PubMed]
8. Sokal, A.; Sauvanet, A.; Fantin, B.; de Lastours, V. Acute Cholangitis: Diagnosis and Management. *J. Visc. Surg.* **2019**, *156*, 515–525. [CrossRef]
9. Tinusz, B.; Szapáry, L.; Paládi, B.; Tenk, J.; Rumbus, Z.; Pécsi, D.; Szakács, Z.; Varga, G.; Rakonczay, Z.; Szepes, Z.; et al. Short-Course Antibiotic Treatment Is Not Inferior to a Long-Course One in Acute Cholangitis: A Systematic Review. *Dig. Dis. Sci.* **2019**, *64*, 307–315. [CrossRef]
10. Gomi, H.; Solomkin, J.S.; Schlossberg, D.; Okamoto, K.; Takada, T.; Strasberg, S.M.; Ukai, T.; Endo, I.; Iwashita, Y.; Hibi, T.; et al. Tokyo Guidelines 2018: Antimicrobial Therapy for Acute Cholangitis and Cholecystitis. *J. Hepatobiliary Pancreat. Sci.* **2018**, *25*, 3–16. [CrossRef]
11. Haal, S.; Ten Böhmer, B.; Balkema, S.; Depla, A.C.; Fockens, P.; Jansen, J.M.; Kuiken, S.D.; Liberov, B.I.; van Soest, E.; van Hooft, J.E.; et al. Antimicrobial Therapy of 3 Days or Less Is Sufficient after Successful ERCP for Acute Cholangitis. *United Eur. Gastroenterol. J.* **2020**, *8*, 481–488. [CrossRef]
12. Satake, M.; Yamaguchi, Y. Three-Day Antibiotic Treatment for Acute Cholangitis Due to Choledocholithiasis with Successful Biliary Duct Drainage: A Single-Center Retrospective Cohort Study. *Int. J. Infect. Dis.* **2020**, *96*, 343–347. [CrossRef] [PubMed]
13. Sawyer, R.G.; Claridge, J.A.; Nathens, A.B.; Rotstein, O.D.; Duane, T.M.; Evans, H.L.; Cook, C.H.; O'Neill, P.J.; Mazuski, J.E.; Askari, R.; et al. Trial of Short-Course Antimicrobial Therapy for Intraabdominal Infection. *N. Engl. J. Med.* **2015**, *372*, 1996–2005. [CrossRef]
14. Loozen, C.S.; Kortram, K.; Kornmann, V.N.N.; van Ramshorst, B.; Vlaminckx, B.; Knibbe, C.A.J.; Kelder, J.C.; Donkervoort, S.C.; Nieuwenhuijzen, G.A.; Ponten, J.E.; et al. Randomized Clinical Trial of Extended Versus Single-Dose Perioperative Antibiotic Prophylaxis for Acute Calculous Cholecystitis. *Br. J. Surg.* **2017**, *104*, e151–e157. [CrossRef] [PubMed]
15. Regimbeau, J.M.; Fuks, D.; Pautrat, K.; Mauvais, F.; Haccart, V.; Msika, S.; Mathonnet, M.; Scotté, M.; Paquet, J.C.; Vons, C.; et al. Effect of Postoperative Antibiotic Administration on Postoperative Infection Following Cholecystectomy for Acute Calculous Cholecystitis: A Randomized Clinical Trial. *JAMA* **2014**, *312*, 145–154. [CrossRef] [PubMed]
16. Masuda, S.; Koizumi, K.; Uojima, H.; Kimura, K.; Nishino, T.; Tasaki, J.; Ichita, C.; Sasaki, A. Effect of Antibiotic Resistance of Pathogens on Initial Antibiotic Therapy for Patients with Cholangitis. *Cureus* **2021**, *13*, e18449. [CrossRef] [PubMed]
17. Kang, C.I.; Sung, Y.K.; Lee, K.H.; Lee, K.T.; Lee, J.K. Clinical Impact of Inappropriate Initial Antimicrobial Therapy on Outcome in Bacteremic Biliary Tract Infections. *Scand. J. Infect. Dis.* **2013**, *45*, 227–234. [CrossRef] [PubMed]
18. Smith, G.B.; Prytherch, D.R.; Meredith, P.; Schmidt, P.E.; Featherstone, P.I. The Ability of the National Early Warning Score (NEWS) to Discriminate Patients at Risk of Early Cardiac Arrest, Unanticipated Intensive Care Unit Admission, and Death. *Resuscitation* **2013**, *84*, 465–470. [CrossRef]

19. Bilben, B.; Grandal, L.; Søvik, S. National Early Warning Score (NEWS) as an Emergency Department Predictor of Disease Severity and 90-Day Survival in the Acutely Dyspneic Patient—A Prospective Observational Study. *Scand. J. Trauma Resusc. Emerg. Med.* **2016**, *24*, 80. [CrossRef]
20. Chen, L.; Zheng, H.; Chen, L.; Wu, S.; Wang, S. National Early Warning Score in Predicting Severe Adverse Outcomes of Emergency Medicine Patients: A Retrospective Cohort Study. *J. Multidiscip. Healthc.* **2021**, *14*, 2067–2078. [CrossRef]
21. Kiriyama, S.; Kozaka, K.; Takada, T.; Strasberg, S.M.; Pitt, H.A.; Gabata, T.; Hata, J.; Liau, K.H.; Miura, F.; Horiguchi, A.; et al. Tokyo Guidelines 2018: Diagnostic Criteria and Severity Grading of Acute Cholangitis (with Videos). *J. Hepatobiliary Pancreat. Sci.* **2018**, *25*, 17–30. [CrossRef] [PubMed]
22. Kogure, H.; Tsujino, T.; Yamamoto, K.; Mizuno, S.; Yashima, Y.; Yagioka, H.; Kawakubo, K.; Sasaki, T.; Nakai, Y.; Hirano, K.; et al. Fever-Based Antibiotic Therapy for Acute Cholangitis Following Successful Endoscopic Biliary Drainage. *J. Gastroenterol.* **2011**, *46*, 1411–1417. [CrossRef] [PubMed]
23. Kanda, Y. Investigation of the Freely Available Easy-to-Use Software 'EZR' for Medical Statistics. *Bone Marrow Transplant.* **2013**, *48*, 452–458. [CrossRef]
24. Van Lent, A.U.; Bartelsman, J.F.; Tytgat, G.N.; Speelman, P.; Prins, J.M. Duration of Antibiotic Therapy for Cholangitis after Successful Endoscopic Drainage of the Biliary Tract. *Gastrointest. Endosc.* **2002**, *55*, 518–522. [CrossRef]
25. Limmathurotsakul, D.; Netinatsunton, N.; Attasaranya, S.; Ovartlarnporn, B. Su1663 An Open-Labeled, Randomized Controlled Trial Comparing between Short Duration and Standard 14 Days Antibiotic Treatments for Acute Cholangitis in Patients with Common Bile Duct Stone after Successful Endoscopic Biliary Drainage. A Preliminary Report. *Gastrointest. Endosc.* **2014**, *79*, AB251. [CrossRef]
26. Gomi, H.; Takada, T.; Hwang, T.L.; Akazawa, K.; Mori, R.; Endo, I.; Miura, F.; Kiriyama, S.; Matsunaga, N.; Itoi, T.; et al. Updated Comprehensive Epidemiology, Microbiology, and Outcomes Among Patients with Acute Cholangitis. *J. Hepatobiliary Pancreat. Sci.* **2017**, *24*, 310–318. [CrossRef]
27. Doi, A.; Morimoto, T.; Iwata, K. Shorter Duration of Antibiotic Treatment for Acute Bacteraemic Cholangitis with Successful Biliary Drainage: A Retrospective Cohort Study. *Clin. Microbiol. Infect.* **2018**, *24*, 1184–1189. [CrossRef]

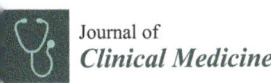

Article

Safe Performance of Track Dilation and Bile Aspiration with ERCP Catheter in EUS-Guided Hepaticogastrostomy with Plastic Stents: A Retrospective Multicenter Study

Ikuhiro Kobori [1,*], Yusuke Hashimoto [2], Taro Shibuki [2], Kei Okumura [2], Masanari Sekine [3], Aki Miyagaki [4], Yoshihiro Sasaki [5], Yuichi Takano [6], Yasumi Katayama [7], Masaru Kuwada [1], Yoshinori Gyotoku [1], Yumi Kusano [1] and Masaya Tamano [1]

1 Department of Gastroenterology, Dokkyo Medical University Saitama Medical Center, Koshigaya 343-8555, Japan
2 Department of Hepatobiliary and Pancreatic Oncology, National Cancer Center Hospital East, Kashiwa 277-8577, Japan
3 Department of Gastroenterology, Jichi Medical University Saitama Medical Center, Saitama 330-0834, Japan
4 Department of Gastroenterology, Toyooka Hospital, Toyooka 668-8501, Japan
5 Department of Gastroenterology, National Organization Disaster Medical Center, Tokyo 190-0014, Japan
6 Department of Gastroenterology, Fujigaoka Hospital, Showa University, Yokohama 227-8501, Japan
7 Endoscopy Center, Dokkyo Medical University Saitama Medical Center, Koshigaya 343-8555, Japan
* Correspondence: viva.s.a.410@gmail.com; Tel.: +81-48-965-1111; Fax: +81-48-965-1169

Abstract: Objectives: Endoscopic-ultrasound-guided hepaticogastrostomy (EUS-HGS) with plastic stent placement is associated with a high incidence of adverse events that may be reduced using an endoscopic retrograde cholangiopancreatography (ERCP) contrast catheter in the track dilation step. In this study, we evaluated the usefulness of track dilation and bile aspiration performed with an ERCP contrast catheter in EUS-HGS with plastic stent placement. Methods: In a multicenter setting, 22 EUS-HGS cases dilated with an ERCP contrast catheter were analyzed retrospectively and compared between a bile aspiration group and no bile aspiration group. Results: Overall, adverse events occurred in three (13.6%) cases of bile leakage, three (13.6%) cases of peritonitis, and one (4.5%) case of bleeding. Comparing patients with and without bile aspiration, 6 of the 11 patients (54.5%) with no bile aspiration had adverse events, whereas only 1 of the 11 patients (9.1%) who had bile aspiration, as much bile as possible, had an adverse event (bleeding). In univariate analysis, the only factor affecting the occurrence of adverse events was bile aspiration whenever possible (odds ratio, 12.0; 95%CI 1.12–128.84). Conclusions: In EUS-HGS with plastic stent placement, track dilation and bile aspiration with an ERCP contrast catheter may be useful in reducing adverse events.

Keywords: endoscopic ultrasonography; endoscopic-ultrasound-guided biliary drainage; endoscopic-ultrasound-guided hepaticogastrostomy; bile aspiration

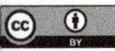

1. Introduction

The endoscopic-ultrasound-guided biliary drainage (EUS-BD) procedure has become widely used in recent years [1–5] but no consensus has yet been established regarding aspects such as puncture site, type of dilator, and type of stent [6–8]. Endoscopic-ultrasound-guided hepaticogastrostomy (EUS-HGS) is an EUS-BD procedure that comprises four steps: bile duct puncture, guidewire passage, track dilation, and stent placement. The occurrence of postoperative adverse events such as bile leakage following EUS-HGS is more frequent in cases with the placement of a plastic stent than in cases where a self-expandable metallic metal stent (SEMS) is used [9]. In the case of an SEMS, even if the track dilation is greater than the outer diameter of the sheath before stent deployment, the stent will eventually expand beyond the dilation diameter and thus prevent bile leakage, whereas a plastic stent is more likely to leak bile when the track is dilated beyond the stent diameter. Therefore, when using plastic stents in EUS-HGS, it is preferable to use a bougie dilator, which dilates equivalently to the stent diameter, rather than a balloon catheter, which dilates beyond the stent diameter. The usefulness of bile aspiration prior to stent placement during EUS-HGS, especially bile aspiration of 10 mL or more, has recently been reported [10]. Although most of the stents in that report were SEMSs, bile aspiration may also be desirable in EUS-HGS with plastic stent placement. To aspirate a large amount of bile, it is necessary to dilate the bile duct with a bougie dilator and then place a regular endoscopic retrograde cholangiopancreatography (ERCP) contrast catheter into the bile duct for aspiration. However, if the pressure in the bile duct remains high, leakage of bile can be expected between dilation and placement of the regular ERCP contrast catheter. Ideally, bile would be aspirated directly using the bougie dilator, but its very thin tip, designed to facilitate tracking, [11] makes it unsuitable for aspiration. One solution to this problem is to use an ERCP contrast catheter. The use of a regular ERCP contrast catheter as the dilation device may reduce procedure time and cost as well as further reduce the risk of biliary leakage, as it eliminates the need to insert a bougie dilator or other dilation device. In this study, we investigated the usefulness of using an ERCP contrast catheter for dilatation and bile aspiration in EUS-HGS with plastic stent placement.

2. Materials and Methods

2.1. Study Design

This was a retrospective multicenter study of patients with biliary obstruction who had undergone EUS-HGS between April 2015 and December 2021 at any of six participating facilities in Japan. The study was approved by the review board at each respective institution and was conducted in accordance with the tenets of the Helsinki Declaration. EUS-HGS was performed according to the indications at each institution, and we retrospectively reviewed patients who underwent track dilation with an ERCP contrast catheter and plastic stent placement (Figure 1). The primary outcome was the rate of adverse events after plastic stent placement. The secondary outcomes were the cause of recurrent biliary obstruction (RBO), time to recurrent biliary obstruction (TRBO), and functional success. RBO was defined as the recurrence of obstructive jaundice and/or cholangitis due to stent occlusion or migration. TRBO was defined as the length of time between stent placement and the occurrence of RBO. Functional success was defined as: (1) a 50% decrease in or normalization of the serum total bilirubin level within 14 days of stent placement; (2) in the case of cholangitis without elevation of the serum total bilirubin level, an improvement of cholangitis. Adverse events other than RBO were categorized as post-procedure complications, which included bile leakage, peritonitis, bleeding, perforation, pancreatitis, cholecystitis, aspiration pneumonia, liver abscess, mediastinal emphysema, and pneumoperitoneum. These complications were categorized as early (within 30 days) or late (at 31 days or later). The time point of adverse events was defined as the point when symptoms associated with these conditions were observed. The adverse events were classified and graded according to the American Society for Gastrointestinal Endoscopy Workshop reports [12]. Peritonitis was diagnosed on the basis of clinical peritoneal inflammation. Bile leakage was defined as the patient presenting with new fluid collection around the EUS-HGS stent outside the stomach and the liver, confirmed by CT (Figure 2).

The study also examined adverse events categorized into two groups: with bile aspiration (as much bile as possible was aspirated) and without bile aspiration (bile was not aspirated prior to plastic stenting). Bile aspiration was performed only at specific study centers. Regardless of the degree of bile duct dilatation (total bilirubin level), bile aspiration was performed starting at a certain date with the expectation of reducing complications.

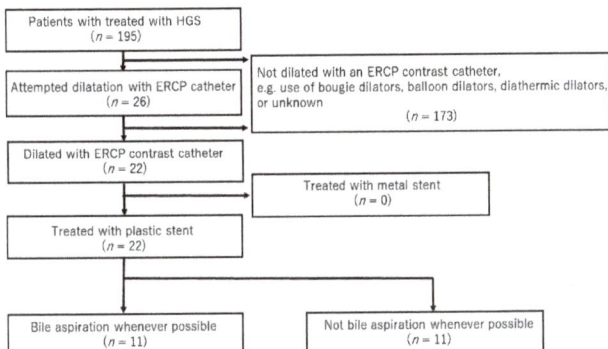

Figure 1. Flowchart of the study design. Abbreviations: ERCP, endoscopic retrograde cholangiopancreatography; HGS, hepaticogastrostomy.

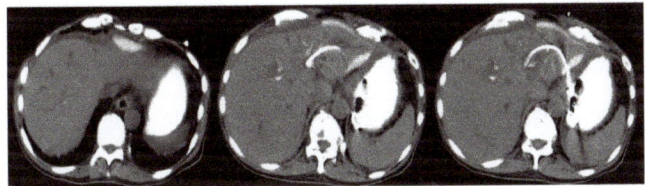

Figure 2. CT scan image showing bile leak. Contrast medium is filling the stomach. Leakage of contrast medium can be seen near the stenting site.

2.2. Patients

Of all patients with biliary obstruction who had undergone EUS-HGS between April 2015 and December 2021, 22 were treated with track dilation by an ERCP contrast catheter and placement of a plastic stent. Biliary obstruction was diagnosed based on the clinical, laboratory, radiographic, and pathological findings. Distal biliary obstruction was defined as a site of stenosis at least 2 cm away from the liver hilum. EUS-HGS was indicated for patients in whom it was difficult to reach the papilla due to gastrointestinal obstruction or surgically altered anatomy, and those in whom it was difficult to cannulate the bile duct even if the papilla was reached. Cases of benign as well as malignant disease were included. Patients who underwent biliary drainage as well as initial drainage were included. Performance status refers to the Eastern Cooperative Oncology Group performance status [13].

2.3. Procedures

We used a linear echoendoscope for EUS-HGS (GF-UCT 240 or GF-UCT 260, Olympus Medical Systems, Tokyo, Japan; EG 580 UT, Fujifilm Corp., Tokyo, Japan). The left lobe of the liver was observed by echoendoscope, and the intrahepatic bile duct was punctured and contrast-enhanced using a 19- or 22-gauge needle. After placement of a guidewire in the bile duct, a tapered-tip single-lumen ERCP contrast catheter (ERCP Catheter, 1.6~2.3 mm, MTW Endoskopie, Wesel, Germany) was introduced to dilate the track, and finally a plastic stent was placed (Figures 3 and 4). In cases where bile was aspirated, the bile was aspirated as much as possible after track dilation with an ERCP catheter, and often more than 20 mL was aspirated. We performed cholangiography after aspirating the bile as much as possible. Then, except for hilar stenosis, after cholangiography was performed, aspiration was performed again until there was no more contrast media, and then a stent was placed. In a case of hilar stenosis, cholangiography was performed, followed by another small volume aspiration, and a stent was placed with contrast remaining. Two types of plastic stents were used: Through & Pass Type-IT (7-Fr, 14 cm, Gadelius Medical, Tokyo, Japan; Figure 5a) and Quick Place V (7-Fr, 11 cm, 15 cm, Olympus Medical Systems, Tokyo, Japan; Figure 5b). The stent length was determined by the cholangiographic findings. Procedure time was calculated from insertion of the echoendoscope into the mouth to its removal. If the track was difficult to dilate with an ERCP contrast catheter, a bougie dilator (ES Dilator, Zeon Medical Co., Tokyo, Japan) was used [11], and the rate of bougie dilator use was additionally studied. Antegrade stent placement was performed using an uncovered SEMS or a plastic stent prior to EUS-HGS stent placement. The decision regarding antegrade stent placement was at the discretion of the endoscopist.

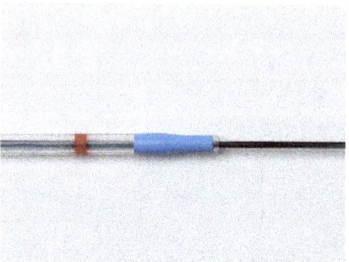

Figure 3. Tapered-tip single-lumen ERCP contrast catheter.

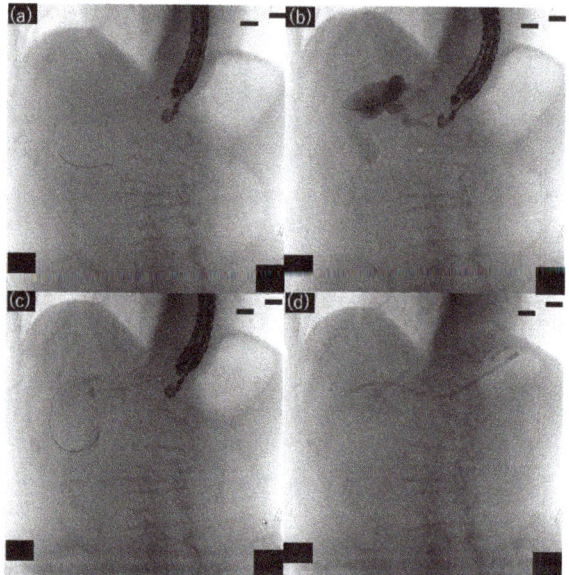

Figure 4. Fluoroscopic images showing hepaticogastrostomy. (**a**) Bile duct puncture and guidewire passage, (**b**) track dilation and cholangiography with an ERCP contrast catheter, (**c**) bile aspiration with an ERCP contrast catheter, (**d**) stent placement.

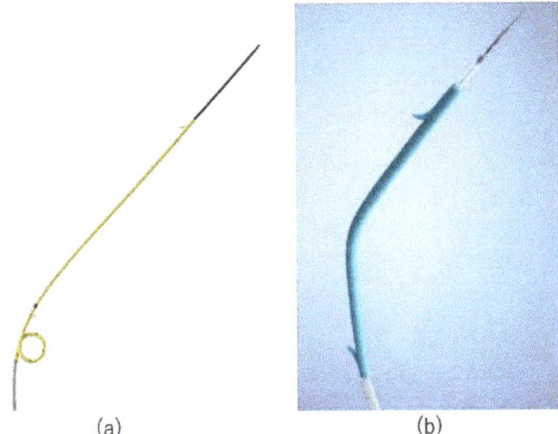

Figure 5. Plastic stent. (**a**) Through & Pass Type-IT (7-Fr, 14 cm, Gadelius Medical, Tokyo, Japan). (**b**) Quick Place V (7-Fr, Olympus Medical Systems, Tokyo, Japan).

2.4. Follow-Up

Patients were followed up at each facility until death or until the date of last known survival; or in the case of benign disease, until the cause of the benign disease was corrected and the EUS-HGS route stent was no longer needed and removed. Computed tomography was performed when adverse events were suspected based on the clinical symptoms or blood tests.

2.5. Statistical Analysis

All statistical analyses were performed using StatFlex Ver. 6 (Artec Inc., Osaka, Japan). TRBO was estimated using the Kaplan–Meier method. Patients who had stent removal or died without RBO were treated as censored cases. Factors affecting adverse events were assessed using univariate logistic regression analysis. Candidate factors affecting adverse events included age, performance status, puncture site, preoperative cholangitis, bile aspiration, antegrade stent placement, and procedure time. $p < 0.05$ was considered to indicate statistical significance.

3. Results

3.1. Patient Characteristics

The patient characteristics are summarized in Table 1. The site of biliary obstruction was distal in 14 patients (63.6%), hilar in 5 patients (22.7%), and anastomotic in 3 patients (13.6%). Four patients (18.2%) had cholangitis prior to the EUS-HGS procedure.

Table 1. Patient characteristics.

Characteristic	Value
Age, y	72 (47–90)
Sex, male/female	12/10
Cause of biliary obstruction	
Gastric cancer	9 (40.9)
Pancreatic cancer	6 (27.3)
Bile duct cancer	3 (13.6)
Duodenal cancer	2 (9.1)
Intrahepatic gallstone	1 (4.5)
Stenosis of choledochojejunostomy	1 (4.5)
Performance Status	

Table 1. Cont.

Characteristic	Value
0	6 (27.3)
1	9 (40.9)
2	2 (9.1)
3	5 (22.7)
Site of biliary obstruction	
Distal	14 (63.6)
Hilar	5 (22.7)
Anastomotic	3 (13.6)
Indication of EUS-HGS	
Difficulty reaching the papilla	12 (54.5)
Surgically altered anatomy	7 (31.8)
Difficulty cannulating the bile duct	3 (13.6)
Presence of cholangitis before EUS-HGS	4 (18.2)

n = 22. Data are expressed as the median (range) or number (%). Continuous variables are presented as the median (range), categorical variables as the absolute number (percentage). Abbreviation: EUS-HGS, endoscopic-ultrasound-guided hepaticogastrostomy.

3.2. Outcomes

Table 2 summarizes the procedure outcomes, and Table 3 summarizes the clinical outcomes. Regarding aspiration of bile prior to plastic stent placement, bile was not aspirated in 11 patients (50.0%), and as much bile as possible was aspirated in 11 patients (50.0%). A conventional dilatation device was used in four patients in whom track dilation was difficult using an ERCP contrast catheter. Track dilation was achieved using an ERCP contrast catheter in 22 of the 26 patients (84.6%).

Table 2. Procedure outcomes.

	Value
Procedure time (min)	45.5 (15–90)
Puncture needle used	
19-gauge	21 (95.5)
22-gauge	1 (4.5)
Puncture site	
B2	15 (68.2)
B3	7 (31.8)
Types of plastic stents	
Through & Pass Type-IT	19 (86.4)
Quick Place V	3 (13.6)
Antegrade stent placement	4 (18.2)
Bile aspiration whenever possible	
No	11 (50)
Yes	11 (50)

n = 22. Data are expressed as the median (range) or number (%). Continuous variables are presented as the median (range), categorical variables as the absolute number (percentage).

Table 3. Clinical outcomes.

	n (%)
Functional success	20 (90.9)
Recurrent biliary obstruction	7 (31.8)
Occlusion	6 (27.3)
Sludge formation	4 (18.2)
Other	2 (9.1)
Migration (toward the gastric side)	1 (4.5)
Adverse events other than recurrent biliary obstruction	

Table 3. Cont.

	n (%)
Early adverse events	7 (31.8)
Bile leakage	3 (13.6)
Peritonitis	3 (13.6)
Bleeding	1 (4.5)
Late adverse events	0 (0)

n = 22.

Functional success was achieved in 20 patients (90.9%). The median duration of observation was 68.5 (range, 12–610) days, and 18 patients (81.8%) died during the observation period. The cause of death was progression of the primary disease in 17 patients and a cause other than the primary disease in 1 patient. No death was attributed to EUS-HGS.

RBO was observed in seven patients (35.0%). The cause of RBO was sludge formation in four patients, migration (toward the gastric side) in one patient, and another cause in two patients. Two patients underwent stent exchange on days 112 and 119, prior to the onset of RBO, and were treated as censored for statistical purposes. Median TRBO was 365 (range, 3–382) days (Figure 6).

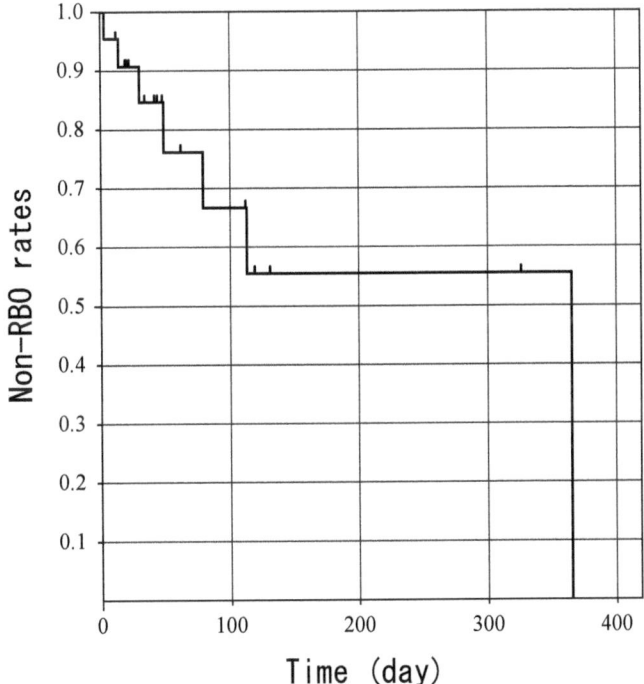

Figure 6. Kaplan–Meier curve of time to recurrent biliary obstruction. The small vertical bars indicate censored patients.

Adverse events other than RBO included bile leakage in three patients (13.6%), peritonitis in three patients (13.6%), and bleeding in one patient (4.5%), all of which were mild, occurred early, and were relieved by conservative treatment. In a comparison of patients with and without bile aspiration prior to plastic stenting, 6 of the 11 patients (54.5%) who did not have bile aspiration had adverse events, whereas only 1 of the 11 patients (9.1%) who had bile aspiration, as much bile as possible, had an adverse event (bleeding). Table 4 summarizes the patient characteristics and outcomes with and without bile aspiration whenever possible. Univariate analyses were performed for factors affecting adverse events (Table 5). Bile aspiration, as much bile as possible, was associated with the occurrence of AEs in the univariate analysis.

Table 4. Patient characteristics and outcomes with and without bile aspiration whenever possible.

Bile Aspiration Whenever Possible	Yes (n = 11)	No (n = 11)
Preprocedural cholangitis (n)	3	1
Procedure time (min)	47 (27–89)	42 (15–90)
Time that the bile aspiration takes (min)	13 (5–20)	
Antegrade stent placement (n)	2	2
Adverse events other than recurrent biliary obstruction (n)	1	6
Bile leakage (n)	0	3
Peritonitis (n)	0	3
Bleeding (n)	1	0

Continuous variables are presented as the median (range), categorical variables as the absolute number.

Table 5. Factors affecting adverse events.

	Univariate Analysis OR (95%CI)	p Value
Age (years)		0.29
<75	1	
≥75	2.86 (0.42–19.65)	
Performance status		0.25
0–1	1	
2–4	0.46 (0.02–2.67)	
Puncture site		0.45
B2	1	
B3	0.48 (0.07–3.19)	
Preprocedural cholangitis		0.75
Yes	1.50 (0.13–17.67)	
No	1	
Bile aspiration whenever possible		0.04
No	12.0 (1.12–128.84)	
Yes	1	
Antegrade stent placement		0.40
Yes	2.60 (0.28–23.81)	
No	1	
Procedure time (min)		0.65
<44.5	1	
≥44.5	1.52 (0.25–9.29)	

Abbreviations: OR, odds ratio; CI, confidence interval.

4. Discussion

Although the use of plastic stents in EUS-HGS has been reported to carry risk for bile leakage [9], the results of our study suggest that biliary aspiration prior to plastic stent placement may considerably reduce the risk of bile leakage and other adverse events. The usefulness of biliary aspiration in EUS-HGS has been reported [10]. The paper reported that biliary aspiration of 10 mL or more during HGS reduces adverse events, and the stents used were metallic stents in 70% and plastic stents in 30% of cases. We believe we have demonstrated that similar results can be obtained even when limited to EUS-HGS with plastic stents. If bile aspiration is performed with an ERCP contrast catheter after track dilation when intraductal biliary pressure is high, bile may leak out during device exchange, and, therefore, the timing of bile aspiration should be simultaneous with track dilation. However, as bile aspiration is difficult to achieve with specialized dilatation devices or balloon catheters with tapered tips, it makes the most sense to use an ERCP contrast catheter that can dilate the track and aspirate bile at the same time. Although it is possible to aspirate bile with a puncture needle prior to track dilation, it is anticipated that a large amount of bile aspiration will cause the bile duct to narrow, which may cause the puncture needle to be pulled out of the bile duct and subsequent guidewire insertion to be difficult. In the present study, we were able to dilate the track and aspirate bile with the ERCP contrast catheter in 84.6% of patients, which is considered a good result. It is worth attempting this technique before using a dedicated fistula-dilating device. We are working to improve tracking of the ERCP contrast catheter using new catheters with a firm, straight tip and by the operator applying slight tension to the guidewire when tracking with the ERCP contrast catheter. In addition, the bile duct should be punctured from B2 whenever possible, as this allows the guidewire and instruments to be inserted in a straight line and improves tracking performance. In the present study, puncture was from B2 in 15 patients (68.2%), which is a large number.

Unlike metal stents, plastic stents do not shorten. There are also plastic stents available for EUS-HGS with pigtail-type stent ends on the gastric side [14], which minimizes the possibility of serious adverse events such as gastric stent end migration into the abdominal cavity [15]. In the present study, there was no instance of gastric stent end migration into the abdominal cavity. Shorter stent patency is a concern in EUS-HGS with plastic stents compared to metal stents [1,16]. In the majority of cases, however, the stent occlusion occurs when the fistula has already formed, and unlike metal stents with uncovered stent ends on the liver side [17], the stent can be removed and replaced with a new stent in the event of stent occlusion. Even in the event of stent occlusion, it is often not a clinical or technical problem, as the stent can be safely replaced. In addition, as bile aspiration during EUS-HGS may significantly control adverse events, it appears that EUS-HGS with a plastic stent is suitable for the purpose of ensuring safe fistula formation. In patients who undergo transpapillary bile duct stenting using the usual ERCP technique, periodic stent replacement before RBO is often performed and is considered useful in actual clinical practice, especially in cases of hilar stenosis. In the EUS-HGS route, periodic replacement of the plastic stent before RBO may be also an option.

EUS-HGS using metal stents with a thin delivery system that eliminates the track dilation procedure has recently been reported in many cases [18] and is expected to reduce the adverse events associated with shorter examination time. However, it is difficult to perform bile aspiration before stenting with this technique and caution is required, especially in cases of cholangitis, because undrained infected bile may remain and cause prolonged cholangitis if the metal stenting results in obstruction of the bile duct regional branch [19]. Based on the present results, we believe that stent placement after bile aspiration is desirable. However, track dilation with an ERCP contrast catheter was difficult in a small number of our cases, and we hope that a dedicated EUS-HGS device that facilitates track dilation and allows bile aspiration will be introduced in the future.

There are several limitations to this study, including its small sample size and retrospective study design. Therefore, selection bias may not be excluded. Some adverse events may have been missed because CT was not performed in all patients on the day after EUS-HGS. The exact amount of bile aspirated is unknown because there is no accurate description of the amount of bile aspirated. It is impossible to give a clear figure for how much should be aspirated, which may reduce reproducibility. In addition, the success rate of track dilation by ERCP contrast catheter may be lower than the present results because a dedicated fistula dilation device might have been used from the beginning if we had expected that track dilation by ERCP contrast catheter would be difficult. Further verification in randomized controlled trials is required in the future.

5. Conclusions

In EUS-HGS with plastic stent placement, track dilation and bile aspiration with an ERCP contrast catheter may be useful in reducing adverse events. Although it cannot be applied to all cases, it can be applied to quite a large number of cases, and we believe it is worth a try.

Author Contributions: Conceptualization, I.K. and Y.H.; methodology, I.K. and Y.H.; formal analysis, Y.K. (Yasumi Katayama); investigation, I.K., Y.H., T.S., K.O., M.S., A.M., Y.S., Y.T., M.K., Y.G., Y.K. (Yumi Kusano) and M.T.; data curation, I.K.; writing—original draft preparation, I.K.; writing—review and editing, I.K.; supervision, Y.H. and Y.K. (Yasumi Katayama); project administration, I.K. All authors have read and agreed to the published version of the manuscript.

Funding: This research received no external funding.

Institutional Review Board Statement: The study was conducted according to the guidelines of the Declaration of Helsinki and approved by the Institutional Review Board of Dokkyo Medical University Saitama Medical Center (approval No. 20131, approval date 24 February 2021) and the review boards at each institution.

Informed Consent Statement: As this is a retrospective study using information contained in medical charts and computerized records, informed consent was obtained from all individual participants included in the study through the opt-out method on our hospital website and in-hospital posting. The ethics committee approved this.

Data Availability Statement: Not applicable.

Acknowledgments: We would like to thank all of the patients involved in this study.

Conflicts of Interest: The authors declare no conflict of interest.

References

1. Isayama, H.; Nakai, Y.; Itoi, T.; Yasuda, I.; Kawakami, H.; Ryozawa, S.; Kitano, M.; Irisawa, A.; Katanuma, A.; Hara, K.; et al. Clinical practice guidelines for safe performance of endoscopic ultrasound/ultrasonography-Guided biliary drainage: 2018. *J. Hepato-Biliary-Pancreat. Sci.* **2019**, *26*, 249–269. [CrossRef] [PubMed]
2. Giovannini, M.; Moutardier, V.; Pesenti, C.; Bories, E.; Lelong, B.; Delpero, J. Endoscopic ultrasound-Guided bilioduodenal anastomosis: A new technique for biliary drainage. *Endoscopy* **2001**, *33*, 898–900. [CrossRef] [PubMed]
3. Itoi, T.; Sofuni, A.; Itokawa, F.; Tsuchiya, T.; Kurihara, T.; Ishii, K.; Tsuji, S.; Ikeuchi, N.; Umeda, J.; Moriyasu, F.; et al. Endoscopic ultrasonography-Guided biliary drainage. *J. Hepato-Biliary-Pancreat. Sci.* **2010**, *17*, 611–616. [CrossRef] [PubMed]
4. Baars, J.E.; Kaffes, A.J.; Saxena, P. EUS-Guided biliary drainage: A comprehensive review of the literature. *Endosc. Ultrasound* **2018**, *7*, 4–9. [CrossRef] [PubMed]
5. Adler, D.; Dhindsa, B.; Mashiana, H.; Dhaliwal, A.; Mohan, B.; Jayaraj, M.; Sayles, H.; Singh, S.; Ohning, G.; Bhat, I. EUS-Guided biliary drainage. A systematic review and meta-Analysis. *Endosc. Ultrasound* **2020**, *9*, 101–109. [CrossRef] [PubMed]
6. Minaga, K.; Ogura, T.; Shiomi, H.; Imai, H.; Hoki, N.; Takenaka, M.; Nishikiori, H.; Yamashita, Y.; Hisa, T.; Kato, H.; et al. Comparison of the efficacy and safety of endoscopic ultrasound-Guided choledochoduodenostomy and hepaticogastrostomy for malignant distal biliary obstruction: Multicenter, randomized, clinical trial. *Dig. Endosc.* **2019**, *31*, 575–582. [CrossRef] [PubMed]
7. Sanz, M.D.B.; Nájera-Muñoz, R.; de la Serna-Higuera, C.; Fuentes-Valenzuela, E.; Fanjul, I.; Chavarría, C.; García-Alonso, F.J.; Sanchez-Ocana, R.; Carbajo, A.Y.; Bazaga, S.; et al. Lumen apposing metal stents versus tubular self-Expandable metal stents for endoscopic ultrasound-Guided choledochoduodenostomy in malignant biliary obstruction. *Surg. Endosc.* **2021**, *35*, 6754–6762. [CrossRef] [PubMed]
8. Dhir, V.; Bale, A. EUS-Guided Hepatico-Gastrostomy: To Dilate or Not to Dilate? *Dig. Dis. Sci.* **2022**. [CrossRef]
9. Khashab, M.A.; Messallam, A.A.; Penas, I.; Nakai, Y.; Modayil, R.J.; De la Serna, C.; Hara, K.; El Zein, M.; Stavropoulos, S.N.; Perez-Miranda, M.; et al. International multicenter comparative trial of transluminal EUS-Guided biliary drainage via hepatogastrostomy vs. choledochoduodenostomy approaches. *Endosc. Int. Open* **2016**, *4*, E175–E181. [CrossRef] [PubMed]
10. Ishiwatari, H.; Satoh, T.; Sato, J.; Kaneko, J.; Matsubayashi, H.; Yabuuchi, Y.; Kishida, Y.; Yoshida, M.; Ito, S.; Kawata, N.; et al. Bile aspiration during EUS-Guided hepaticogastrostomy is associated with lower risk of postprocedural adverse events: A retrospective single-Center study. *Surg. Endosc.* **2021**, *35*, 6836–6845. [CrossRef]
11. Kanno, Y.; Ito, K.; Koshita, S.; Ogawa, T.; Masu, K.; Masaki, Y.; Noda, Y. Efficacy of a newly developed dilator for endoscopic ultrasound-Guided biliary drainage. *World J. Gastrointest. Endosc.* **2017**, *9*, 304–309. [CrossRef] [PubMed]
12. Cotton, P.B.; Eisen, G.M.; Aabakken, L.; Baron, T.H.; Hutter, M.M.; Jacobson, B.C.; Vargo, J.J. A lexicon for endoscopic adverse events: Report of an ASGE workshop. *Gastrointest. Endosc.* **2010**, *71*, 446–454. [CrossRef] [PubMed]
13. Oken, M.M.; Creech, R.H.; Tormey, D.C.; Horton, J.; Davis, T.E.; McFadden, E.T.; Carbone, P.P. Toxicity and response criteria of the Eastern Cooperative Oncology Group. *Am. J. Clin. Oncol.* **1982**, *5*, 649–655. [CrossRef] [PubMed]

14. Umeda, J.; Itoi, T.; Tsuchiya, T.; Sofuni, A.; Itokawa, F.; Ishii, K.; Tsuji, S.; Ikeuchi, N.; Kamada, K.; Tanaka, R.; et al. A newly designed plastic stent for EUS-Guided hepaticogastrostomy: A prospective preliminary feasibility study (with videos). *Gastrointest. Endosc.* **2015**, *82*, 390–396.e392. [CrossRef] [PubMed]
15. Martins, F.P.; Rossini, L.G.; Ferrari, A.P. Migration of a covered metallic stent following endoscopic ultrasound-Guided hepaticogastrostomy: Fatal complication. *Endoscopy* **2010**, *42*, E126–E127. [CrossRef] [PubMed]
16. Harai, S.; Hijioka, S.; Nagashio, Y.; Ohba, A.; Maruki, Y.; Sone, M.; Saito, Y.; Okusaka, T.; Fukasawa, M.; Enomoto, N. Usefulness of the laser-Cut, fully covered, self-Expandable metallic stent for endoscopic ultrasound-Guided hepaticogastrostomy. *J. Hepato-Biliary-Pancreat. Sci.* **2022**. [CrossRef] [PubMed]
17. Nakai, Y.; Isayama, H.; Yamamoto, N.; Matsubara, S.; Ito, Y.; Sasahira, N.; Hakuta, R.; Umefune, G.; Takahara, N.; Hamada, T.; et al. Safety and effectiveness of a long, partially covered metal stent for endoscopic ultrasound-Guided hepaticogastrostomy in patients with malignant biliary obstruction. *Endoscopy* **2016**, *48*, 1125–1128. [CrossRef] [PubMed]
18. Park, D.H.; Lee, T.H.; Paik, W.H.; Choi, J.-H.; Song, T.J.; Lee, S.S.; Seo, D.-W.; Lee, S.K.; Kim, M.-H. Feasibility and safety of a novel dedicated device for one-Step EUS-Guided biliary drainage: A randomized trial. *J. Gastroenterol. Hepatol.* **2015**, *30*, 1461–1466. [CrossRef] [PubMed]
19. Hara, K.; Yamao, K.; Mizuno, N.; Hijioka, S.; Imaoka, H.; Tajika, M.; Tanaka, T.; Ishihara, M.; Okuno, N.; Hieda, N.; et al. Endoscopic ultrasonography-Guided biliary drainage: Who, when, which, and how? *World J. Gastroenterol.* **2016**, *22*, 1297–1303. [CrossRef] [PubMed]

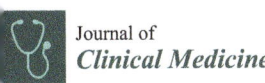

Article

The Feasibility of Whole-Liver Drainage with a Novel 8 mm Fully Covered Self-Expandable Metal Stent Possessing an Ultra-Slim Introducer for Malignant Hilar Biliary Obstructions

Saburo Matsubara *, Keito Nakagawa, Kentaro Suda, Takeshi Otsuka, Masashi Oka and Sumiko Nagoshi

Department of Gastroenterology and Hepatology, Saitama Medical Center, Saitama Medical University, Saitama 350-8550, Japan
* Correspondence: saburom@saitama-med.ac.jp; Tel.: +81-49-228-3400 (ext. 7839); Fax: +81-49-226-5284

Abstract: Background: In the case of an unresectable malignant hilar biliary obstruction (MHBO), the optimal drainage method has not yet been established. Recently, an 8 mm, fully covered, self-expandable metal stent (FCSEMS) with an ultra-slim introducer has become available. In this article, the results of whole-liver drainage tests using this novel FCSEMS for MHBO are reported. Methods: Unresectable MHBOs up to Bismuth IIIa with strictures limited to the secondary branches were eligible. The proximal end of the stent was placed in such a way as to avoid blocking the side branches, and the distal end was placed above the papilla when possible. Consecutive patients treated between April 2017 and January 2021 were retrospectively analyzed. The technical and functional success rates, rates and causes of recurrent biliary obstruction (RBO), time to RBO (TRBO), revision for RBO, and adverse events (AEs) were evaluated. Results: Eleven patients (Bismuth I/II/IIIa: 1/7/3) were enrolled. Two stents were placed in nine patients and three were placed in two patients. Both the technical and functional success rates were 100%. RBO occurred in four (36%) patients due to sludge formation. Revision was performed for three patients, with the successful removal of all stents. The median TRBO was 187 days, and no late AEs other than the RBO occurred. Regarding the distal position of the stent, the RBO rate was significantly lower (14.3% vs. 75%, $p = 0.041$) and the cumulative TRBO was significantly longer (median TRBO: not reached vs. 80 days, $p = 0.031$) in the case of the placement above the papilla than the placement across the papilla. Conclusion: For unresectable MHBOs of Bismuth I, II, and IIIa, whole-liver drainage with a novel 8 mm FCSEMS possessing an ultra-slim introducer was feasible and potentially safe, with favorable stent patency. Placement above the papilla might be preferable to placement across the papilla.

Keywords: malignant hilar biliary obstruction; endoscopic biliary drainage; fully covered self-expandable metal stent

1. Introduction

Endoscopic retrograde cholangiopancreatography (ERCP) is the gold standard for the drainage of unresectable malignant hilar biliary obstructions (MHBOs) [1–3]. Although there have been a number of studies regarding the type of stent and the drainage area, the optimal drainage method has not yet been established [4–7]. Uncovered self-expandable metal stents (UCSEMSs) have a longer patency period than plastic stents (PSs) due to their larger diameter [7,8], but recurrent biliary obstruction (RBO) can still often occur because of recent advances in chemotherapy that have prolonged survival. It is problematic that UCSEMSs cannot be removed, as this can make revision difficult when RBO occurs.

Fully covered self-expandable metal stents (FCSEMSs) are removable and potentially have a longer patency period than UCSEMSs through the prevention of tumor ingrowth, whereas their placement across the side branches may result in liver abscesses [9]. In recent years, several retrospective studies have been performed using thinner, 6 mm FCSEMSs. However, the development of liver abscesses could not be eliminated, and the patency

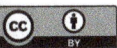

was not satisfactory [10,11]. When FCSEMSs are placed in the hilar region, it seems that whole-liver drainage using multiple stents should be performed to avoid blocking the side branches [9]. Nevertheless, the introducer of the FCSEMSs used in these studies was 8-Fr, making it difficult to implant multiple stents, particularly more than three.

Recently, a novel FCSEMS (HANAROSTENT Benefit; Boston Scientific Japan, Tokyo, Japan) with a 5.9-Fr ultra-slim introducer attached to a 0.025-inch guidewire was launched (Figure 1). Two introducers can be inserted into the scope channel simultaneously, facilitating the placement of multiple stents side by side. Furthermore, the stent diameter is 8 mm, which might provide a better patency than 6 mm FCSEMSs [9]. This study was conducted in order to evaluate the safety and efficacy of whole-liver drainage using this novel 8 mm FCSEMS in patients with unresectable MHBO.

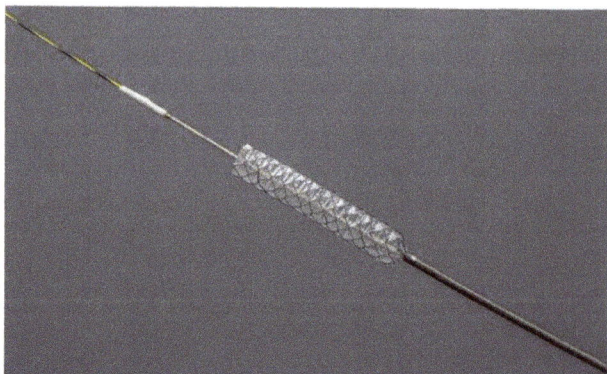

Figure 1. HANAROSTENT Benefit (Boston Scientific Japan, Tokyo, Japan). The fully covered, braided-type, self-expandable metal stent of 8 mm diameter with an ultra-slim introducer of 5.9-Fr. (image provided by Boston Scientific Japan).

2. Patients and Methods

2.1. Patients

This was a single center, retrospective cohort study using prospectively collected ERCP data, conducted at Saitama Medical Center, Saitama Medical University. We extracted data on consecutive cases, in whom whole-liver drainage was attempted using the 8 mm FCSEMS between April 2017 and January 2021. Eligibility for this procedure included unresectable MHBO of Bismuth types [12] I, II, and IIIa, in which strictures were limited to the secondary branches (the main trunk of the right anterior branch and right posterior branch). Bismuth IV and IIIa with strictures beyond the third branches were excluded because they require more than four stents for whole-liver drainage. More than four 8 mm SEMSs placed side by side could be dangerous because of the overexpansion of the bile ducts; thus, the number of stents was limited to three. In addition, Bismuth IIIb was excluded because the secondary branch of the left lobe (segment 4) is usually thin and short, making it difficult to place the 8 mm FCSEMS in the appropriate position. Patients with a surgically altered anatomy, excepting Billroth I reconstruction, were excluded. Written informed consent for the procedure was obtained from all patients prior to ERCP. The data acquisition and analysis were performed in compliance with protocols and approved by the Ethical Committee of Saitama Medical Center, Saitama Medical University (ethical approval number 2534). Informed consent for the present study was withdrawn by opting out.

2.2. Procedures

During ERCP, patients were sedated with midazolam and pethidine hydrochloride while in the prone position. A therapeutic duodenoscope (TJF-260V or TJF-Q290V; Olympus Medical Systems, Tokyo, Japan) with a 4.2 mm accessory channel was used for all patients.

A standard ERCP catheter with a 0.025-inch guidewire (EndSelector; Boston Scientific Japan, or VisiGlide2; Olympus Medical Systems) was applied for the biliary cannulation and passage through the stricture to access the target branch. If the desired branch could not be approached, a 0.025-inch hydrophilic guidewire (Radifocus; Terumo Cop., Tokyo, Japan) was employed.

Prior to the stent deployment, 0.025-inch guidewires were placed in all the target branches. In the case of Bismuth I or II, two introducers were inserted simultaneously into the bilateral hepatic ducts, and stents were released one by one to ensure that their proximal ends did not exceed both hepatic ducts (Figure 2). In the case of Bismuth IIIa, three stents were placed in the main trunk of the right anterior branch, the main trunk of the right posterior branch, and the left hepatic duct. For the placement of three stents, since three introducers cannot be inserted simultaneously, one stent was placed first, and then the remaining two introducers were inserted simultaneously. This is because if two stents were placed first, it would be difficult to insert the third introducer. Finally, two stents were released one by one, taking care not to block the side branches (Figure 3). The stents were placed above the papilla if the distal end of the stricture was more than 2 cm from the papilla; otherwise, the stents were placed across the papilla. Stent lengths of 60 mm, 80 mm, 100 mm, and 120 mm were available, and the appropriate length was selected for each case. In cases where the stents were placed across the papilla, endoscopic sphincterotomy was performed.

At the end of the procedure, a catheter was inserted into all the stents and contrast imaging was performed to ensure that all the branches were contrasted.

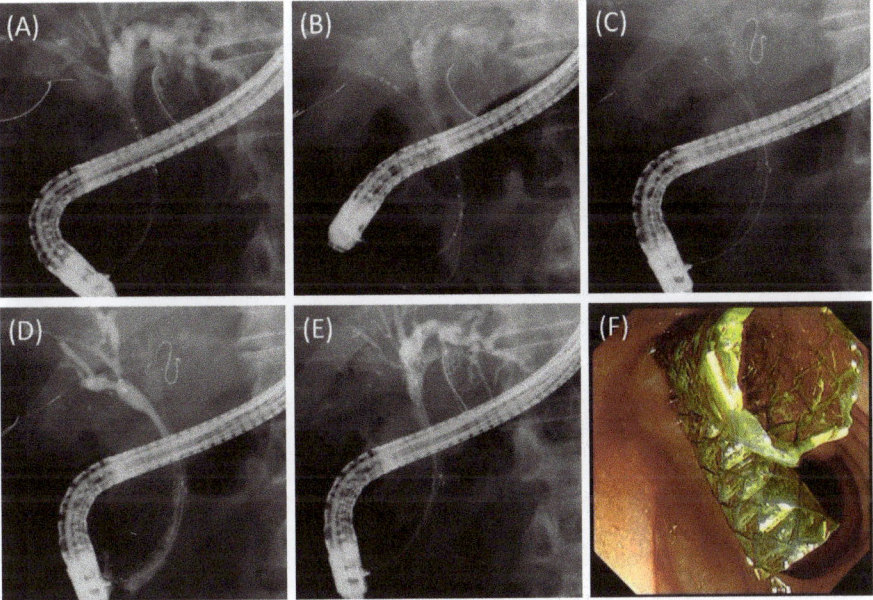

Figure 2. Deployment of two 8 mm FCSEMSs. (**A**) Two introducers were simultaneously inserted into the bile duct. (**B**) One stent was deployed in the left hepatic duct across the papilla. (**C**) Another stent was deployed in the right hepatic duct across the papilla. (**D**) Cholangiography after stent placement depicted all intrahepatic branches of the right hepatic lobe. (**E**) Cholangiography after stent placement depicted all intrahepatic branches of the left hepatic lobe. (**F**) Endoscopic view of two stents across the papilla.

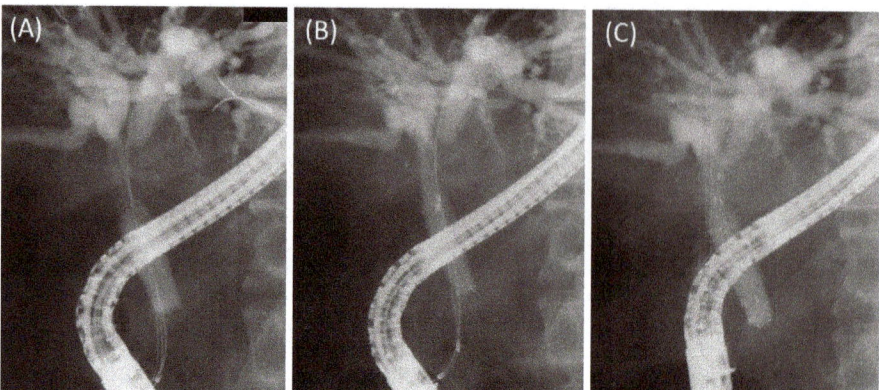

Figure 3. Deployment of three 8 mm FCSEMSs. (**A**) After placing three guidewires in the right anterior, right posterior, and left lateral branches, one introducer was inserted into the right posterior branch. (**B**) Following stent placement in the right posterior branch above the papilla, two introducers were inserted though the side of the first stent. (**C**) Finally, three stents were placed above the papilla without blocking the side branches.

2.3. Outcome Measures and Definitions

We evaluated the technical success rate, functional success rate, early (up to 14 days) and late adverse events (AEs), RBO rate, causes of RBO, time to RBO (TRBO), methods and success rate of the revision for RBO, and survival. Subgroup analyses of the stent position (above or across the papilla) and timing (with or without prior RBO) were also performed in regard to the RBO. Technical success was defined as the placement of all the stents in the intended positions. AEs were defined and graded according to the lexicon of the American Society for Gastrointestinal Endoscopy [13]. A liver abscess was defined as a new fluid collection in the liver upon imaging, with fever. The definitions of the functional success rate and RBO were in accordance with the TOKYO criteria 2014 [14]. The TRBO was defined as the time from the placement of the 8 mm FCSEMSs to RBO occurrence.

2.4. Statistical Analyses

Descriptive continuous variables were presented as numbers (percentages) or medians (ranges). Statistical comparisons were performed with Fisher's exact test for discrete variables and with the Mann–Whitney U test for continuous variables. The Kaplan–Meier method was used to estimate the cumulative TRBO and overall survival (OS). Deaths without RBO were treated as censored at the time of death in TRBO. The log-rank test was used to compare the TRBO in the subgroup analyses, and p-values of 0.05 or less were considered statistically significant. The follow-up data were gathered until November 2021. All statistical analyses were performed with EZR Ver. 1.52 (Saitama Medical Center, Jichi Medical University, Saitama, Japan) [15], which is a graphical user interface for R (the R Foundation for Statistical Computing, Vienna, Austria).

3. Results

3.1. Patient Characteristics

Eleven patients were enrolled in this study. Causes of MHBO included gallbladder cancer in four patients, bile duct cancer in four patients, pancreatic cancer in one patient, lymph node metastasis from colon cancer in one patient, and malignant lymphoma in one patient, as shown in Table 1. In terms of the Bismuth classification, type II was the most common, with seven cases, followed by three cases of type IIIa and one case of type I. Bismuth type I is a pancreatic body cancer involving the perihilar region. Four patients underwent whole-liver drainage with 8 mm FCSEMSs at index ERCP, while the other seven patients had previously undergone biliary drainage with PSs, naso-biliary tubes (NBTs), or other FCSEMSs. Of these seven patients, four had experienced RBO prior to the placement of the 8 mm FCSEMSs.

Table 1. Patient characteristics.

Age, years	81 (60–85)
Sex, male	9 (81.8)
Primary cancer	
Gallbladder	4 (36.4)
Bile duct	4 (36.4)
Pancreas	1 (9.1)
Colon	1 (9.1)
Malignant lymphoma	1 (9.1)
Bismuth classification	
I	1 (9.1)
II	7 (63.6)
IIIa	3 (27.3)
Prior drainage	7 (63.6)
Prior RBO	4 (36.4)
Chemotherapy	6 (54.5)

Numbers are shown as numbers (%) or medians (ranges).

3.2. Details and Outcomes of the Procedures

Table 2 shows the details and outcomes of the procedures. In one case of Bismuth IIIa, cholangiography showed that communication was preserved between the right anterior and posterior branches; thus, two stents were placed in the bilateral hepatic ducts. Therefore, the placement of two stents was attempted in nine patients, and the placement of three stents was attempted in the remaining two patients, which were successful in all cases. Functional success was achieved in all cases. Stents were placed above the papilla in seven patients and across the papilla in four patients. The dilation of the stricture with an 8 mm balloon catheter was required in one patient subjected to three-stent placement. Early AEs developed in two patients with mild pancreatitis, which were resolved conventionally.

Table 2. Procedure details and outcomes.

Technical success	11 (100)
Functional success	11 (100)
CBD diameter, mm	8 (6–12)
Number of stents	
2	9 (81.8)
3	2 (18.2)
Stent length	
60 mm	12
80 mm	11
100 mm	1
Stent position	
Above the papilla	7 (63.6)
Across the papilla	4 (36.4)
Dilation of the stricture	1 (9.1)
Procedure time, mins	62 (30–84)
Early Aes	
Pancreatitis (mild)	2 (18.2)

Numbers are shown as numbers (%) or medians (ranges). CBD, common bile duct; AE, adverse event.

3.3. Long-Term Outcomes

Long-term outcomes of the study patients are shown in Table 3. The median follow-up period (range) was 207 days (47–378 days). RBO due to sludge occurred in four patients. Of these, revision was performed in three patients (two with across-the-papilla placement, one with above-the-papilla placement), while one patient did not undergo revision due to his poor general condition caused by the progression of the primary cancer. In the revision, all stents were successfully removed using rat-tooth forceps or a snare through the accessory channel, even in the case with above-the-papilla placement (Figure 4). The median TRBO (95% CI, confidence interval) was 187 days (49 days—NA, not applicable).

Table 3. Long-term outcomes.

Follow-up period, days	207 (47–378)
RBO	
All pts (*n* = 11)	4 (36.4)
Pts with stents above the papilla (*n* = 7)/across the papilla (*n* = 4)	1 (14.3)/3 (75)
Pts without prior RBO (*n* = 7)/with RBO (*n* = 4)	1 (14.3)/3 (75)
Causes of RBO	
Sludge	4
TRBO, days (95% CI)	
All pts (*n* = 11)	187 (49—NA)
Pts with stents above the papilla (*n* = 7)/across the papilla (*n* = 4)	NA (131—NA)/80 (49—NA)
Pts without prior RBO (*n* = 7)/with RBO (*n* = 4)	NA (187—NA)/80 (49—NA)
Revision for RBO	3 (27.3)
Exchange for 8 mm FCSEMSs	2
Exchange for NBTs	1
Late AEs other than RBO	0
OS, days (95% CI)	275 (82—NA)

Numbers are shown as numbers (%) or medians (ranges). RBO, recurrent biliary obstruction; Pt, patient; TRBO, time to recurrent biliary obstruction; NA, not applicable; FCSEMS, fully covered self-expandable metal stent; NBT, naso-biliary tube; AE, adverse event; OS, overall survival.

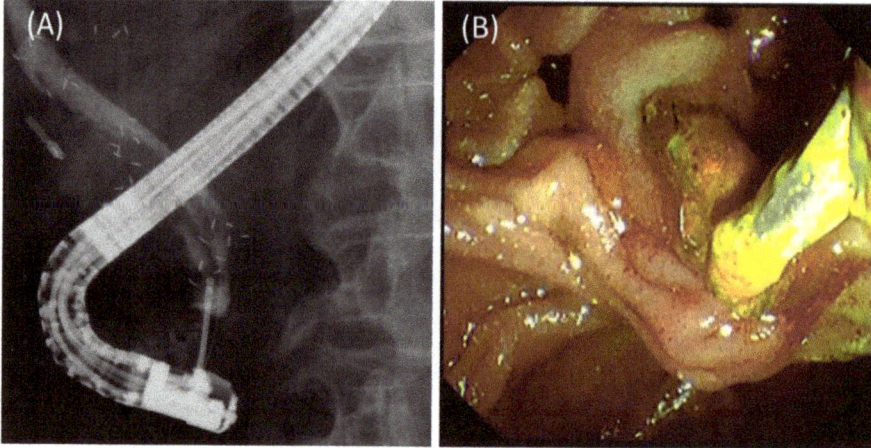

Figure 4. Revision for stent occlusion due to sludge in the case of three stent placements above the papilla. (**A**) Rat-tooth forceps were inserted into the bile duct and used to grasp the distal end of one stent. (**B**) Endoscopic view of the retrieval of the stent, grasped by the forceps.

In the subgroup analyses, the RBO rate was significantly lower (14.3% vs. 75%, $p = 0.041$) and the cumulative TRBO was significantly longer (median TRBO (95% CI): NA (131 days—NA) vs. 80 days (49 days—NA), $p = 0.031$) in the case of the above-the-papilla placement than in the across-the-papilla placement. Regarding prior RBO, the RBO rate was significantly lower (14.3% vs. 75%, $p = 0.041$) and the cumulative TRBO was significantly longer (median TRBO (95% CI): NA (187 days—NA) vs. 80 days (49 days—NA), $p = 0.005$) in patients without prior RBO than in those with prior RBO. There were no late AEs other than RBO, including stent migration.

During the study period, seven patients (63.6%) died due to the progression of the primary cancer. The median OS (95% CI) was 275 days (82 days—NA). Kaplan–Meier curves for the cumulative TRBO and OS are shown in Figure 5.

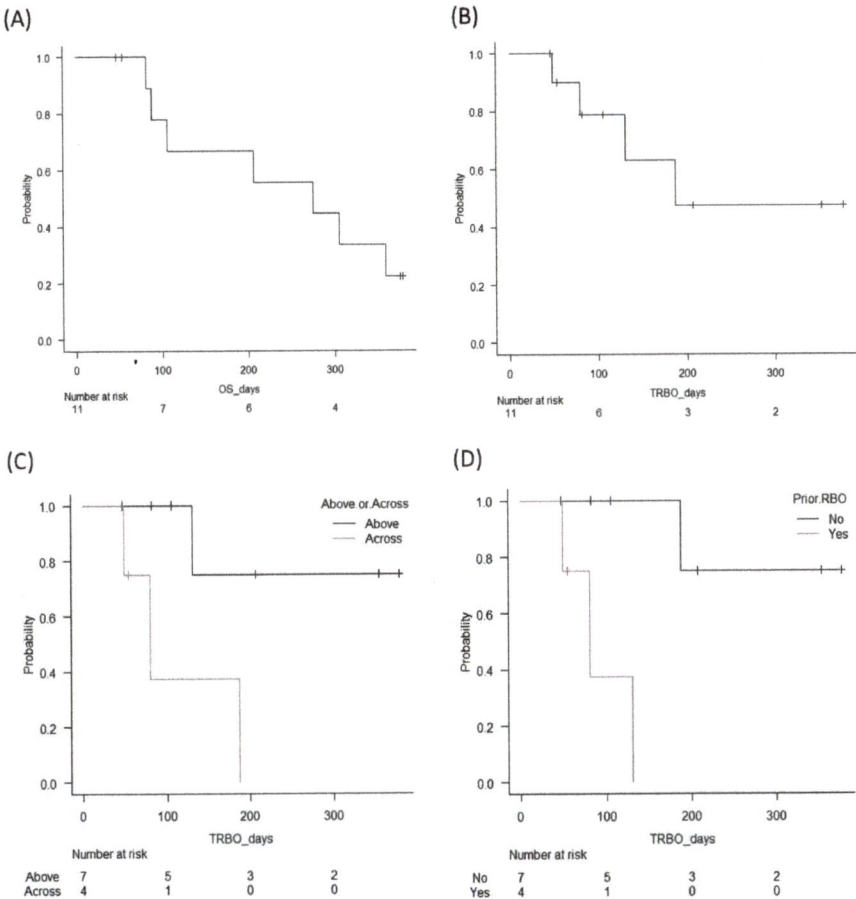

Figure 5. Kaplan–Meier curves for the stent patency and survival. (**A**) Overall survival (OS). Median OS was 275 days. (**B**) Time to recurrent obstruction (TRBO). Median TRBO was 187 days. (**C**) Comparison of TRBO in above and across the papilla placements. Median TRBO was significantly longer (not applicable vs. 80 days, $p = 0.031$) in above-the-papilla placement than the across-the-papilla placement. (**D**) Comparison of TRBO in cases with or without prior RBO. Median TRBO was significantly longer (not applicable vs. 80 days, $p = 0.005$) in patients without prior RBO than in those with prior RBO.

4. Discussion

In the present study, whole-liver drainage with novel 8 mm FCSMESs for unresectable MHBOs of Bismuth type I, II, or IIIa was feasible and safe and yielded a reasonably favorable TRBO of six months. In addition, it was shown that TRBO was significantly longer in the case of the above-the-papilla placement than in the across-the-papilla placement.

In the case of palliative drainage for unresectable MHBOs, UCSMESs have been shown to have a longer patency than PSs [7,8]. In terms of the drainage area, it has been shown that drainage of more than 50% of the liver volume is associated with not only stent patency but also a better prognosis [16], and some recent studies, including an RCT, have shown that bilateral drainage is superior to unilateral drainage for stent patency [4,8]. Given recent improvements in the performance of UCSEMSs, bilateral drainage using UCSEMSs is considered the current standard of care [17,18]. However, since UCSEMSs cannot be removed, revision, with respect to multiple implanted UCSEMSs, in complex MHBO is often problematic when RBO occurs. It is also often impossible to access the undrained area where cholangitis develops. In the case of chemotherapy, it is important to avoid the interruption of chemotherapy due to RBO or cholangitis so as to maintain the treatment intensity. In addition, if conversion to surgery becomes possible after the lesion shrinks, unremovable UCSEMSs may be a hindrance to surgery. For these reasons, there are those who believe that it is better to use PSs instead of UCSEMSs for patients undergoing chemotherapy and to replace the stent periodically [19–21].

However, the increased number of ERCPs is problematic in terms of the patient burden and cost. Therefore, some retrospective studies were conducted using removable 6 mm FCSEMSs, expected to show a longer patency than PSs. Inoue et al. reported the application of 6 mm FCSMESs to 30 patients with Bismuth II-IV MHBO, with technical success in 28 cases (93%). One stent was placed in 10 patients and two were placed in 18 patients, with median TRBOs of 152 days and 142 days, respectively. Liver abscesses were observed in two patients (7%), and the stent was removed in one patient [10]. Yoshida et al. performed 16 procedures of 6 mm FCSMES placement in 10 patients with Bismuth II-IV MHBO, with technical success in 15 patients (94%), and two stents were placed in all the patients. The median TRBO was 113 days, and liver abscesses were observed in two patients (13%) [11]. The stent introducers used in these studies were as thick as 8-Fr, which made it impossible, in some cases, to insert a second stent even after the balloon dilation of the stricture. On the other hand, the introducer of the 8 mm FCSEMS was as thin as 5.9-Fr, facilitating successful stent placement in all patients, including three stents. The dilation of the stricture was performed in only one case. Liver abscess is a serious life-threatening AE, as well as a long-term interrupter of chemotherapy, and it should be avoided. However, even with their relatively thin diameters, the 6 mm FCSEMSs caused liver abscesses by obstructing the side branches. In the present study, no liver abscesses occurred, even though 8 mm FCSESMs were used, because they were placed without blocking the side branches. The TRBO in the present study was favorable compared to those of previous studies. The reason for this may be due to the larger diameter of the stent or the absence of Bismuth IV cases.

In bilateral drainage using UCSEMSs for MHBO, 8 mm stents are often used. Since FCSEMSs of the same diameter were used in the present study, we expected a longer patency period compared to UCSEMSs through the prevention of tumor ingrowth. However, the median TRBO for bilateral drainage using UCSEMSs in prospective studies was 200–300 days [4,7,22], which is better than the outcome of the present study. The advantage of FCSEMSs is that they prevent tumor ingrowth, but migration and sludge formation are drawbacks [23]. Because of their equal influences, the TRBOs of FCSEMSs and UCSEMSs are comparable in the case of distal MBO (DMBO) [24]. However, in MHBO, FCSEMS occlusion due to sludge is more likely to occur because of the use of longer and thinner stents than in DHBO, while ingrowth into the UCSEMs could be somewhat controlled with advances in chemotherapy, leading to a longer TRBO in the case of UCSEMSs. In fact, RBO due to sludge was much more common in the present study (36%) than that reported for FCSEMSs in DMBO. Another possible reason for the shorter TRBO in the present study, compared to that reported for UCSEMSs in MHBO, was that one-third of patients had prior RBO. In MHBO, prior cholangitis or RBO is considered a risk factor for early stent occlusion, which is thought to be due to residual sludge in the intrahepatic bile ducts [25]. In fact, patients with prior RBO had high RBO rates and shorter TRBOs than those without prior TRBO in the present study. Furthermore, the fact that one-third of the patients underwent across-the-papilla placement may also be the reason for the shorter TRBO in the present study, compared to that reported for UCSEMSs in MHBO. Above-the-papilla placement is expected to reduce the RBO by sludge formation due to less reflux of the intestinal fluid, and this possibility has been demonstrated in the case of PSs [26]. Since UCSEMSs are less likely to be occluded by sludge, there was no difference in TRBO between the placements above and across the papilla [27]. However, as FCSEMSs have a high risk of sludge formation, it is theoretically better to use above-the-papilla placement, as demonstrated in the present study. While we cannot be sure, based on the small number of cases, the TRBO of the 8 mm FCSEMSs with above-the-papilla placement might be better than that of UCSEMSs.

AEs occurred in two patients (18%) with mild pancreatitis. One patient underwent above-the-papilla placement, which was probably caused by ERCP itself. The other showed a case of two stents placed across the papilla. All four patients with across-the-papilla stenting had two stents placed, and one of them (25%) developed pancreatitis. In previous reports, in a total of 26 patients with two 6 mm CSEMSs placed across the papilla, no pancreatitis was observed [11,28]. The reason for the relatively high incidence of pancreatitis in the present study is not clear, but the difference in the diameter of stents may be the cause. In a report by Ishigaki et al., using two 8 mm UCSEMSs placed side by side across the papilla, the incidence of pancreatitis was 29%, which was similar to ours [29]. However, most of their cases were moderate, while our case was mild. High axial force is believed to be a cause of pancreatitis after SEMS [30], and the 8 mm FCSEMSs had a lower axial force than WallFlex (Boston Scientific Japan), used by Ishigaki et al., which may have resulted in the lower severity of the pancreatitis. In addition, the fact that FCSEMSs can be removed when necessary is a major advantage.

The present study has several limitations. Firstly, it was a single center, retrospective study. Therefore, selection bias and reporting bias could not be eliminated. Secondly, only a small number of cases were included, with no comparison cases. Thirdly, only cases up to Bismuth III were included, and more advanced cases were excluded. Consequently, the generalization of this method is restricted.

In conclusion, whole-liver drainage with a novel 8 mm FCSEMS possessing an ultra-slim introducer of 5.9-Fr was feasible and potentially safe and might have favorable stent patency for unresectable MHBOs of Bismuth I, II, and IIIa. Further investigations based on prospective designs involving large cohorts at multiple centers are warranted.

Author Contributions: Conceptualization, S.M.; methodology, S.M.; software, S.M.; validation, S.M., S.N., K.N., K.S., T.O. and M.O.; formal analysis, S.M.; investigation, S.M.; writing—original draft preparation, S.M.; writing—review and editing, S.N.; visualization, S.M.; supervision, S.N.; project administration, S.M. All authors have read and agreed to the published version of the manuscript.

Funding: This review received no external funding.

Institutional Review Board Statement: The study was conducted in accordance with the Declaration of Helsinki, and approved by the Institutional Review Board of Saitama Medical Center, Saitama Medical University (study no: 2534, date of approval: 23 June 2022).

Informed Consent Statement: Patient consent was waived due to opting out.

Acknowledgments: We are grateful to Tetsuro Fujita and Koji Yakabi for their assistance.

Conflicts of Interest: The authors declare no conflict of interest.

References

1. Larghi, A.; Tringali, A.; Lecca, P.G.; Giordano, M.; Costamagna, G. Management of Hilar Biliary Strictures. *Am. J. Gastroenterol.* **2008**, *103*, 458–473. [CrossRef] [PubMed]
2. Rerknimitr, R.; Angsuwatcharakon, P.; Ratanachu-Ek, T.; Khor, C.J.L.; Ponnudurai, R.; Moon, J.H.; Seo, D.W.; Pantongrag-Brown, L.; Sangchan, A.; Pisespongsa, P.; et al. Asia-Pacific consensus recommendations for endoscopic and interventional management of hilar cholangiocarcinoma. *J. Gastroenterol. Hepatol.* **2013**, *28*, 593–607. [CrossRef] [PubMed]
3. Dumonceau, J.M.; Tringali, A.; Papanikolaou, I.S.; Blero, D.; Mangiavillano, B.; Schmidt, A.; Vanbiervliet, G.; Costamagna, G.; Devière, J.; García-Cano, J.; et al. Endoscopic biliary stenting: Indications, choice of stents, and results: European Society of Gastrointestinal Endoscopy (ESGE) Clinical Guideline–Updated October 2017. *Endoscopy* **2018**, *50*, 910–930. [CrossRef] [PubMed]

4. Lee, T.H.; Kim, T.H.; Moon, J.H.; Lee, S.H.; Choi, H.J.; Hwangbo, Y.; Hyun, J.J.; Choi, J.-H.; Jeong, S.; Kim, J.H.; et al. Bilateral versus unilateral placement of metal stents for inoperable high-grade malignant hilar biliary strictures: A multicenter, prospective, randomized study (with video). *Gastrointest. Endosc.* **2017**, *86*, 817–827. [CrossRef]
5. Hakuta, R.; Kogure, H.; Nakai, Y.; Kawakami, H.; Maguchi, H.; Mukai, T.; Iwashita, T.; Saito, T.; Togawa, O.; Matsubara, S.; et al. Unilateral versus Bilateral Endoscopic Nasobiliary Drainage and Subsequent Metal Stent Placement for Unresectable Malignant Hilar Obstruction: A Multicenter Randomized Controlled Trial. *J. Clin. Med.* **2021**, *10*, 206. [CrossRef] [PubMed]
6. Meybodi, M.A.; Shakoor, D.; Nanavati, J.; Ichkhanian, Y.; Vosoughi, K.; Brewer Gutierrez, O.I.; Kalloo, A.N.; Singh, V.; Kumbhari, V.; Ngamruengphong, S.; et al. Unilateral versus bilateral endoscopic stenting in patients with unresectable malignant hilar obstruction: A systematic review and meta-analysis. *Endosc. Int. Open* **2020**, *8*, E281–E290. [CrossRef]
7. Mukai, T.; Yasuda, I.; Nakashima, M.; Doi, S.; Iwashita, T.; Iwata, K.; Kato, T.; Tomita, E.; Moriwaki, H. Metallic stents are more efficacious than plastic stents in unresectable malignant hilar biliary strictures: A randomized controlled trial. *J. Hepato-Biliary-Pancreatic Sci.* **2012**, *20*, 214–222. [CrossRef]
8. Xia, M.-X.; Cai, X.-B.; Pan, Y.-L.; Wu, J.; Gao, D.-J.; Ye, X.; Wang, T.-T.; Hu, B. Optimal stent placement strategy for malignant hilar biliary obstruction: A large multicenter parallel study. *Gastrointest. Endosc.* **2019**, *91*, 1117–1128.e9. [CrossRef]
9. Costamagna, G.; Tringali, A. Can we insert a covered stent, partially or not, in case of hilar biliary stenosis? *Endosc. Int. Open* **2017**, *5*, E1218–E1219. [CrossRef]
10. Inoue, T.; Okumura, F.; Naitoh, I.; Fukusada, S.; Kachi, K.; Ozeki, T.; Anbe, K.; Iwasaki, H.; Mizushima, T.; Kobayashi, Y.; et al. Feasibility of the placement of a novel 6-mm diameter threaded fully covered self-expandable metal stent for malignant hilar biliary obstructions (with videos). *Gastrointest. Endosc.* **2016**, *84*, 352–357. [CrossRef]
11. Yoshida, T.; Hara, K.; Imaoka, H.; Hijioka, S.; Mizuno, N.; Ishihara, M.; Tanaka, T.; Tajika, M.; Niwa, Y.; Yamao, K. Benefits of side-by-side deployment of 6-mm covered self-expandable metal stents for hilar malignant biliary obstructions. *J. Hepato-Biliary-Pancreatic Sci.* **2016**, *23*, 548–555. [CrossRef] [PubMed]
12. Bismuth, H.; Nakache, R.; Diamond, T. Management Strategies in Resection for Hilar Cholangiocarcinoma. *Ann. Surg.* **1992**, *215*, 31–38. [CrossRef] [PubMed]
13. Cotton, P.B.; Eisen, G.M.; Aabakken, L.; Baron, T.H.; Hutter, M.M.; Jacobson, B.C.; Mergener, K.; Nemcek, A., Jr.; Petersen, B.T.; Petrini, J.L.; et al. A lexicon for endoscopic adverse events: Report of an ASGE workshop. *Gastrointest. Endosc.* **2010**, *71*, 446–454. [CrossRef] [PubMed]
14. Isayama, H.; Hamada, T.; Yasuda, I.; Itoi, T.; Ryozawa, S.; Nakai, Y.; Kogure, H.; Koike, K. Tokyo criteria 2014 for transpapillary biliary stenting. *Dig. Endosc.* **2014**, *27*, 259–264. [CrossRef]
15. Kanda, Y. Investigation of the freely available easy-to-use software 'EZR' for medical statistics. *Bone Marrow Transplant.* **2013**, *48*, 452–458. [CrossRef]
16. Vienne, A.; Hobeika, E.; Gouya, H.; Lapidus, N.; Fritsch, J.; Choury, A.D.; Chryssostalis, A.; Gaudric, M.; Pelletier, G.; Buffet, C.; et al. Prediction of drainage effectiveness during endoscopic stenting of malignant hilar strictures: The role of liver volume assessment. *Gastrointest. Endosc.* **2010**, *72*, 728–735. [CrossRef]
17. Tringali, A.; Boskoski, I.; Costamagna, G. Endoscopic Stenting in Hilar Cholangiocarcinoma: When, How, and How Much to Drain? *Gastroenterol. Res. Pract.* **2019**, *2019*, 5161350. [CrossRef]
18. Lee, T.H.; Moon, J.H.; Park, S. Biliary stenting for hilar malignant biliary obstruction. *Dig. Endosc.* **2019**, *32*, 275–286. [CrossRef]
19. Nagino, M.; Hirano, S.; Yoshitomi, H.; Aoki, T.; Uesaka, K.; Unno, M.; Ebata, T.; Konishi, M.; Sano, K.; Shimada, K.; et al. Clinical practice guidelines for the management of biliary tract cancers 2019: The 3rd English edition. *J. Hepato-Biliary-Pancreatic Sci.* **2020**, *28*, 26–54. [CrossRef]
20. Qumseya, B.J.; Jamil, L.H.; Elmunzer, B.J.; Riaz, A.; Ceppa, E.P.; Thosani, N.C.; Buxbaum, J.L.; Storm, A.C.; Sawhney, M.S.; Pawa, S.; et al. ASGE guideline on the role of endoscopy in the management of malignant hilar obstruction. *Gastrointest. Endosc.* **2021**, *94*, 222–234.e22. [CrossRef]
21. Choi, J.H.; Lee, S.H.; You, M.S.; Shin, B.-S.; Choi, Y.H.; Kang, J.; Jang, S.; Paik, W.H.; Ryu, J.K.; Kim, Y.-T. Step-wise endoscopic approach to palliative bilateral biliary drainage for unresectable advanced malignant hilar obstruction. *Sci. Rep.* **2019**, *9*, 13207. [CrossRef] [PubMed]
22. Lee, T.H.; Moon, J.H.; Choi, J.-H.; Lee, S.H.; Lee, Y.N.; Paik, W.H.; Jang, D.K.; Cho, B.W.; Yang, J.K.; Hwangbo, Y.; et al. Prospective comparison of endoscopic bilateral stent-in-stent versus stent-by-stent deployment for inoperable advanced malignant hilar biliary stricture. *Gastrointest. Endosc.* **2019**, *90*, 222–230. [CrossRef] [PubMed]
23. Isayama, H.; Komatsu, Y.; Tsujino, T.; Sasahira, N.; Hirano, K.; Toda, N.; Nakai, Y.; Yamamoto, N.; Tada, M.; Yoshida, H.; et al. A prospective randomised study of "covered" versus "uncovered" diamond stents for the management of distal malignant biliary obstruction. *Gut* **2004**, *53*, 729–734. [CrossRef] [PubMed]
24. Tringali, A.; Hassan, C.; Rota, M.; Rossi, M.; Mutignani, M.; Aabakken, L. Covered vs. uncovered self-expandable metal stents for malignant distal biliary strictures: A systematic review and meta-analysis. *Laryngo-Rhino-Otologie* **2018**, *50*, 631–641. [CrossRef]
25. Miura, S.; Kanno, A.; Masamune, A.; Hamada, S.; Hongou, S.; Yoshida, N.; Nakano, E.; Takikawa, T.; Kume, K.; Kikuta, K.; et al. Risk factors for recurrent biliary obstruction following placement of self-expandable metallic stents in patients with malignant perihilar biliary stricture. *Laryngo-Rhino-Otologie* **2016**, *48*, 536–545. [CrossRef]

26. Kurita, A.; Uza, N.; Asada, M.; Yoshimura, K.; Takemura, T.; Yazumi, S.; Kodama, Y.; Seno, H. Stent placement above the sphincter of Oddi is a useful option for patients with inoperable malignant hilar biliary obstruction. *Surg. Endosc.* **2021**, *36*, 2869–2878. [CrossRef]
27. Cosgrove, N.; Siddiqui, A.A.; Adler, D.G.; Shahid, H.; Sarkar, A.; Sharma, A.; Kowalski, T.E.; Loren, D.; Warndorf, M.; Chennat, J.; et al. A Comparison of Bilateral Side-by-Side Metal Stents Deployed Above and Across the Sphincter of Oddi in the Management of Malignant Hilar Biliary Obstruction. *J. Clin. Gastroenterol.* **2017**, *51*, 528–533. [CrossRef]
28. Kitamura, K.; Yamamiya, A.; Ishii, Y.; Mitsui, Y.; Nomoto, T.; Yoshida, H. Side-by-side partially covered self-expandable metal stent placement for malignant hilar biliary obstruction. *Endosc. Int. Open* **2017**, *05*, E1211–E1217. [CrossRef]
29. Ishigaki, K.; Hamada, T.; Nakai, Y.; Isayama, H.; Sato, T.; Hakuta, R.; Saito, K.; Saito, T.; Takahara, N.; Mizuno, S.; et al. Retrospective Comparative Study of Side-by-Side and Stent-in-Stent Metal Stent Placement for Hilar Malignant Biliary Obstruction. *Am. J. Dig. Dis.* **2020**, *65*, 3710–3718. [CrossRef]
30. Kawakubo, K.; Isayama, H.; Nakai, Y.; Togawa, O.; Sasahira, N.; Kogure, H.; Sasaki, T.; Matsubara, S.; Yamamoto, N.; Hirano, K.; et al. Risk factors for pancreatitis following transpapillary self-expandable metal stent placement. *Surg. Endosc.* **2011**, *26*, 771–776. [CrossRef]

MDPI
St. Alban-Anlage 66
4052 Basel
Switzerland
www.mdpi.com

Journal of Clinical Medicine Editorial Office
E-mail: jcm@mdpi.com
www.mdpi.com/journal/jcm

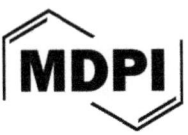

Disclaimer/Publisher's Note: The statements, opinions and data contained in all publications are solely those of the individual author(s) and contributor(s) and not of MDPI and/or the editor(s). MDPI and/or the editor(s) disclaim responsibility for any injury to people or property resulting from any ideas, methods, instructions or products referred to in the content.

www.ingramcontent.com/pod-product-compliance
Lightning Source LLC
LaVergne TN
LVHW070716100526
838202LV00013B/1108